Gymnastics Medicine

Emily Sweeney
Editor

Gymnastics Medicine

Evaluation, Management and Rehabilitation

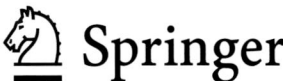

Editor
Emily Sweeney
Department of Orthopedics
University of Colorado School of Medicine
Children's Hospital Colorado
Sports Medicine Center
Aurora, CO
USA

ISBN 978-3-030-26287-7   ISBN 978-3-030-26288-4 (eBook)
https://doi.org/10.1007/978-3-030-26288-4

© Springer Nature Switzerland AG 2020
This work is subject to copyright. All rights are reserved by the Publisher, whether the whole or part of the material is concerned, specifically the rights of translation, reprinting, reuse of illustrations, recitation, broadcasting, reproduction on microfilms or in any other physical way, and transmission or information storage and retrieval, electronic adaptation, computer software, or by similar or dissimilar methodology now known or hereafter developed.
The use of general descriptive names, registered names, trademarks, service marks, etc. in this publication does not imply, even in the absence of a specific statement, that such names are exempt from the relevant protective laws and regulations and therefore free for general use.
The publisher, the authors, and the editors are safe to assume that the advice and information in this book are believed to be true and accurate at the date of publication. Neither the publisher nor the authors or the editors give a warranty, expressed or implied, with respect to the material contained herein or for any errors or omissions that may have been made. The publisher remains neutral with regard to jurisdictional claims in published maps and institutional affiliations.

This Springer imprint is published by the registered company Springer Nature Switzerland AG
The registered company address is: Gewerbestrasse 11, 6330 Cham, Switzerland

Foreword

Gymnastics is an incredibly diverse sport with unique demands that stretch our routinely held sports medicine principles. Each discipline within gymnastics, described in more detail within this book, presents varied biomechanical demands, injury patterns, return-to-play decision-making, and treatment protocols. This highlights the precise need for this book. *Gymnastics Medicine: Evaluation, Management, and Rehabilitation* outlines a comprehensive approach to gymnastics sports medicine care.

I have dedicated much of my career to the health and wellness of gymnasts. It has been a tremendous honor to provide care as a member of the USA Gymnastics medical staff. I have traveled with USA Gymnastics as a team physician for domestic and international events, including as their team physician for the 2016 Rio Olympic Games. These opportunities are ones that I do not take for granted. Why do my colleagues and I dedicate so much of our personal and professional time to advance the medical care of gymnasts? We do it because of the passion we have for the sport, we do it for the athletes, and we do it to support our colleagues.

We have a duty as sports medicine practitioners to provide high-quality, compassionate, and ethical care, to the best of our abilities. Education provides a key avenue to developing this high level of care. I am grateful for the hard work Dr. Sweeney and all the authors have put into the publication of this book. This book serves as a broad and comprehensive overview of all the layers of medical care gymnasts deserve. These include epidemiology of injury, biomechanics, injury profiles, treatment, and rehabilitation.

I have had the pleasure to work with Dr. Sweeney during USA Gymnastics events and have known her to be an excellent clinician who exhibits a strong passion for gymnastics medicine. She has worked tirelessly in her own community but also nationally to advance the care of gymnasts, and I cannot think of a better ambassador to bring this compilation of work to the broader community of sports medicine practitioners. It is my honor to write these words of support. I hope that all healthcare professionals who care for gymnasts take the time to read this book. It serves as an excellent roadmap to inform quality of care for this much deserving population of athletes.

Huntington Beach, CA, USA David W. Kruse, MD
June 18, 2019

Preface

Gymnastics is an amazing sport that encompasses a number of skills and events. To be successful in the sport requires hard work, discipline, excellent time management skills, bravery, and toughness. During my life, I have competed, coached, and judged gymnastics, and now I work as a researcher and pediatric sports medicine physician who frequently cares for gymnasts. I love the sport of gymnastics and am honored to present this medical gymnastics book.

The demands of gymnastics lead to a number of injury patterns and medical conditions. Thus, medical providers who take care of gymnasts should be aware of the unique injuries and issues that face gymnasts. This book provides vital information for physicians, advanced practice providers, physical therapists, athletic trainers, exercise scientists, and mental health professionals who care for gymnasts. By learning more about the nuances of the sport and associated medical issues, the reader will gain an appreciation for the sport and be able to provide better care for all gymnasts. Along with the medical providers noted above, it is my hope that coaches, parents, and gymnasts can also use concepts from this book to decrease injuries and burnout in order to help gymnasts reach their peak potential.

This text covers a number of topics that affect gymnasts. The book starts with an introduction to the history of gymnastics and provides a brief review of the gymnastics disciplines and events. An overview of gymnastics injury epidemiology lays the foundation for the rest of the book. Growth and developmental issues are also covered in this text because many young gymnasts train long hours before or during puberty. Concepts related to the biomechanics of gymnastics, common overuse and acute musculoskeletal injuries, psychological issues, concussions, as well as rehabilitation and return-to-play principles make up the remainder of the book.

This book has been created with the tireless efforts of all of its authors, who are all experts in aspects of gymnastics and sports medicine. Their excellent contributions have made this a comprehensive book that will provide useful information for medical providers and others involved in the care of gymnasts.

In addition to the work of the authors, I must acknowledge a number of other people who assisted in the creation of this book: my parents and siblings who supported my first flips in gymnastics; my gymnastics coaches and teammates; my coworkers at Children's Hospital Colorado and University of Colorado School of Medicine, who have been supportive of my work in gymnastics; my teachers and mentors in medicine who have helped shape me into the physician I am today; and finally, my husband and son. Without the loving support, patience, and feedback of my husband, Scott, this book would not have been possible. Finally, I must recognize my son, Henry, who has brought me boundless joy and love in such a short time. Henry, I hope you are ready to learn more than you ever wanted about gymnastics!

Over the last three decades, I have learned so much about the sport of gymnastics. It has taught me a number of life lessons that I carry with me today. I hope that, through this text, I am able to provide useful medical educational material and, more importantly, to give others an appreciation for the sport and its athletes.

Aurora, CO, USA   Emily Sweeney, MD

Contents

1	**History and Overview of Gymnastics Disciplines** .... Kasia Kilijanek and Kristen Sanchez	1
2	**Epidemiology of Gymnastics Injuries** .... Sigrid F. Wolf and Cynthia R. LaBella	15
3	**Biomechanics of Gymnastics** .... Edward Nyman Jr.	27
4	**Growth and Development in Gymnastics** .... Lauren Klein Ritchie, Natalie Ronshaugen, and Jennifer Sygo	55
5	**Psychological Aspects of Injury in Gymnastics** .... Jamie L. Shapiro, Michelle L. Bartlett, and Leah E. Lomonte	75
6	**Medical Illness in Gymnasts** .... Aubrey Armento and Emily Sweeney	101
7	**Head and Neck Injuries in Gymnasts** .... Christine Eng and Steven Makovitch	119
8	**Spine Injuries in Gymnasts** .... Steven Makovitch and Christine Eng	135
9	**Upper Extremity Injuries in Gymnasts** .... Leah G. Concannon, Melinda S. Loveless, and Sean T. Matsuwaka	177
10	**Lower Extremity Injuries in Gymnasts** .... Nicole B. Katz, Ellen Casey, Alexia G. Gagliardi, and Jay C. Albright	209

11	**Rehabilitation of Gymnasts**	233
	David Tilley and David A. James	
12	**Return to Play in Gymnastics**	291
	Marla Ranieri, Morgan Potter, Melissa Mascaro, and Marsha Grant-Ford	

Index 345

Contributors

Jay C. Albright, MD University of Colorado School of Medicine, Children's Hospital Colorado, Aurora, CO, USA

Aubrey Armento, MD University of Colorado, School of Medicine, Aurora, CO, USA

Children's Hospital Colorado, Sports Medicine Center, Aurora, CO, USA

Michelle L. Bartlett, PhD West Texas A&M University, Canyon, TX, USA

Ellen Casey, MD Department of Physiatry, Hospital for Special Surgery, New York, NY, USA

Leah G. Concannon, MD Department of Rehabilitation Medicine, University of Washington, Seattle, WA, USA

Christine Eng, MD Harvard Medical School, Department of Physical Medicine and Rehabilitation, Spaulding Rehabilitation Hospital, Charlestown, MA, USA

Alexia G. Gagliardi, BA Children's Hospital Colorado, Aurora, CO, USA

Marsha Grant-Ford, PhD ATC Montclair State University, Montclair, NJ, USA

David A. James, PT, DPT, OCS, SCS University of Colorado School of Medicine, Physical Therapy Program, Aurora, CO, USA

Nicole B. Katz, BS Lewis School of Medicine at Temple University, Philadelphia, PA, USA

Kasia Kilijanek, DPT Children's Hospital Colorado, Sports Medicine Center, Aurora, CO, USA

Cynthia R. LaBella, MD Institute for Sports Medicine, Ann & Robert H. Lurie Children's Hospital of Chicago, Chicago, IL, USA

Leah E. Lomonte, MA University of Denver, Denver, CO, USA

Melinda S. Loveless, MD Department of Rehabilitation Medicine, University of Washington, Seattle, WA, USA

Steven Makovitch, DO Harvard Medical School, Department of Physical Medicine and Rehabilitation, Spaulding Rehabilitation Hospital, Charlestown, MA, USA

Melissa Mascaro, MD CAQSM Family and Sports Medicine Institute of NJ, Summit, NJ, USA

Sean T. Matsuwaka, MD Department of Rehabilitation Medicine, University of Washington, Seattle, WA, USA

Edward Nyman Jr., PhD College of Health Professions, The University of Findlay, Findlay, OH, USA

Morgan Potter, BA Department of Physical Therapy, University of Delaware, Newark, DE, USA

Marla Ranieri, PT, DPT OCS Drayer Physical Therapy, Flanders, NJ, USA

Lauren Klein Ritchie, MD University of Colorado School of Medicine, Aurora, CO, USA

Children's Hospital Colorado, Aurora, CO, USA

Natalie Ronshaugen, MD Children's Hospital & Medical Center, Omaha, NE, USA

University of Nebraska Medical Center, Omaha, NE, USA

Kristen Sanchez, DPT Cascade Sports Injury Prevention and Physical Therapy LLC, Lakewood, CO, USA

Jamie L. Shapiro, PhD University of Denver, Denver, CO, USA

Emily Sweeney, MD Department of Orthopedics, University of Colorado School of Medicine, Children's Hospital Colorado, Sports Medicine Center, Aurora, CO, USA

Jennifer Sygo, MSc, RD, CSSD Cleveland Clinic Canada, Toronto, ON, Canada

Gymnastics Canada – Women's Artistic Program, Gloucester, ON, Canada

David Tilley, PT, DPT, SCS, CSCS Champion Physical Therapy and Performance, Waltham, MA, USA

Sigrid F. Wolf, MD Institute for Sports Medicine, Ann & Robert H. Lurie Children's Hospital of Chicago, Chicago, IL, USA

Chapter 1
History and Overview of Gymnastics Disciplines

Kasia Kilijanek and Kristen Sanchez

1.1 A Brief History of Gymnastics

The word "gymnastics" comes from the Greek word "gymnos," meaning "to exercise naked" [1, 2]. Gymnastics and the development of the sport can be traced back to 776 BC when men and women participants were depicted in paintings vaulting over horses and swords [1, 2]. It was thought to be an exhibitionary demonstration of athleticism with a resemblance to wrestling and was used for entertainment value. Despite anecdotal reports of gymnastics competitions, there are no official record of gymnasts competing in the Ancient Olympic Games.

1.1.1 The Early Years of Gymnastics

During the era of the Roman Empire, gymnastics was used as a method of training for other sports and became an important part of military training [1–3]. Interestingly, the only known apparatus at that time was the wooden horse, as seen in Fig. 1.1 [1]. During the Renaissance, writers began to emphasize the importance of physical strength and encourage youth to participate in climbing and movement for overall health [1, 2]. Many of the skills they performed were influenced by ancient gymnastics movements. The resurgence of fitness routines during this period was thought to influence the pioneers of the sport, including Johann Friedrich Jahn (1778–1852) of

K. Kilijanek (✉)
Children's Hospital Colorado, Sports Medicine Center, Aurora, CO, USA
e-mail: Kasia.Kilijanek@childrenscolorado.org

K. Sanchez
Cascade Sports Injury Prevention and Physical Therapy LLC, Lakewood, CO, USA
e-mail: Kristen@csinjuryprevention.com

© Springer Nature Switzerland AG 2020
E. Sweeney (ed.), *Gymnastics Medicine*,
https://doi.org/10.1007/978-3-030-26288-4_1

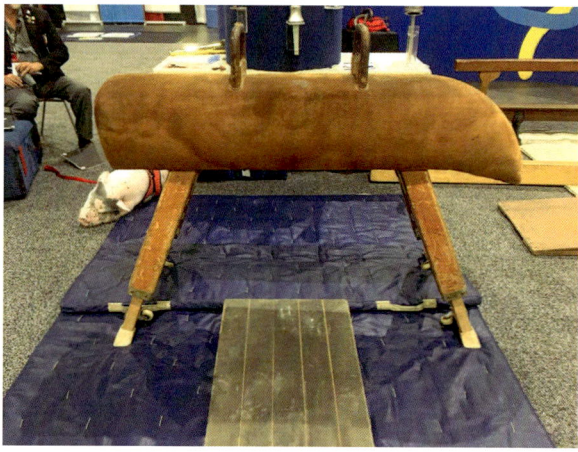

Fig. 1.1 Pommel horse. Initially the horse was wooden but more modern versions are covered in leather

Germany and Pehr Henrik Ling of Sweden, who are often credited with being the founders of modern gymnastics. Jahn founded the gymnastics club movement, opening his first gymnastics club for youth and adults in 1811 [4]. He was a part of the German military at the time and created workout routines with various apparatuses to improve the strength and mental stamina of soldiers [1, 4]. For example, his bar routines involved repetitive dipping motions to increase strength as opposed to the normal gliding and kipping we know today. Jahn is often regarded as "the father of the sport of gymnastics" for his work and invention of the parallel bars, high bar, and still rings [1–3, 5]. Rudimentary versions of these apparatuses can be seen in Fig. 1.2.

Pehr Henrik Ling was a founder of a teacher-training in 1813 that created gymnastics-specific exercises thought to be of medical benefit for the athlete [5]. The apparatus known today as the floor exercise was developed from Ling's callisthenic exercises and used clubs, wands, and dumbbells as shown in Fig. 1.3 [5]. The works of Jahn and Ling were revolutionary for their time and combined Swedish calisthenics, German aerobics, heavy lifting, and organized routines. Over time, Jahn and Ling's influence spread throughout Europe and to North America.

1.1.2 The Later Years (1825–1972)

By 1825, the first three gymnasiums were opened in the United States by three German refugees: Charles Beck, Charles Follen, and Francis Leiber [1, 2]. Each had trained under Jahn learning his style of gymnastics [1]. Interestingly, the gymnastics they taught in the United States was slow to gain traction. Many speculated that the slow growth was likely due to the heavy emphasis on strength (from the original intent to build strong soldiers). Thus, over the next 30 years, many regarded gymnastics as a hobby rather than a sport [1, 3, 6].

The return of the Olympics in 1896 was pivotal for gymnastics. Gymnastics was one of the nine sports eligible for competition, though it was unregulated at the time

Fig. 1.2 Parallel bars used in men's artistic gymnastics

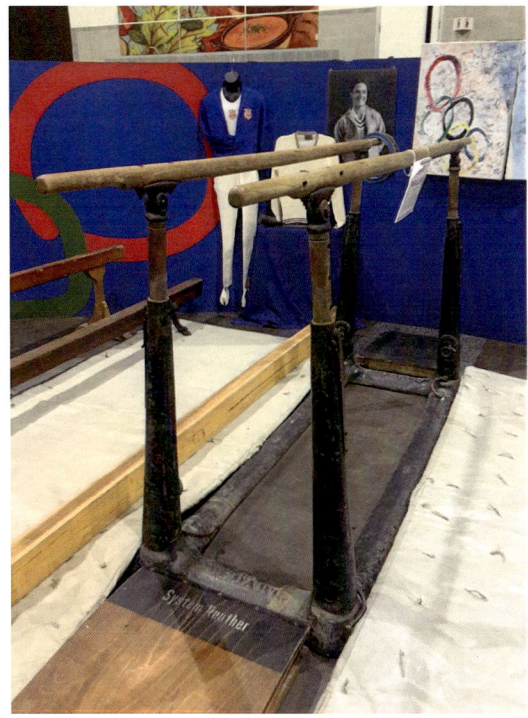

Fig. 1.3 Equipment used in early gymnastics events

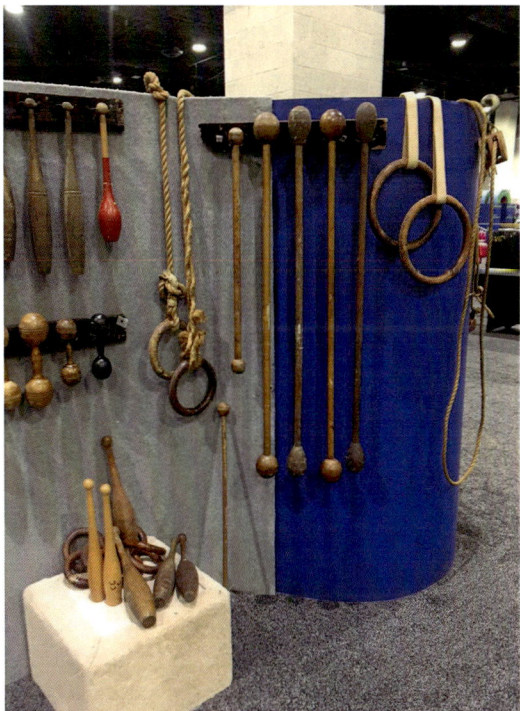

[1, 7]. Events would change without agreement in an attempt to demonstrate the overall best athlete and not the best gymnast. Because of the lack of regulation, events over the next few decades changed frequently and, at times, included long jump, high jump, heavy throwing, parallel bars, high bars, and pommel horse [1–3]. Civilians could participate without training and compete to demonstrate their fitness. In response to the poorly managed competitions, the Federation of International Gymnastics (FIG) and the International Olympic Committee (IOC) put in place more rules for the 1912 Olympics [1, 2, 8]. Under these new regulations, there were many changes to the sport during the first part of the twentieth century. For example, in 1928, women were allowed to compete in gymnastics during the Olympics, although not as individual athletes [1]. In 1932, tumbling and floor routines were introduced as part of the competition [1]. The 1952 Olympics are often marked as the modernization of gymnastics [1]. It was at this time that Soviet Union dominated almost every individual Men's and Women's event. Throughout the next two decades, gymnastics was still a relatively unpopular sport. Then, at the 1972 Olympics, gold medalist Olga Korbut from the Soviet Union became a sports sensation. Her gymnastics performance helped spark interest in the sport around the world [9]. Since then, gymnastics has been one of the most popular Olympic sports.

1.1.3 Today's Regulations

Today, the highest governing body for gymnastics recognized by the IOC is still the FIG [6]. Each country runs their gymnastics programs slightly differently. In the United States, USA Gymnastics (USAG) was recognized by the FIG in 1970 to create rules and policies to prepare athletes to be eligible for competition at a world-class level through national team tracks and developmental categories [8].

The structure of the agencies and governing bodies of gymnastics largely influences training policies of gyms, the values of coaches and gymnasts, safety, and the progression of athletes through levels. USAG has levels that span across all disciplines with slight variability between each. The Junior Olympic (JO) national team track includes levels 1 through 10 and Junior and Senior Elite. The lower levels are typically the "compulsory levels," and then gymnasts progress to the upper "optional levels." Compulsory levels are created to teach the foundational skills and strength of gymnastics with standardized routines. Optional-level athletes have freedom of skill selection for their competitive skill level. The JO track is also designed to prepare gymnasts for the national and international competitions within their discipline.

To allow for a more inclusive participation, USAG also created the Xcel Program to encourage participation in gymnastics with less demanding training hours. Currently artistic women's, artistic men's, and rhythmic gymnastics have added Xcel to their competitive levels. Athletes can compete in Bronze, Silver, Gold, Platinum, and Diamond levels. Other recreational leagues exist, typically at a state level in the United States, that have various rules and regulations. Many states also have high school gymnastics programs; the rules for these programs vary from state to state. The National Collegiate Athletic Association (NCAA) also has men's and women's artistic gymnastics.

1.2 Disciplines

Gymnastics includes eight different disciplines including women's artistic gymnastics, men's artistic gymnastics, acrobatic gymnastics, tumbling and trampoline, rhythmic gymnastics, aerobic gymnastics, Gymnastics for All, and parkour. Each discipline within the FIG is broken down into eligibility, levels, general skills required, and gender participation. Although each discipline looks fundamentally different, the basics of tumbling, flexibility, and strength training are the foundation for all. The differences between sports become more apparent at the competitive compulsory and optional levels. Because women's and men's artistic gymnastics are the most popular disciplines in the U.S., many of the concepts in this book refer to these athletes in particular. However, it is important to note that there is overlap between many of the disciplines. Therefore, a number of ideas referring to artistic gymnasts throughout this book can be applied to all gymnasts.

1.2.1 Women's Artistic Gymnastics

Women's artistic gymnastics is the most popular discipline in the gymnastics world. It initially debuted in the Olympics in 1928 [6]. Women's artistic events include vault, uneven parallel bars, balance beam, and floor exercise. Though some of the events and rules are similar to men's artistic gymnastics, there are also unique aspects that have created a sport specifically for women [6].

The vault requires a sprint and a forward or backwards entry onto a springboard. The athlete then launches off the springboard onto the vault, allowing for propulsion off of the vault into another flip and/or twist. The uneven parallel bars require upper extremity strength and dynamic stability to perform a continuous series of swinging elements, handstands, release moves, and a dismount. The dismount can involve great height that allows for multiple flips and twists. The balance beam apparatus is a wooden beam, covered in suede, minimally padded, and is 10 cm (4 inches) wide, 5 m (16.4 feet) long, and 125 cm (4.1 feet) high [6]. This event requires precision and control to perform choreographed dance, turns, leaps, tumbling, and a dismount without falling. The floor exercise uses the standard 12-by-12 m spring-loaded floor [6]. For women, floor exercise requires a well-choreographed routine of seamless dance, leaps, and tumbling set to wordless music. This event allows for creativity, personality, and variability of skills that demonstrate the athlete's power, flexibility, and grace.

Because of the increasing popularity and advancements in coaching over the years, women's artistic gymnastics has allowed for incredible advancements in the difficulty of skills. In all events, women are performing skills that are higher and involve more twists and flips than could have been conceived in the early years. Many of the skills that women were performing in the early Olympics are now basic skills for lower to mid-level gymnasts.

Routines are created based on the requirements set for each level. Level 1–5 gymnasts all compete the same "compulsory" routines, whereas the "optional" levels 6–10 allow for individualized routines but still have a set of requirements that must be met in order to have the highest starting value. The Code of Points is the rule book that describes the rules and requirements for each level. The starting value for each routine is the predetermined score that the routine is worth based on the sum of each skill value to be performed, to a maximum of 10.0 [10]. Judges deduct points based on errors in artistry, execution, composition, and technique [6, 10]. In the optional levels, the gymnasts may receive bonus points for performing more difficult skills and combinations.

In 2006, the FIG began using a new scoring system for elite gymnasts. This system has a difficulty and execution score but it no longer limits the maximal points to 10.0. The athlete receives an "E" or execution score based on her performance quality of skills and their deductions. The highest possible "E" score is 10.0. The gymnast also receives a "D" or difficulty score that is based on the summation of her most difficult skills in the routine. The two scores are added together to give the gymnast one final score [6, 10].

1.2.2 Men's Artistic Gymnastics

Men's artistic gymnastics is similar to women's artistic gymnastics but has some different events and requirements. Because of the upper extremity dominance in men's artistic gymnastics, male gymnasts require extreme shoulder strength and stability. The six men's events include the floor exercise, pommel horse, still rings, vault, parallel bars, and high bar.

The floor exercise for men requires a sequence of acrobatic tumbling, jumps, circles, or flairs, a balance element on one leg or arm, and a static strength hold on the upper extremities [11]. Though men's floor does not typically utilize music or choreography, the transitional skills must be performed with rhythm and harmony [11]. The pommel horse is an upper extremity dominant event and is often considered the most difficult event [11]. The pommel horse itself is 115 cm (3.8 feet) high, 35 cm (13.8 inches) wide, and 160 cm (5.25 feet) long with two handles evenly spaced on the top [11]. This event requires the gymnasts to perform rhythmic, continuous circles on their arms while maintaining adequate hip and foot height. Handstands, flairs, and scissors, as well as various traveling movements across the apparatus, allow for bonus points [11]. The still rings require incredible upper body strength and stability [11]. The goal is to perform the swinging, handstands, and 2-second holds while keeping the rings in place. Similar to the women, the vault requires the male gymnast to sprint and jump onto a spring board, allowing for propulsion from his hands off of the vault to perform various twists or flips. The parallel bars stand 195 cm (6.4 feet) high and is an event that utilizes swinging, flight, and static strength holds that are performed above, between, or below the parallel bars. The dismount is commonly performed to the side [11]. The high bar event is made of a 275-cm (9 feet)-high 1-inch-diameter metal bar upon which gymnasts perform swinging and flight elements that create difficulty when executed in series. The athletes swing forward, backward, or on a single arm and often perform pirouettes and release moves. Gymnasts score difficulty points for high-flying release skills and dismounts involving multiple twists and flips [11]. Overall, the levels and scoring system for men's gymnastics is similar to women's artistic gymnastics.

1.2.3 Acrobatic Gymnastics

Acrobatic gymnastics began with sanctioned competitions in 1973 in the United States. By 1998, when the FIG recognized acrobatic gymnastics as a discipline to include for the World Championships, there were 54 countries affiliated [8]. In 2018, there were 134 countries involved in acrobatic gymnastics [8]. Acrobatic gymnastics has international competitions sanctioned by the FIG including World Championships, World Cup, and World Games [8].

The sport combines both dynamic and static elements along with artistry and partnership. The partnership distinguishes this discipline from any other. There are five possible groupings, including women's pair, women's trio, mixed pair (male base and female flyer), men's pair, and men's four. There are one, two, or three "bases" and one "top" or "flyer." The athletes compete on a standard 12-by-12-m spring floor, consistent with artistic gymnastics. Figure 1.4a, b show a women's pair group performing different variations of balance elements.

The JO program for acrobatic gymnastics begins with compulsory levels 5 through 7, and optional levels 8 through Senior Elite. In acrobatic gymnastics, groups are awarded points for the routines based on their performance in three categories: difficulty, execution, and artistry. Athletes compete one to three routines including dynamic, balance, or combined.

As acrobatic gymnastics becomes more popular, it is important for healthcare providers to understand some of the basic skills required for these gymnasts. For example, flexibility is often emphasized for the flyers, whereas a base's job is to provide stability and power for their partner. The optional levels of acrobatic gymnastics require various handstand transition shapes, and multiple saltos (no-handed flips). It is also important to note the high degree of aesthetics valued in acrobatic gymnastics, putting the athletes at high risk for impaired eating behaviors compared to age-matched peers [7]. Additionally, the level of flexibility required for these athletes should be considered for management of musculoskeletal conditions.

Fig. 1.4 Acrobatic gymnastics women's pairs showing strength, flexibility, and balance. (**a**) Acrobatic gymnastics women's pair demonstrating a balance element. (**b**) Acrobatic gymnastics women's pair demonstrating a balance element with a "base" and "flyer"

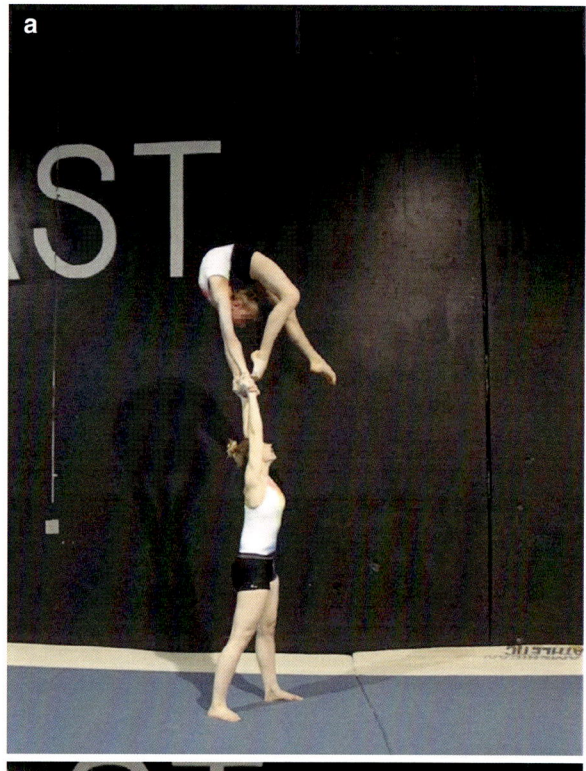

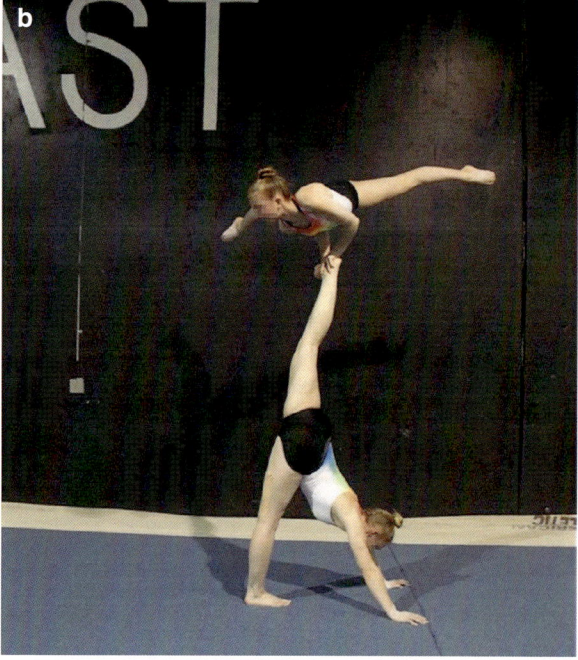

1.2.4 Tumbling and Trampoline (T&T)

Trampoline gymnastics, or tumbling and trampoline (T&T) as it is known in the United States, is organized as a part of USAG and the FIG. Greg Neeson from the United States was thought to be the first creator of the trampoline in 1936; however it was not until 1976 when trampoline was recognized as an official sport in the United States [8]. The year 2000 was the first Olympic year for trampoline [6]. Power tumbling is currently not considered an Olympic sport, but is part of the competitive T&T program in the United States.

Athletes may compete in individual trampoline, synchronized trampoline, double mini-trampoline, and tumbling. Individuals can compete in as few as one event or may perform up to all four events. Currently, trampoline gymnastics is a part of the Olympic Games, World Games, World Cups, and Trampoline World Championships.

Individual trampoline is a series or routine of several saltos, twists, and jumps. Athletes are awarded points based on difficulty level and execution of the skills. The height of each skill is an important factor in trampoline work, along with horizontal displacement of the jumps. Athletes lose points based on distance traveled from the center mark. Synchronized trampoline elements are performed side by side and are judged on synchronicity along with all of the other criteria evaluated in individual trampoline.

Double-mini is performed by both men and women; it consists of two jumps performed on the designated areas of the trampoline and require a safe landing onto the landing mat. The initial jump is called the "mount" that takes you to the spotter area, followed by a dismount skill to the ground.

Tumbling, or power tumbling, is competed by both men and women on a rod floor connected to a landing mat. A rod floor is often used as a training tool for other disciplines due to the level of bounce it provides for athletes. It is made of steel frames and fiberglass rods closely linked together; therefore, it provides more return of energy than the spring floor used by artistic gymnasts. The musculoskeletal demands are most similar to that of an artistic gymnast who competes on floor.

In the JO or national team track for T&T, athletes can begin competing at age 6 and are divided into age categories. Trampoline athletes advance through the levels by demonstrating safety and competence of the previous level. Levels 1 through 7 athletes compete compulsory routines and levels 8 through 10 and elite compete one compulsory and one optional routine.

Skills performed in the trampoline events don't require the extreme flexibility or mobility that the other disciplines do. Rather, power, and the ability to generate and maintain force, momentum, and height are valued for these competitors. Although these athletes must be able to achieve full tuck, pike, and layout shapes to achieve high scores, they are not often required to demonstrate unilateral flexibility or the extreme back extension required in rhythmic, acrobatic, and artistic gymnasts.

1.2.5 Rhythmic Gymnastics

Rhythmic gymnastics is also a part of USAG and organized under the umbrella of the FIG. It is strongly influenced by classical ballet and combines dance with various apparatuses or equipment [1, 6, 12]. In addition, there is a thought to be a large influence from Swedish free-moving styles of dance [8]. Competitive rhythmic gymnastics began in 1940 in the Soviet Union [8]. The FIG adopted Rhythmic gymnastics in 1963.

Rhythmic gymnasts compete on a 13-by-13-m spring floor [6]. World-class athletes of rhythmic gymnastics are eligible to compete in the Olympic Games, World Championships, World Cup, World Challenge Cup, and the World Games. This is the only sport in the FIG where women are the only gender who are eligible to compete.

Similar to the other disciplines, USAG had designed the levels of rhythmic gymnastics to allow for development of the basic fundamental elements in levels 3 through 6. Gymnasts learn how to utilize hand-held apparatuses with pre-determined choreography and routines. Levels 7 through 10 and Junior and Senior Elite are optional levels and allow for more freedom of choreography through creative combinations of elements with artistry. Every year, the apparatuses the athletes utilize rotate between the rope, hoop, ball, clubs, and ribbon. Athletes may compete as individuals, but are also eligible to compete in a group of five gymnasts. They may compete with the same apparatus or "mixed" apparatus.

Gymnasts are awarded points based on the difficulty of the elements, execution, and overall artistry. Dance and aesthetic lines are highly valued in rhythmic gymnastics. The degree of flexibility required by these athletes is unparalleled to the other disciplines within the FIG. Although bilateral coordination is a skill that is encouraged early in training, athletes typically have a dominate kicking, leaping, and turning leg. This often creates an imbalance of passive and active strength and flexibility. High degrees of lumbar, thoracic, shoulder, wrist, and cervical mobility are required for the optional and advanced levels.

The heavy influence of the Soviet Union in the creation and development of this sport also leads to a high level of pressure for a unique and slender somatotype for aesthetic appeal. Medical providers should be aware that rhythmic gymnasts have high levels of impaired eating behaviors [12–14].

1.2.6 Aerobic Gymnastics

Aerobic gymnastics is one of the newest disciplines to be sanctioned by the FIG. Although USAG supports its growth, it is not one of the governing bodies. Aerobic gymnastics developed from the growth of aerobics in the United States in the 1980s [6, 8]. The FIG adopted aerobic gymnastics as a competitive sport in

1996. There are currently World Championships, World Games, and World Cup events. In 2017, there were 17 participating countries and 116 athletes in the World Games, making it a small portion of the FIG. Competitors can compete in a group or as individuals. Aerobic gymnasts must demonstrate a fluid routine of flexibility, endurance, strength, and coordination, while demonstrating the seven basic steps of aerobics. These gymnasts demonstrate their ability to generate power from a static position, such as an explosive push-up; however, they are not required to perform backward or forward tumbling series.

1.2.7 Gymnastics for All

Gymnastics for All was officially recognized as its own gymnastics discipline by the FIG in 1984 [6, 14]. This gymnastics discipline is both physical and conceptual, as it offers a variety of movements for all ages, genders, abilities, and cultural backgrounds [6]. It offers an aesthetic experience to both participants and spectators, and it often uses all the gymnastics equipment and apparatuses (i.e., floor, vault, beam, bars, trampoline, ribbons, clubs, hoops, etc.) [6]. Gymnastics for All focuses on the development of general gymnastics skills, fitness, health, movement patterns, and, even daily life skills [14]. Due to the inclusivity of this gymnastics discipline, it has the most participants worldwide compared to the other gymnastics disciplines. Competitive Gymnastics for All athletes may participate in Power TeamGym (levels 1 through 10), acrobatics and tumbling (Novice, Junior and Senior divisions), or World Gym for Life Challenge [6, 14]. Group performances can be as large as thousands of participants and may require large stadiums for performances [6, 14]. Locally, gymnastics facilities participate in hosting exhibitions, festival performances, and end of year shows associated with Gymnastics for All. Internationally, the World Gymnaestrada is held in various countries to allow for small or large group performances from around the world to showcase their talents every 4 years, similar to the Olympics [6, 14]. The physical requirements for these athletes do not typically require the flexibility or acrobatics seen in other disciplines; rather, dance, choreography, and synchronization are the emphasis.

1.2.8 Parkour

Parkour is a sport with growing popularity and media attention and deserves mention in this medical textbook, as some of the movements and injuries are similar to other gymnastics disciplines. In addition, parkour was officially made a discipline of FIG in 2018.

Some will claim that Parkour originated on "the streets"; however, the origination can be traced back to the early 1900s and is rather separate from the origination of gymnastics. Georges Hébert was a French Naval officer who created a physical regimen he called "the Natural Method," which involved training the ten useful skills of walking, running, jumping, climbing, swimming, throwing, lifting, self-defense, quadrupedal movement, and balance [15, 16]. Hébert's motto was: "étra fort pour étre utile," which translates to "be strong to be useful" [16]. His work was inspired by how well the natives of Martinique were able to overcome obstacles in their path as they were fleeing from the eruption of Mount Pelée in 1902 [15, 16]. He compared the movements of the fleeing Europeans, who appeared to have "lost" their ability to efficiently and effectively move, to the native's ability to run, climb, jump, or swim to safety to save their lives [15, 16]. Hébert's physical regimen and the use of obstacle courses became the basis for French military training during World War I [15, 16].

David Belle was another originator tied to the world of parkour [16]. He was the son of a French fireman, Raymond Belle [16]. David was inspired by his father's training in the French fire brigade to perfect his own Natural Method skills and then later with his friends in his teens [16]. In 1997, his talented group of friends were asked to perform at a live event in Paris and called themselves the Yamisaki [16]. From here on, parkour began to gain popularity throughout the world and in the media [16].

FIG officially voted in parkour as their eighth discipline in 2018 [6], though it is controversial among many "traceurs" whether parkour belongs to the gymnastics world or not. In fact, large parts of the parkour community that are not involved in the FIG adamantly demand that "we are not gymnastics," in response to FIG's slogan "we are gymnastics" when the FIG began to sponsor parkour competitions in 2018, beginning with the first FIG World Cup series [15, 17]. Parkour associations, such as the International Parkour Federation (IPF), American Parkour (APK), Sport Parkour League, and World Freerunning Parkour Federation [15], have been established for years, have created parkour coaching certifications, and have held informal competitions and showcases prior to the FIG's involvement with parkour. While official competitions have only existed within the last 5–10 years, some parkour athletes do not believe that parkour should become a competitive sport and see it as more of an "art" similar to dance.

Modern techniques for parkour, such as flips, vaults, and swinging on bars, are similar to that in gymnastics; however, there are specific movements, apparatuses, and skills unique to the parkour world. The kinds of movements utilized depend on which event is being performed. The events that FIG has created are called Speedrun and Freestyle, but other parkour associations may include a Skill event and other variations [6, 15]. The obstacle course style has been defined as getting from point A to point B in the most *efficient* way possible, including running, climbing, swinging, jumping, and leaping to, from, under, or over obstacles in the way [15]. Conversely, Freerunning can be described as getting from point A to point B in the most *creative* way possible [15]. Because of the novelty of competition in this sport, the events may be different depending on the league, governing body of the competition, and advancements in the sport.

1.2.9 Cirque

Cirque gymnastics is hybrid of gymnastics and performing arts that is not organized through a single sanctioned governing body, but deserves mention in this medical textbook as these athletes commonly have competitive gymnastics backgrounds and their livelihoods are often based on their performance. Cirque events and apparatuses may include, but are not limited to aerial silks, hand balancing, lyra, straps, cyr wheel, and trapeze. At this time, there is no formal body to regulate or set criteria for judging standards leaving room for interpretation of each of these apparatuses. Therefore, healthcare providers may face unique challenges for each cirque athlete's level of training, preferred apparatuses, experience, and background.

1.3 Conclusion

Gymnastics has changed significantly over the last few centuries. It is important for the medical team to have a basic understanding of the different disciplines of gymnastics as well as the unique injuries that are common to athletes in each discipline. In addition, since the rules and procedures for gymnastics frequently change, research and education must continue in order to provide the best evidence-based approaches to the care of all gymnasts. The following chapters will examine the various medical issues that are seen in gymnasts including common psychological and orthopedic problems.

References

1. Goodbody J. The illustrated history of gymnastics. London: Stanley Paul & Co. Ltd; 1982.
2. Krüger M. Body culture and nation building: the history of gymnastics in Germany in the period of its foundation as a nation-state. Int J Hist Sport. 1996;13(3):409–17. https://doi.org/10.1080/09523369608713957.
3. Fullman J. The Olympics: ancient to modern. 1st ed. London: Wayland; 2017.
4. The Editors of Encyclopaedia Britannica. Friedrich Ludwig Jahn. Encyclopædia Britannica. 2018. https://www.britannica.com/biography/Friedrich-Ludwig-Jahn. Accessed 15 Feb 2019.
5. Frederick AB. Gymnastics. Encyclopædia Britannica. 2018. https://www.britannica.com/sports/gymnastics#ref700591. Accessed 15 Feb 2019.
6. Federation Internationale de Gymnastique. About the FIG: history. Available from: http://www.gymnastics.sport/site/. Accessed 3 Jan 2019.
7. Salbach H, Klinkowski N, Pfeiffer E, Lehmkuhl U, Korte A. Body image and attitudinal aspects of eating disorders in rhythmic gymnasts. Psychopathology. 2007;40(6):388–93. Epub 2007 Jul 25. PubMed PMID: 17652951.
8. USA Gymnastics. About USA Gymnastics. Available from: http://usagym.org. Accessed 19 Dec 2018.
9. Olga's Achievements. Olga Korbut. 2012. http://olgakorbut.com/olgas-achievements/. Accessed 15 Feb 2019.

10. USA Gymnastics. FIG elite/International Scoring. https://usagym.org/pages/events/pages/fig_scoring.html.
11. USA Gymnastics. Men's artistic gymnastics event descriptions. Gymnastics 101. https://usagym.org/pages/gymnastics101/men/events.html. Accessed 15 Feb 2019.
12. Klinkowski N, Korte A, Pfeiffer E, Lehmkuhl U, Salbach-Andrae H. Psychopathology in elite rhythmic gymnasts and anorexia nervosa patients. Eur Child Adolesc Psychiatry. 2008;17(2):108–13. Epub 2007 Sep 10. PubMed PMID: 17846815.
13. Silva MG, Silva HH, Paiva T. Sleep duration, body composition, dietary profile and eating behaviours among children and adolescents: a comparison between Portuguese acrobatic gymnasts. Eur J Pediatr. 2018;177(6):815–25. https://doi.org/10.1007/s00431-018-3124-z. Epub 2018 Mar 3. PubMed PMID: 29502302.
14. Gymnastics Ireland. Gymnastics for all | Disciplines. https://www.gymnasticsireland.com/disciplines/gymnastics-for-all. Accessed 15 Feb 2019.
15. World Freerunning Parkour Federation. A brief & basic history of parkour. https://wfpf.com/history-parkour/. Accessed 15 Feb 2019.
16. Henry M. The parkour roadmap. Herndon: Mascot Books; 2017.
17. APK American Parkour. We are not gymnastics. 2019. http://americanparkour.com/news/we-are-not-gymnastics/. Accessed 15 Feb 2019.

Chapter 2
Epidemiology of Gymnastics Injuries

Sigrid F. Wolf and Cynthia R. LaBella

2.1 Introduction

Gymnastics is a popular sport both in the United States (USA) and internationally. According to the Federation Internationale de Gymnastique or the International Gymnastics Federation (FIG), approximately 50 million people worldwide participate regularly in club gymnastics [1]. In the United States, approximately 3.3% (estimated 984,000) of children ages 6–12 participate in gymnastics on a regular basis [2]. Gymnastics contains eight disciplines: Men's Artistic, Women's Artistic, Rhythmic, Trampoline, Acrobatic, Aerobic, Gymnastics for All, and Parkour [3]. In the United States, athletes can participate in a variety of settings including club/USA Gymnastics Junior Olympic (USAG JO) program, high school teams, National Collegiate Athletic Association (NCAA) teams, national/international elite level, and the Olympics.

2.2 Participation Estimates

Gymnastics participation is growing in the United States. USA Gymnastics (USAG) reports 125,216 athlete members in its most recent count, increased by over 400% from approximately 30,000 athletes in 1980 [4].

S. F. Wolf (✉) · C. R. LaBella
Institute for Sports Medicine, Ann & Robert H. Lurie Children's Hospital of Chicago, Chicago, IL, USA
e-mail: sfwolf@luriechildrens.org; CLabella@luriechildrens.org

2.2.1 Club

There are no published estimates for club-level gymnastics participation. Many club gymnasts participate in the USAG program; however, there are other local and state-based club programs in which some gymnasts participate. Therefore, estimates for participation are difficult to obtain.

2.2.2 High School

In the 2017–2018 school year, 18,867 female and 1,715 male gymnasts competed for their high school teams [5].

2.2.3 NCAA

At the collegiate level, there are currently 1,447 female and 343 male NCAA gymnasts, and 61 Division I (DI), 7 Division II (DII), and 15 Division III (DIII) schools offering women's gymnastics. Only 15 DI and one DIII college offer men's gymnastics. NCAA gymnastics participation has decreased by nearly 50% since the early 1980s when 2,063 female gymnasts participated at 179 colleges and 1,367 male gymnasts participated at 79 colleges. The average college squad size has increased from 10.7–12.9 women and 15.1–17.8 men in 1982 to 18.3–19.6 women and 21.3–23 men in 2018 [6].

2.2.4 Elite

At the elite level, FIG estimates a total of 31,700 athletes including 7,839 male gymnasts and 16,624 female gymnasts are competing at an international level. The breakdown by disciplines is shown in Table 2.1 [7]. Approximately 320 gymnasts across all gymnastics disciplines compete at each Olympic Games [1].

Table 2.1 Number of FIG gymnasts competing internationally [7]

Men's artistic gymnastics	3653
Women's artistic gymnastics	3821
Rhythmic gymnastics	6375
Trampoline gymnastics	7225
Acrobatic gymnastics	4830
Aerobic gymnastics	5754
Parkour	42

2.3 Injury Epidemiology Data Limitations

Gymnastics injury epidemiology is difficult to study for a number of reasons. First, most of the existing research studies are small and rarely include male gymnasts. Second, it is difficult to define the terms "gymnastics" and "injury" consistently. Gymnastics is a heterogeneous sport composed of many different activities and disciplines performed by people of all ages and levels ranging from young children practicing gymnastic skills at home to young adult Olympians.

Moreover, gymnastics rules, equipment, and training methods have evolved over the past few decades making prior research less applicable for today's gymnasts. The term "injury" is defined in many different ways in the literature including self-reported injury, seeking evaluation by a medical provider, reported pain, emergency room visits, time lost, modified practice, etc. These definitions each have limitations, particularly in that many gymnasts continue modified training while injured and do not report their injuries consistently. Complicating matters further, most clubs do not have medical providers or athletic trainers to verify and record injuries. In one prospective study of elite and subelite gymnasts, the athletes retrospectively reported only 54% of the injuries found prospectively during the same time period [8]. Finally, there is a paucity of data collection and information on injuries by gymnastics organizations. These challenges highlight the need for a national, centralized database to record gymnastics injuries, particularly at the club level.

2.4 Injuries in Gymnastics

2.4.1 Overall Injuries

At some point, most gymnasts will suffer an injury [9]. The overall injury rate in gymnasts is 1.4 injuries per 1000 hours of training in men and 1.5 per 1000 hours in women, although estimates vary ranging from 1.08 to 50.3 per 1000 hours [3, 10]. Put differently, across all age groups, male gymnasts are estimated to have 678 injuries per 1000 athletes per year, and female gymnasts have 306 injuries per 1000 athletes per year [3]. Increasing training hours and higher levels of gymnastics are associated with increased injury incidence and severity [1, 3]. Among all disciplines, artistic gymnasts have the highest rates of injury with reported rates ranging from 1.6 to 4.1 per 1000 hours of training [1, 3].

2.4.2 Injury Types

Across all gymnastics populations, sprains and strains are the most common injury types. Extremity injuries comprise approximately 75% of all gymnastics injuries, and ankle sprain is the most common diagnosis in every level (Table 2.2) [3].

Table 2.2 Most common gymnastics injury types for all levels combined [3]

Injury type	Percentage
Strains/sprains	36%
Fractures/stress fractures	10%
Abrasions/contusions/inflammation/lacerations	8%
Concussion	8%
Bursitis	5%
Other/incomplete recording	33%

2.4.3 Gender Differences

Male Gymnasts Upper extremity injuries are more common in male gymnasts comprising 43% of injuries. This is unsurprising since male gymnasts use apparatuses, such as rings and pommel horse, that demand more use of the upper body. The shoulder is usually cited as the most commonly injured body part, although the hand/wrist is reported as the most common in some studies [9–11]. Other frequently injured body parts include the lower extremity (34%), torso/spine (12%), and head/neck (5%) [3].

Female Gymnasts Lower extremity injuries are more common in female gymnasts, comprising 51% of injuries. Ankle and foot injuries are the most frequent [3, 12]. Upper extremity injuries make up another 31%—largely hand and wrist injuries [3, 9]. Torso and spine injuries account for 13% which are primarily low back injuries including spondylolysis, vertebral body fractures, discogenic pain, and spondylogenic back pain [3, 13]. Head and neck injuries account for 1% of reported injuries.

2.4.4 Level Differences for Injuries

The frequency and type of injuries that occur in gymnastics vary based on level and discipline. Table 2.3 outlines injury rates.

Club Club-level gymnasts are infrequently studied. Available studies represent a variety of disciplines, levels, and training hours which are not always clearly delineated, making it difficult to reliably compare them to other gymnast groups. Research suggests that they suffer more injuries than their non-athletic peers [14]. Injury estimates range from 0.52 to 4.1 injuries per 1000 hours of gymnastics exposure [8, 10, 15]. Club-level female gymnasts older than 10 years or participating 16 or more hours per week have higher rates of injury [15, 16]. Following this trend, injury rates are lower overall in club gymnasts than in collegiate gymnasts [10]. One small study of 64 gymnasts found that injured subelite gymnasts are more likely than injured elite gymnasts to miss training sessions rather than modify practice [15].

Table 2.3 Injury rates at different gymnastics levels

Level	Injury rate
Club/JO	0.52–4.1 injuries per 1000 hours
Women's High School	1.09–2.38 injuries per 1000 athlete exposures (AEs)
Women's NCAA Collegiate	10.4 injuries per 1000 AEs
Men's NCAA Collegiate	8.78 injuries per 1000 AEs
Olympic Female	86.4 injuries per 1000 gymnasts
Olympic Male	79.9 injuries per 1000 gymnasts
All levels Combined Female	1.5 injuries per 1000 hours
All levels Combined Male	1.4 injuries per 1000 hours

Across all club levels, the most commonly injured body part is the lower extremity, accounting for 54–70% of injuries (most commonly the ankle). Upper extremity injuries comprise 17–25% of injuries (most commonly the wrist). Spine/trunk injury estimates vary from 0% to 43% of injuries—the majority of which are lower back injuries [9]. Strains and sprains are the most frequent injury type, although stress fractures, mostly in the low back and foot, have been found to occur in one out of six club gymnasts during their lifetime participation. Moreover, 30% of club gymnasts report suffering at least one concussion during their career [15]. Risk factors for injury in club gymnasts include supervision by less experienced coaches, fewer hours preparing for competition, and lower overall levels of physical fitness [8].

High School High schools seldom have gymnastics teams. Injury estimates are from the National High School Sports-Related Injury Surveillance Study and only reflect girls' gymnastics [17]. High school gymnastics injury rates range from 1.09 to 2.38 injuries per 1000 athlete exposures (AEs), compared to 1.97 to 2.17 injuries per 1000 AEs for all high school sports combined. For comparison, men's high school football injury rates reported during the same time period range from 3.50 to 3.81 per 1000 AEs, men's wrestling 1.98 to 2.50 per 1000 AEs, and women's soccer 1.93 to 2.42 per 1000 AEs. The most common injury types in female high school gymnasts are strains and sprains. Other common injuries include concussions, fractures, and contusions. Ankle sprain/strain is the most common diagnosis accounting for 14–39% of recorded injuries followed by knee injuries at 14–21%. 3.4–11.9% of all injuries required surgery [17]. Of note, available data from this database are incomplete with up to 50% of high school gymnast's injury diagnoses not recorded each year. This may be because many high school gymnastics programs train off-site at a nearby club, and therefore the athletes may not be reporting their injuries to their school's athletic trainer.

NCAA Collegiate Women's gymnastics has the highest overall injury rate among women's NCAA sports at 10.4 injuries per 1000 AEs, double the overall average injury rate for NCAA women's sports. The only college sport with a higher injury rate is men's wrestling at 13.1 per 1000 AEs. For comparison, NCAA men's football has an average 9.2 per 1000 AEs. Women's soccer has a higher competition injury rate than female gymnastics at 17.2 per 1000 AEs versus 13.2 per 1000 AEs [18].

Men's NCAA gymnastics has 8.78 injuries per 1000 AEs [11]. Male gymnasts suffer fewer major injuries that result in missed participation time or that require surgery compared to their female counterparts [11].

Among collegiate gymnasts, freshman-eligible gymnasts suffer the most injuries [11]. Division I gymnasts have higher rates of injury than Division II and III gymnasts (relative risk = 1.62) [19]. The most frequently injured body part in collegiate female gymnasts is the ankle, followed by the knee, lower leg/Achilles, trunk/low back, and foot [12, 19]. Most common injury types are sprains (20.3%) and strains (18.7%) [19]. The knee is the most common location of severe injury with 21% of reported knee injuries requiring surgery—mostly for anterior cruciate ligament tears [19]. There is a paucity of data on concussion and low back injuries at the NCAA level. We theorize that this is because of less awareness of these injuries in years past.

Elite/Olympic Elite gymnasts, particularly those competing at an international level, have more frequent injuries than lower level gymnasts [3]. Their injuries last longer than in subelite gymnasts, and injured athletes are more likely to modify training sessions rather than miss practice [8]. During the Olympics, female and male gymnasts have similar injury rates at 86.4 injuries per 1000 female gymnasts and 79.9 injuries per 1000 male gymnasts. Overall injury rates are 84 injuries per 1000 gymnasts with 38% of these injuries leading to time loss [1]. This injury rate is lower than many other Olympic sports including hockey, handball, and taekwondo which all have >150 injuries per 1000 athletes [1]. Nevertheless, women's artistic gymnastics injury incidence has increased over the past three Olympic games [1]. The youngest and oldest gymnasts have the highest injury rates at the Olympics. Experts suspect that this is the result of poor conditioning and immature musculoskeletal systems in the youngest gymnasts and weaker musculoskeletal tissues in the oldest gymnasts [1].

Strains and sprains account for 36% of Olympic gymnastics injuries, followed by contusions (10%), fractures (7%), and concussions (3%) [1, 3]. The most commonly injured body part is the lower limb (63%), followed by the trunk (23%), upper limb (14%), lumbar spine (14%), and foot (12.8%). As with all other gymnastics levels, ankle sprain is the most common diagnosis overall and the most common injury leading to time loss from Olympic competition [1, 3].

2.4.5 Injury Differences Between Disciplines

Most gymnastics research focuses on women's artistic gymnastics, so it is difficult to compare discipline injury rates. Among the Olympic disciplines, men's and women's artistic gymnastics have higher injury rates than rhythmic gymnastics; trampoline gymnastics has the lowest injury rate [1]. The reported injury rate in club rhythmic gymnastics is 1.08/1000 hours exposure which is similar to reported rates in club artistic gymnasts. The most commonly injured body parts in rhythmic gymnastics are the ankle (39%) and low back (22%) [14]. Similar injury patterns have been found in high-level, Scandinavian, TeamGym gymnasts [20]. Among trampoline gymnasts, the lower limb, spine, and upper limb are injured most frequently, and the most common diagnosis is knee sprain [21]. Acrobatic gymnasts suffer mostly lower limb injuries but have more upper limb injuries compared to trampoline gymnasts [21]. This is likely due to increased use of upper body in acrobatic gymnastics for the gymnasts to support themselves and others compared to trampoline gymnastics which primarily loads the lower body.

2.4.6 Acute Versus Overuse Injuries

There is an increased rate of overuse injuries compared to acute injuries as gymnasts progress to higher levels of competition because of the increased hours, intensity, and repetition of movements needed to perfect more complicated skills [8, 9, 22]. Wrist and low back injuries occur more often from overuse compared to ankle injuries which usually occur acutely [9]. At the artistic gymnastics club level, one study of 96 gymnasts, levels 4–10, estimated 1.8 overuse injuries per 1000 hours with the lower back being most frequently injured [15]. There was no data at the high school level for overuse injuries, but 16% of injuries were reported to be recurrent [17]. In NCAA female gymnasts, 30% of injuries were categorized as overuse, most commonly ankle, lower leg, and Achilles injuries [19]. At the elite level, chronic injuries account for the majority of injuries (64–75%) [8, 22].

2.4.7 Catastrophic Injuries

High School Gymnasts Despite the high overall number of gymnastics injuries, very few are catastrophic injuries, i.e., leading to severe injury (such as fractured cervical vertebra), permanent severe functional disability, or death. Over the past 35 years, high school gymnasts have had an average of 1.24 traumatic catastrophic injuries per 100,000 female gymnasts, and 3.4 per 100,000 male gymnasts. Of these, only one traumatic fatality occurred which was in a male high school gymnast. For comparison, the high school sports with the highest traumatic catastrophic injury rates were cheerleading (3.66/100,000 for males, 3.26/100,000 females), football (2.68/100,000), and ice hockey (2.58/100,000) [23].

Collegiate Gymnasts At the college level, catastrophic injuries are more frequent. Female gymnasts have an average of 3.83 catastrophic injuries per 100,000 participants, while males have 16.41 injuries per 100,000 participants. There have been no recorded fatalities from traumatic injuries at the college level. The other college sports with high catastrophic injury rates are women's skiing (11.4/100,000), men's football (10.0/100,000), men's ice hockey (8.8/100,000), men's skiing (4.7/100,000), and equestrian (4.1/100,000). Given the small numbers of high school and collegiate male gymnasts, these numbers should be interpreted with caution [23].

Club and Olympic Gymnasts There have been no recorded catastrophic injuries in gymnasts in the past three summer Olympics [1]. Unfortunately, there is no centralized database to evaluate catastrophic, traumatic injuries for club/USAG JO program gymnastics.

2.5 Emergency Department Evaluation of Injuries

Estimated numbers of emergency department (ED) visits for gymnastics injuries are high, with an incidence of 4.8 injuries per year requiring ED visits per 1000 gymnasts ages 6–17 [24]. Many of these injuries occur at home in younger children practicing unsupervised gymnastics. Lower extremity sprains and strains are the most common injury types for adolescents ages 12–17 (52% of all injuries), while younger children ages 6–11 are more likely to suffer upper extremity fractures and dislocations (50% of all injuries). Of gymnastics injuries treated in the ED, 2.6% result in hospital admission—92% for fractures and dislocations [24]. The overall breakdown of diagnoses is shown in Table 2.4. One limitation of this data set is that it may be less precise given the setting.

2.6 Why Are Gymnasts Injured So Frequently?

At all levels, gymnastics has one of the highest injury rates among girls' sports [25]. Gymnasts must practice intensely for long hours to become successful. Elite gymnasts train for 21–37 hours per week 11–12 months per year [1, 24]. They have an early age of entry and specialization defined as "participation in a single sport at the exclusion of other sports" [26]. Other factors contributing to its high injury rate include peak age of competition during teen years, high-impact movements, and increasing skill difficulty to progress between levels [9, 19, 24]. Most gymnasts still have immature musculoskeletal systems which increases their risk for injury to their growth cartilage, articular cartilage, and bones, especially during growth spurts [1, 9]. Other factors that have been found to increase injury risk include ignoring early signs of overuse injuries, increased life stress, and negative state of mood such as fear [19, 20].

Table 2.4 Most common gymnastics-related injury types in children treated in emergency departments [24]

Diagnosis	Injury prevalence (%)
Strains/sprains	44.3
Fractures/dislocations	30.4
Abrasions/contusions	15.6
Lacerations/avulsions	3.7
Concussion/closed head injury	1.7
Others	4.3

2.7 Injury Mechanisms

2.7.1 Biomechanics

There are multiple proposed mechanisms for the most common injuries in gymnastics. Across all levels, injuries occur most frequently during tumbling and dismount/landing [3, 9, 12, 19, 20]. Front and back handsprings and saltos/flips are the most common skills leading to injury [10]. There are multiple risk factors hypothesized to contribute to injury, including small landing mat size and spaces between mats, explosive movements, repetitive forces and movements, joint overload, and hyperextension [3, 19]. Skill difficulty increases with level, and judges reward more difficult routines leading athletes to push their limits and perform higher risk skills [3, 19].

Altered or poor biomechanics also increase injury risk. Poor biomechanics can result from practicing while injured or having poor fall mechanics such as tensing up and using the arms to brace for a fall [19, 24]. Lower extremity injuries, especially ankle injuries, most commonly occur during floor exercises and landing [12]. Insufficient rotation can change the angle at which the feet and ankles strike the floor leading to injuries [3, 12, 19]. Low back injuries are thought to be secondary to repetitive flexion, hyperextension, rotation, and compression of the spine—particularly with vaults, dismounts, and somersaults [9, 12]. Adjustments to landing biomechanics to prevent under-rotation of the feet/ankles and decreasing back hyperextension may decrease injury rates [3].

2.7.2 Differences Between Apparatuses

At all levels, approximately one in three female gymnastics injuries occur during floor exercise because gymnasts spend the most time on the floor during warm-up and practice [12, 15, 17]. In NCAA female athletes, contusions are most common on the balance beam, while most shoulder injuries occur on the uneven bars [19]. Interestingly, the most common mechanism for concussion is contact with a surface (i.e., mat) on the uneven bars [19].

2.8 Timing of Injuries

2.8.1 Practice Versus Competition

Competition is a high-risk time for gymnastics injuries. Although more overall injuries occur during practice, competition injury rates are 2–6 times higher per exposure time, and competition injuries tend to be more severe [1, 3, 10, 12, 15, 18, 19]. In high school gymnasts, injury rates during competition are nearly double those of practice rates [17]. In NCAA gymnasts, competition injury rates are estimated 1.7 times higher, and gymnasts are six times more likely to suffer knee internal derangement and nearly three times more likely to sprain an ankle ligament during competition [12, 19].

2.8.2 Season

Peak emergency room visits for gymnastics injuries occur in fall and spring, corresponding with high school and club competition seasons [24]. There is mixed data on whether the most injuries occur in the beginning, middle, or end of a gymnastics session [9, 20]. Some studies show that injuries occur more frequently during preseason when gymnasts have recently returned from a vacation or are preparing their routines and learning new skills [9, 12, 20].

2.9 Next Steps

Gymnastics injury epidemiology studies are limited by changes in the sport, the focus on female artistic gymnasts, small heterogeneous study populations, and recall bias. In particular, further efforts should be made to study long-term outcomes for gymnastics injuries, the effects of rule and equipment changes, concussions, club-level gymnasts, and male gymnasts. A centralized injury and safety database is needed to enhance understanding of gymnastics injury epidemiology and better protect gymnasts from harm.

References

1. Edouard P, Steffen K, Junge A, Leglise M, Soligard T, Engebretsen L. Gymnastics injury incidence during the 2008, 2012 and 2016 Olympic Games: analysis of prospectively collected surveillance data from 963 registered gymnasts during Olympic Games. Br J Sports Med. 2018;52(7):475–81.
2. Project Play [Internet]. 2018. Available from: https://www.aspenprojectplay.org/kids-sports-participation-rates/.
3. Thomas RE, Thomas BC. A systematic review of injuries in gymnastics. Phys Sportsmed. 2019;47:96–121.
4. USA Gymnastics Statistics. Membership categories breakdown [updated September, 2016]. Available from: https://usagym.org/PDFs/About USA Gymnastics/Statistics/stats-memshipcategories.pdf.
5. The National Federation of State High School Associations. 2017–2018 high school athletics participation survey [Internet]. [cited 11/5/2018]. Available from: https://www.nfhs.org/ParticipationStatistics/ParticipationStatistics/.

6. NCAA. NCAA sports sponsorship and participation rates database. Available from: http://www.ncaa.org/about/resources/research/ncaa-sports-sponsorship-and-participation-rates-database.
7. Federation Internationale De Gymnastique Population. Available from: http://www.gymnastics.sport/site/pages/about-population.php.
8. Kolt GS, Kirkby RJ. Epidemiology of injury in elite and subelite female gymnasts: a comparison of retrospective and prospective findings. Br J Sports Med. 1999;33(5):312–8.
9. Caine DJ, Nassar L. Gymnastics injuries. Med Sport Sci. 2005;48:18–58.
10. Hart E, Meehan WP 3rd, Bae DS, d'Hemecourt P, Stracciolini A. The young injured gymnast: a literature review and discussion. Curr Sports Med Rep. 2018;17(11):366–75.
11. Westermann RW, Giblin M, Vaske A, Grosso K, Wolf BR. Evaluation of men's and women's gymnastics injuries: a 10-year observational study. Sports Health. 2015;7(2):161–5.
12. Marshall SW, Covassin T, Dick R, Nassar LG, Agel J. Descriptive epidemiology of collegiate women's gymnastics injuries: National Collegiate Athletic Association Injury Surveillance System, 1988-1989 through 2003-2004. J Athl Train. 2007;42(2):234–40.
13. Micheli LJ. Back injuries in gymnastics. Clin Sports Med. 1985;4(1):85–93.
14. Cupisti A, D'Alessandro C, Evangelisti I, Umbri C, Rossi M, Galetta F, et al. Injury survey in competitive sub-elite rhythmic gymnasts: results from a prospective controlled study. J Sports Med Phys Fitness. 2007;47(2):203–7.
15. O'Kane JW, Levy MR, Pietila KE, Caine DJ, Schiff MA. Survey of injuries in Seattle area levels 4 to 10 female club gymnasts. Clin J Sport Med. 2011;21(6):486–92.
16. Saluan P, Styron J, Ackley JF, Prinzbach A, Billow D. Injury types and incidence rates in pre-collegiate female gymnasts: a 21-year experience at a single training facility. Orthop J Sports Med. 2015;3(4):2325967115577596.
17. High School RIO Convenience Summary Reports 2008–2012 [Internet]. The National High School Sports-Related Injury Surveillance Study. 2008–2012 [cited 11/11/2018]. Available from: http://www.ucdenver.edu/academics/colleges/PublicHealth/research/ResearchProjects/piper/projects/RIO/Pages/Study-Reports.aspx.
18. Kerr ZY, Marshall SW, Dompier TP, Corlette J, Klossner DA, Gilchrist J. College sports-related injuries—United States, 2009-10 through 2013-14 academic years. MMWR Morb Mortal Wkly Rep. 2015;64:1330–6.
19. Kerr ZY, Hayden R, Barr M, Klossner DA, Dompier TP. Epidemiology of National Collegiate Athletic Association women's gymnastics injuries, 2009-2010 through 2013-2014. J Athl Train. 2015;50(8):870–8.
20. Harringe ML, Renstrom P, Werner S. Injury incidence, mechanism and diagnosis in top-level teamgym: a prospective study conducted over one season. Scand J Med Sci Sports. 2007;17(2):115–9.
21. Grapton X, Lion A, Gauchard GC, Barrault D, Perrin PP. Specific injuries induced by the practice of trampoline, tumbling and acrobatic gymnastics. Knee Surg Sports Traumatol Arthrosc. 2013;21(2):494–9.
22. Kolar E, Pavletic MS, Smrdu M, Atikovic A. Athletes' perception of the causes of injury in gymnastics. J Sports Med Phys Fitness. 2017;57(5):703–10.
23. NCCSIR. Catastrophic sports injury research thirty-fifth annual report: Fall 1982-Spring 2017 [Internet]. 2017 [cited 11/5/2018]. Available from: nccsir.unc.edu.
24. Singh S, Smith GA, Fields SK, McKenzie LB. Gymnastics-related injuries to children treated in emergency departments in the United States, 1990-2005. Pediatrics. 2008;121(4):e954–60.
25. Caine D, Caine C, Maffulli N. Incidence and distribution of pediatric sport-related injuries. Clin J Sport Med. 2006;16(6):500–13.
26. Bell DR, Post EG, Biese K, Bay C, Valovich McLeod T. Sport specialization and risk of overuse injuries: a systematic review with meta-analysis. Pediatrics. 2018;142(3):e20180657.

Chapter 3
Biomechanics of Gymnastics

Edward Nyman Jr.

3.1 Biomechanics: An Overview

Perhaps no classification of athlete experiences the mechanical perturbation of the musculoskeletal system to the extent reached by the gymnast. In artistic gymnastics, athletes are subject to forces and joint moments that regularly approach, and occasionally exceed, the normal tolerances of hard and soft tissues [1]. Thus, it is requisite that the clinical practitioner responsible for care of such athletes has a sound understanding of the biomechanics of the sport, knowledge of the thresholds for such potentially injurious forces, and an understanding of acute and chronic force mitigation in an effort to prevent and treat injuries in these fortuitous athletes.

Biomechanics encompasses the field of science dedicated to better understanding the kinetics (forces) and kinematics (movements) of the body and their interaction with respect to ambulation, static balance, and dynamic activity. In the fields of sports medicine, orthopedics, and physical therapy, biomechanics informs the practitioner of the tolerable and potentially injurious loads from linear and angular force application perspectives. Knowledge of basic biomechanical constructs may help clinicians better prevent injury and maximize athletic performance.

Given that the gymnast pushes the boundaries of biomechanical tolerances of the body's tissues, it should come as little surprise that the history of the field of biomechanics is fairly well correlated with the sport's origins. While gymnastics was first described as an athletic practice in the times of the ancient Greeks and later Romans [2], so too was the field of biomechanics, as the earliest traces (study of musculoskeletal anatomy) of the discipline dates back to as early as fourth century BC via

E. Nyman Jr. (✉)
College of Health Professions, The University of Findlay, Findlay, OH, USA
e-mail: nyman@findlay.edu

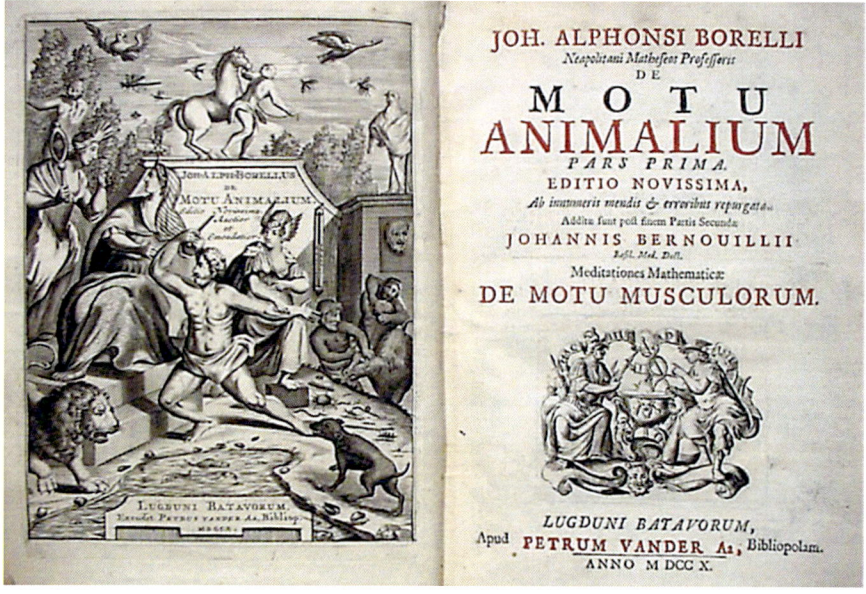

Fig. 3.1 Borelli's (and Aristotle's) *De Motu Animalium* represent some of the earliest roots of the field of biomechanics

Aristotle's *De Motu Animalium* (Fig. 3.1). Leonardo da Vinci and later Giovanni Borelli further catapulted biomechanical research in the fifteenth and seventeenth centuries, respectively [3]. Since then, the field has evolved in leaps and bounds. Ironically, these leaps and bounds may be directly tied to the advancements the sport of gymnastics has experienced, as both entities were well established by the mid-eighteenth century in part due to the efforts of Eadweard Muybridge (a forefather of modern biomechanics) and Pierre de Coubertin (considered the father of the modern Olympic Games).

While the histories of both biomechanics and gymnastics can be individually traced back centuries, relatively more modern ages have continued to see interactions between these entities. While numerous authors have scientifically evaluated gymnastics performance from a sports science, exercise physiology, and biomechanical basis, few have been as active in the space during the late twentieth and early twenty-first centuries as Dr. William Sands (Fig. 3.2). Dr. Sands' work has spanned three decades and has enlightened the coach and practitioner on biomechanical principles and performance enhancement relative to the modern sport. To date, he has published a multitude of empirical research articles relative to the sport of gymnastics – ranging from skill biomechanics to exercise physiology, to electromyography (EMG) – many of which will benefit the clinical practitioner in this field and may be considered requisite reading [4–8].

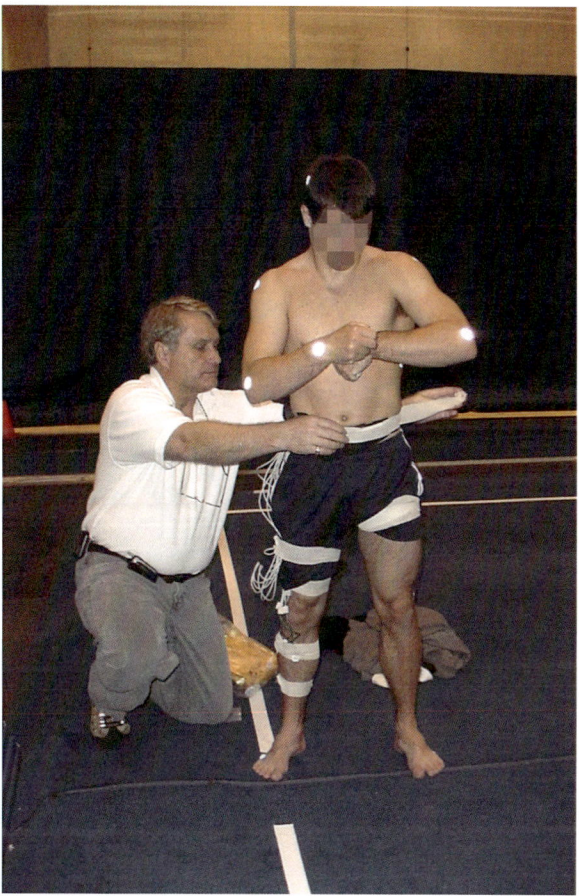

Fig. 3.2 Dr. William Sands conducting EMG analysis on male artistic gymnast

3.2 Clinical Biomechanics for Gymnastics

In an effort to provide the best clinical care for the gymnast, a clear understanding of orthopedic biomechanics and the unique sport-specific biomechanics of the sport is critical. While a few clinical practitioners are highly informed on the contemporary issues of the sport due to a personal history of a high-level of involvement as a gymnast themselves, many first encounter these athletes in the clinic as a student or practicing professional. It may come as no surprise that a fairly high percentage of medical professionals are not extensively informed in the biomechanics of gymnastics and therefore may prescriptively over- or underload the healing structures during return-to-sport protocol phases of healing. While it is beyond the scope of this chapter, and textbook, to provide an in-depth education on gymnastics skill classification, nomenclature, and proper technique, a baseline level of knowledge about the apparatus, competitive events, and some of the more common skills is essential for the practitioner engaging these athletes.

Those practitioners with a background as a gymnast, or who perhaps have a child who currently participates in the sport, have likely corresponded with colleagues in the allied healthcare fields whom assume the demands on the musculoskeletal system for a gymnast may be similar to that of a cheerleader or dancer. While those activities may also experience high forces, and indeed yield a myriad of musculoskeletal injuries, the mechanical demands for other sports cannot necessarily be aggregated and applied to the gymnast. For instance, overhead shoulder complex injuries are frequent in gymnasts [9]. Performance of women's uneven bars, or men's high bar, rings, and parallel bars, yields shoulder injuries that are far more like those experienced by a baseball pitcher or other high angular velocity throwing athlete than that of a cheerleader who experiences a shoulder injury from tumbling activities. While all such injuries may have similar presentations, a clearer understanding of the mechanical loads and high perturbations will better inform the clinician when differentially diagnosing pathologies with mechanism of injury in mind.

Further, when a gymnast performs a high angular velocity "swinging" or "pirouetting" skill (most commonly on high bar for men or uneven bars for women), the "overhead" activity loading force profile (specifically the resultant force vector) may be more like that of an overhead clean and jerk performance in Olympic weightlifting than it is like pitching mechanics. In such an example, acute injury to the glenohumeral joint derived from performance of a "hop full" or transitional release on uneven bars (Fig. 3.3), or a Yurchenko entry on vault, may provide a mechanism of injury consistent with a Bankart lesion due to the force vector at play rather than a SLAP lesion not uncommonly witnessed in high-velocity pitching mechanics. The lesson herein for the practitioner is that "overhead" mechanisms of injury for gymnastics may not "fit into the box" of the more common mechanisms of overhead injury in other common sports. Rendered to its simplest form, the clinicians must check their gut assumptions about mechanisms of injury when these athletes arrive for consultation and remember to ask oneself, "How many of my other athlete-patients spend much of their practice time supporting their full body weight on his or her hands?"

Another reason for the clinician to ensure acquisition of an appropriate knowledge base of the biomechanics of gymnastics is that such baseline knowledge enables the practitioner to be a better consumer of contemporary biomechanics research related to the sport. Such research knowledge acquisition, and any dissemination, therein enhances the evidence-based medicine paradigm. As many current professional journal articles in the field of injury and rehabilitation biomechanics have shifted away from pedagogical kinesiology into mechanical engineering and bioengineering arenas, a requisite baseline knowledge of the physics behind the musculoskeletal system perturbations of the sport is necessary.

Anatomical variability inherent across populations has been well documented. Without doubt, variability in the morphology of joint structures may biomechanically predispose the athlete to higher risk of injury [10, 11]. Such may be the case with

Fig. 3.3 Women's uneven bars performance loads and perturbates the shoulder complex extensively

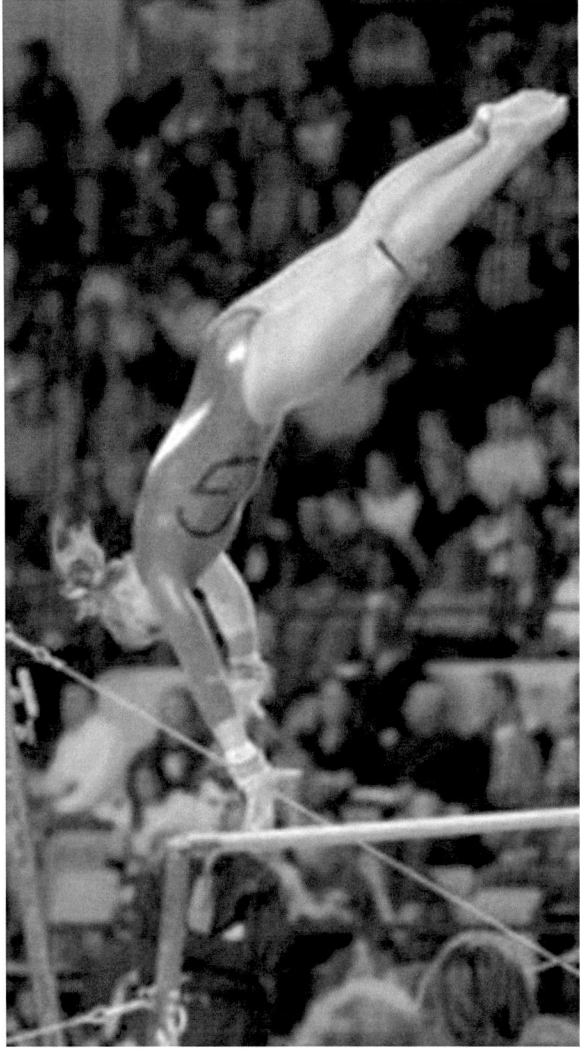

significant version of the acetabulum of the hip of the young gymnast. The biomechanics necessary for participation in gymnastics requires extreme hip range of motion [12]. Those with significant version of the proximal femur or acetabulum (primarily retroversion) may be more likely to experience edge loading of the femoral neck on the acetabular rim and thus, femoacetabular impingement (FAI) is more likely to occur in these individuals [13]. Similar phenomena have been documented for anatomical variability of the glenohumeral joint, tibiofemoral joint, and subtalar joints in the literature. For instance, proximal tibial geometric anomalies, (Fig. 3.4) such as excessive posterior inferior tibial slope, may increase ACL injury risk [9, 14, 15].

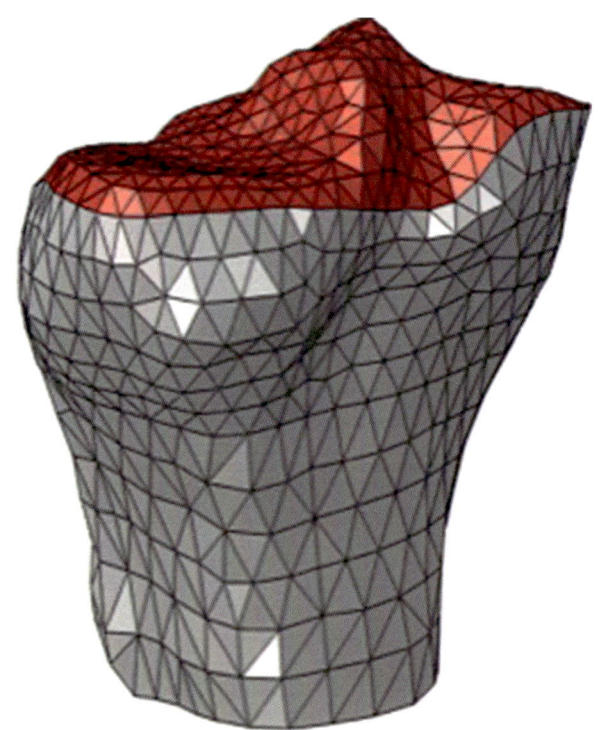

Fig. 3.4 Extensive morphological variability exists for joint contact surfaces. Depicted here is a finite-element computational model of the complex geometry of the proximal tibia

3.3 Foundations of Biomechanics

It may be most fitting to begin a discussion of the biomechanical basics relative to gymnastics with the biomechanical component that initially attracts most television viewers and fans to the sport – the *kinematics* (description of motion). Viewers, participants, and clinicians are commonly in awe of the sport due to the vastly dynamic ranges of motion and strength of the gymnast requisite in performing skills that appear to nearly defy physics. Kinematics refers simply to a *description* of motion. When a researcher or clinician describes a joint's range of motion in degrees (quantitative) or as excessive, lacking, or asymmetrical (qualitative), they are referring to the patient's (or healthy performer's) kinematics. While symmetry may be the most commonly utilized clinical kinematic, other quantitative descriptions are utilized and may be very impactful in clinical practice. These include normative values of range of motion, baseline references (intra-subject), or performance metrics such as linear or angular velocity, acceleration, or displacement.

While beyond the scope of this text for a detailed description, it is helpful for the clinician to review and to understand the *cardinal planes* (from the Latin, *cardinalis*, "to pivot") and associated *axes of rotation* with respect to all joints and body segments such that a valid and reliable convention for such kinematic descriptions can be maintained (Fig. 3.5a). Knowledge of the "right-hand rule" – wherein the

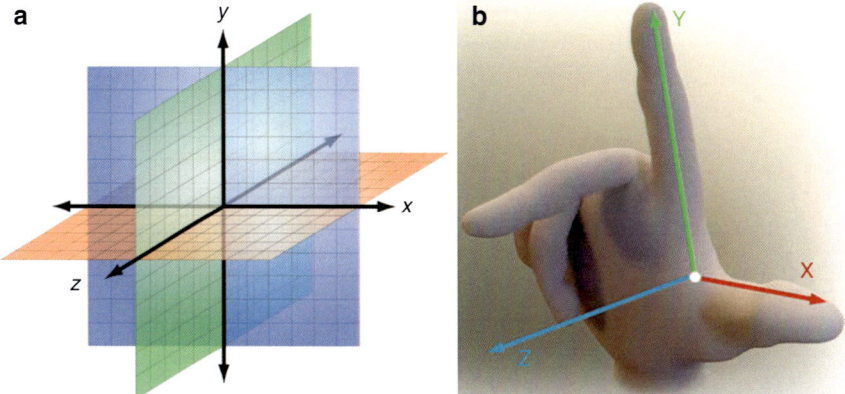

Fig. 3.5 (**a–b**) Cardinal planes, orthogonal axes of motion, and the right-hand rule utilized in biomechanics

direction of the curled fingers of the right hand denote the positive direction of rotation of a joint – is also helpful (Fig. 3.5b). Utilization of such conventions enables simple reference planes for motion. These planes are sagittal, frontal (also known as coronal), and transverse. It may be sufficient for the purposes of this text to remind the reader that establishment of a coordinate reference system (whether relative or fixed reference) is imperative for assessment and monitoring of kinematic values and changes – be they planar joint range of motion, velocity, linear acceleration, or angular acceleration. A common coordinate reference system utilized in human biomechanics is the Cartesian coordinate system (x, y, z).

Kinetics quantify the *forces* acting upon the body. These forces can be linearly directed (such as pressure at the bottom of the foot) or delivered angularly (such as *joint moments* – otherwise known as torques) around a musculoskeletal joint. Common SI units for kinetics therefore include newton (linear force), PSI (pressure), and $N*m^{-1}$ (torque). As with kinematics, quantitative assessment of these metrics may aid prediction, prevention, and rehabilitation efforts of the clinician. Direct application examples include but are not limited to static balance sway (with neurocognitive implications related to concussion), strength, and power (assessable via isokinetic dynamometry assessment of joint torque capability).

The forces described as acting upon the body are commonly referred to as vector forces. A vector includes both magnitude (extent or amount of force) and direction (at what angle relative to a given cardinal plane (or planes) is the force being applied). For instance, when a gymnast's foot makes contact with the vaulting spring board upon initiating an Amanar (round off, back handspring, back layout salto with two and a half twists off the vault table) or Biles (round off, back handspring with half twist onto the vault table, front layout salto with two twists off the vault table), the foot applies force to the board with a particular amplitude in newton but with individually addressable components directed in each of the X, Y, and Z directions.

Mechanical stress and strain are critical concepts for the expression and understanding of the mechanical properties of biological tissues including bone, ligament, and tendon. *Mechanical stress* is a physically quantifiable expression of applied force relative to the cross-sectional area shared by objects in contact with one another. *Mechanical strain* is a measure of deformation of a material and is specifically calculated by evaluating the change in length of an object loaded by applied forces relative to the object's original length. In evaluating the characteristics and mechanical performance envelopes of various types of biological materials within the human musculoskeletal system, the relationship between mechanical stress and strain of such materials informs the *material properties* of the structure or substance. A commonly referred to material property is the modulus of elasticity (otherwise known as Young's modulus). *Young's modulus* (E) is equal to the initial linear slope of the stress–strain curve of a material placed under loading conditions (Fig. 3.6). Matching of the materials properties (including, but not limited to, Young's modulus) for orthopedic hardware, graft materials, and fracture fixation materials to that of the biologic structures undergoing healing may limit deleterious effects of excessive *stress-shielding* and may also inform the healing and rehabilitation processes.

In order to calculate such properties, an appreciation for tension, compression, and bending loads is also imperative. *Tension* can be defined as a "pulling" force applied to a material in an effort to elongate the structure. *Compression* is in essence the polar opposite of tension and can be simply defined as a "pushing" force applied (often applied axially or perpendicular to the long axis) in an effort to shorten the length of a structure.

Shear force represents force applied parallel to the surfaces in contact with one another. An example of shear force is the anterior translation of the proximal tibia adjacent to the femoral condyles during performance of a Lachman's (anterior translation) test performed during clinical assessment of ACL integrity. Finally, *bending* occurs when an object (such as a long bone) sustains tension on one side of its neutral axis and compression on the other side. In bioengineering research, it has been determined that bones, particularly long bones, are most susceptible to fracture from applied bending moments with the fracture propagation typically initiated on the tension side of the neutral axis [3].

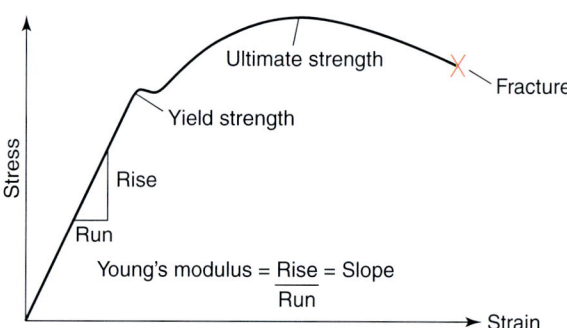

Fig. 3.6 Stress versus strain plot for a biologic material with Young's (elastic) modulus noted

Any discussion of the basics of biomechanics must include a thorough description of the body as a *system of levers*. Indeed, from a musculoskeletal perspective, the body is simply a system of long, short, or irregularly shaped levers that are angularly or linearly displaced by the force generated by a muscle or group of muscles.

Movement of limb segments via internal muscle contractions must often overcome externally applied forces or other resistive constructs. Further complicating such efforts is the fact that, generally, the *moment arm* component for the internally generated joint torques is relatively short as compared with that of the external (resistive) moment arm. As such, humans – including gymnasts – are at considerable mechanical disadvantage from a torque perspective. This disadvantage, however, comes with a positive trade-off: that of exceptional range of motion. This is the cost and privilege of the third-class *lever system* – a category into which the majority of our joints fall.

When the clinician contemplates the biomechanical loads of the limb segments and joints, both qualitative and quantitative data may be considered. From a biomechanical perspective, though seemingly more tools (hardware and software) are available to the practitioner each year, full-scale adoption of quantitative assessment tools has yet to come to fruition. As such, even in our modern age, qualitative assessment and record-keeping still constitute a majority of clinically tracked biomechanical data. Reasons for this may include the cost-prohibitive, time-inefficient, and requisite training time investments – and further complicated by poor reimbursement parameters – for the use of such nascent technology. Many clinicians across specialties therein defer to less precise (and potentially less valid and reliable) tools because of a level of comfort and consistency with respect to currently deployed methodology. This current practice, however, makes large-scale ("big-data") sharing of patient data trends more difficult by a significant order of magnitude. Future research into improving the rate of adoption and consistent utilization of objective quantitative assessment tools may benefit the care of these athletes.

Inside the musculoskeletal system of the athlete, intra-joint articular contact surfaces undergo significant loading during gymnastics performance. In order to further understand the forces a gymnast's joints withstand, it is important to first review the biomechanical principles relative to such loading. A brief glance back a few paragraphs should rekindle the concepts of mechanical stress and strain as well as tension and compression. Joint *contact stress* (stress between components in contact with one another) and *joint congruency* ("goodness of fit" between components in contact with one another) may be viewed as inversely related to one another. A poor match between the radii of curvature of one joint structure (the head of the humerus) with its articular surface (the glenoid fossa of the scapula) due to anatomical variability (such as an excessively shallow fossa – as depicted in Fig. 3.7) can predispose the gymnast to chronic instability and pathology such as a labral tear.

When one considers the three-dimensional articular surface area of contact between two bones interacting at a joint, it should be clear that when the applied force is held constant, a decrease in total articular contact area will yield a higher stress concentration, while an increase in contact area will result in a decrease in

Fig. 3.7 Representative MR image of a female gymnast depicting shallow glenoid fossa morphology

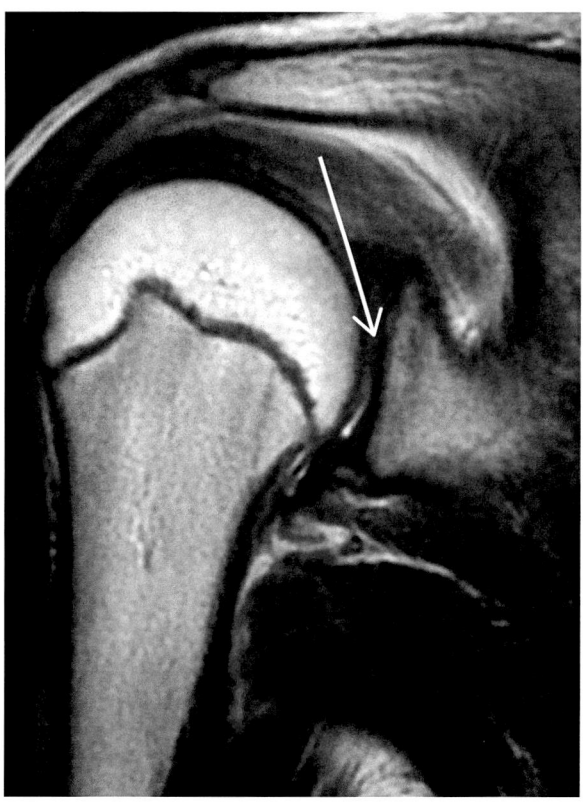

stress concentration. Henceforth, any congenitally inherent or transient acute pathology to the articular contact surfaces of a joint can yield an undesirable decrease in shared surface contact area. In the hip, for example, the calculable radii of curvature of the acetabulum and femoral head may be close approximations of one another or quite different (pathological). Joint congruency of the dynamically active joint, however, is not fixed, as the extent of congruency depends on the weight-bearing status as well as co-contraction of surrounding musculature. At the hip, for example, the weight-bearing associated with stance increases the congruency of the joint as the joint is loaded.

In open-chain activities, such as performing a leg kick or leg swing, as the limb segment accelerates, the centrifugal forces acting upon the joint, as well as factors associated with soft tissue constructs, can decrease the level of congruency of the joint. *Close-packed* positions relative to joint congruency refer to those dynamic agonistic and antagonistic co-contraction scenarios ("loaded" or "weight-bearing"), whereas *open-packed* refers to those open-chain dynamic free ("non-weight-bearing") limb movements.

As a gymnast interacts with the outside environment (namely the equipment and matting), reaction forces consistent with Newton's laws are continuously being applied from the gymnast to the environment (equipment) and back again. These continuous athlete–environment interactions can be measured quantitatively. One commonly measured and studied interaction is ground reaction force (GRF) which consists of tri-axial components, the largest of which is typically relegated to the vertical (GRFz) component (Fig. 3.8).

The concepts of impulse, momentum, and force mitigation must also be present in mind when considering the mechanical loading of the musculoskeletal system of the gymnast. *Impulse* is defined as the change in momentum of an object relative to the time over which a force acts upon it. *Momentum* is simply defined as the product of the mass of an object and its velocity. An important relationship is therefore present between impulse and momentum such that *impulse* is always equal to the change in momentum of a mechanical system.

Mitigation of an applied force (impulse) is manipulated constantly by the gymnastics performer in their efforts to minimize peak force through the biological structures of the body upon landing skills such as dismounts. Simultaneous flexion of the ankles (dorsiflexion), knees, and hips upon making contact with the ground after performing a high-velocity airborne skill distributes the total momentum over time such that the peak value is minimized (ideally staying below the threshold for mechanical failure, i.e., injury). One would be remiss to not turn attention at this point to chronic-loading-related *material fatigue*. Repeated *sub*-failure-threshold

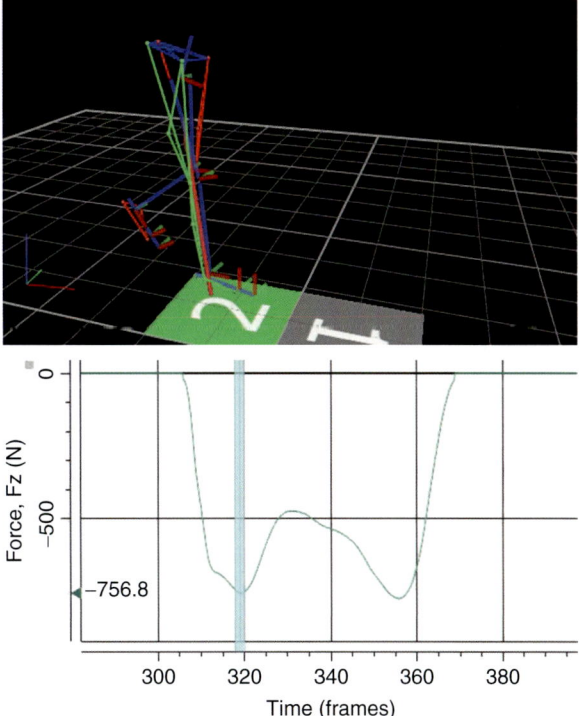

Fig. 3.8 Representative ground reaction force (GRFz) for athlete moving across the floor

loading and unloading of biological materials lowers the threshold for acute mechanical failure. This is akin to repetitive bending and straightening of a metal paperclip. In such an example – as has been experienced by nearly anyone who has "fidgeted" with a paperclip in his or her hand – after a series of subacute bending moments in opposing directions (bend and straighten the said paperclip repeatedly) placed upon the metal strand, failure ultimately occurs at a torque far lower than that which would have been required previous to the chronic loading condition (such as trying to snap the paperclip with one sudden bending torque). The best clinical example of this is the gymnast with a stress fracture. Repeated stress on part of the bone eventually leads to a fracture that can occur even with a low-energy mechanism.

In wrapping up biomechanical basics, consideration of bone remodeling is requisite. In accordance with *Wolff's law*, the bone (and other stressed biomaterials) remodels relative to the stress and strain which it is chronically exposed [16, 17]. Henceforth, chronic overloading may be injurious, but prolonged bouts of unloading may have a deleterious and unintended effect, should the recovering athlete return to sport too rapidly [1]. This is too often seen when an athlete is "cleared" by a medical professional to fully return to a sport such as gymnastics without a carefully developed "return-to-play" gradual transition protocol, such as that recently outlined by Sweeney and colleagues [18].

3.4 Perturbation of the Musculoskeletal System Specific to Gymnastics

Comparison of the biomechanical loads on the body during gymnastics practice and competition between male and female gymnasts is not as simple as adjusting for mass or scale. Without a doubt, sex-divergent mechanical and other physiological properties are a factor in the mechanical performance, loading, perturbation, and recovery of the bodies between male and female gymnasts [19]. Unlike most athletic activities, however, these differences are equaled – if not surpassed – by differences in biomechanical loads imposed by equipment, matting, technical performance rules, and other factors that differ between disciplines in gymnastics [20, 21]. A gymnastics floor exercise routine, for instance, though performed on the same mechanical surface (carpet-covered foam over a spring deck) requires far different metabolic and mechanical components even for age-, height-, mass-, and skill-level matched gymnasts of difference sexes. Women's floor exercise constitutes approximately 60–90 seconds of performance to musical accompaniment and requires continuous movement choreography in addition to their balance, strength, and dynamic tumbling skills, whereas men perform much more direct balance, strength, and tumbling skills without extensive choreographic movement nor musical accompaniment and for 20–25% shorter total duration.

In artistic gymnastics, men perform on vault, high bar, parallel bars, rings, pommel horse, and floor exercise, whereas women perform on vault, uneven bars, balance beam, and floor exercise. Different events and judging constraints are present for rhythmic, acrobatic, and trampoline – all of which are considered as their own gymnastics-related competitive disciplines (see Chap. 1 for more details on the different disciplines). While each of these specific events and specific disciplines present different biomechanical challenges for the gymnasts, some common movement paradigms can be characterized.

3.4.1 Running in Gymnastics

As male and female gymnasts typically train and compete without footwear, shock attenuation and force transfer occur without the augmentation witnessed in most other sports. This is an important consideration for the clinician as any assessed mechanical faults (i.e., those diagnosed in gait analysis) are more difficult to correct in the barefoot athlete. Further complicating the matter is that gymnasts may utilize different foot–ground contact strategies in training and performance of different events and for different skill performance within the same events. Additionally, as in track and field or distance running, two gymnasts within the same discipline may indeed adopt different foot contact strategies when performing the same skill.

In general, the barefoot gymnast runs in a manner fairly comparable to that of a track sprinter as the overwhelming predominance of running in the sport is short duration at moderate to high speeds. Many short runs are utilized and may range from 3 (beam, uneven bars mounts, or floor) to 12 (vault) steps. The center of pressure for these running approaches, particularly in the more elite gymnast, is shifted toward the ball of the foot and away from the rearfoot – resulting in a mid-to-forefoot ground contact mechanics.

3.4.2 Jumping in Gymnastics

As aforementioned, the gymnast commonly performs high-intensity, short-duration jumping in a barefoot condition. Examples include jumping to mount an apparatus and very rapid ground contact jumping from the vaulting board or off of the floor exercise or beam apparatus surface to perform a leap, jump, or salto (with or without twists) before landing in a controlled fashion. The minimal ground contact time necessitated to transfer energy to the apparatus and rapidly back to the athlete in order to create lift and rotation yields a resultantly high impulse [22, 23]. Recall that force applied to a surface creates an impulse that changes the momentum of the gymnast. Henceforth, a gymnast experiences a very short but *high* peak force during such "jumping" takeoffs [24].

3.4.3 Landing in Gymnastics

Gymnastics is well known by the media and fans for its "stuck landing." In an effort to perfectly control ("stick") the landing upon completion of a floor exercise tumbling pass, vault, or apparatus dismount, nearly the polar opposite of the rapid ground contact required to generate maximum lift or rotation in the jumping example above becomes the objective. Such a landing requires a significant *increase* in ground contact time achieved by near-simultaneous flexion of the trunk, hips, knees, and ankles (dorsi-flexion) such that the force is mitigated over a longer period of time [9, 25, 26]. Landing forces, especially those experienced upon landing on vault and via dismounts from uneven bars, high bar, and rings, approach and sometimes exceed, *by a factor of 18 to 30 times body weight* or higher [1]. These forces can exceed hard and soft tissue tolerances potentially resulting in acute injury [9, 27]. Repeated bouts of such landings experienced during practice may increase the likelihood of chronic mechanical stress-imposed injury [9, 28, 29]. Asymmetry, particularly of the lower extremity, upon landings is associated with landing-related injuries [30, 31] and is widely seen in gymnasts of all levels on many events including vault landings (Fig. 3.9). Such asymmetry may interplay with intrinsic aberrant neuromuscular motor pattern behavior upon landing such as dynamic valgus collapse of the knee resulting in ACL rupture or other lower extremity injuries [32–35].

Renewed attention to landing rules have induced some judging changes to allow – if not reward – increased flexion angles (without scoring deduction) and a slight widening of the feet which may help reduce lower extremity injury. This is of great interest to researchers and clinicians seeking to minimize risk of musculoskeletal injury in the sport. Historically, more abrupt landings with legs and hips in greater extension were sought after and rewarded for their aesthetic appeal [9]; fortunately, this has recently begun to change via less rigid judging deductions relative to landing form in the contemporary sport.

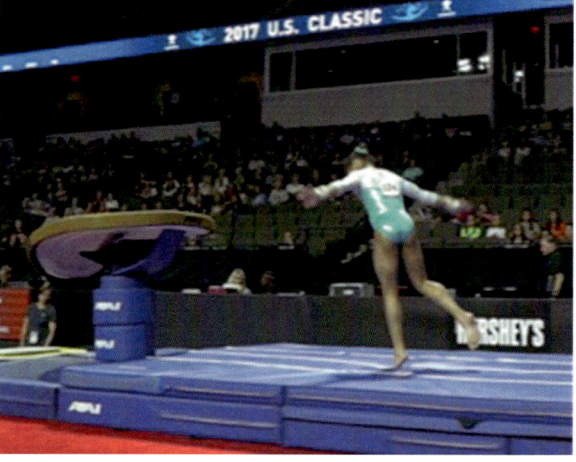

Fig. 3.9 Elite women's gymnastics vault landing phase. Note the limb asymmetry

3.4.4 Airborne Saltos and Twisting Skills in Gymnastics

Once a gymnast becomes airborne – regardless of the discipline or event – his or her ability to seemingly defy Newtonian physics becomes apparent. While no magic is indeed performed wherein the laws of physics are actually violated, the musculoskeletal demands to make these athletic feats a reality require very high levels of core strength and the learned motor ability (acquired from hundreds, if not thousands, of repetitions of skill attempts) to manipulate their *moment of inertia.*

It may come as no surprise that the highly successful gymnast is typically much shorter than their colleagues in sports such as basketball or volleyball. Shorter limbs and torso lengths enhance one's ability to benefit from moment of inertia changes – a trait commonly shared with gymnasts' counterparts in diving. As a gymnast begins to leave the ground or apparatus following rapid ground contact, he or she typically completes a very high velocity extension in length of his or her body – in essence accelerating their center of mass as completely as possible toward vertical. As the total angular momentum for the airborne skill is constant once in the air, highly rehearsed manipulation of body positioning is relied upon to vary the angular velocity of planned longitudinal or transverse axis rotations [36]. Nearly immediately after completing the ground takeoff extension position, the gymnast will then maximally, or near maximally, shorten the moment of inertia around his or her axes of rotation (which axis is dependent upon whether the gymnast seeks to perform a salto or twist – *or both at the same time*). Such manipulation of the center of gravity relative to the center of mass of the athlete is commonly known in the gymnastics and trampoline environments as a "cat twist" technique.

3.4.5 Arm-Supported Skill Performance in Gymnastics

On all arm support events, the entire shoulder complex, elbow, and wrist can be exposed to very high stress concentrations, hard and soft tissue structural impingement, and resultant joint surface edge-loading that can result in acute or chronic musculoskeletal injury. Men's rings (Fig. 3.10) and women's uneven bars are

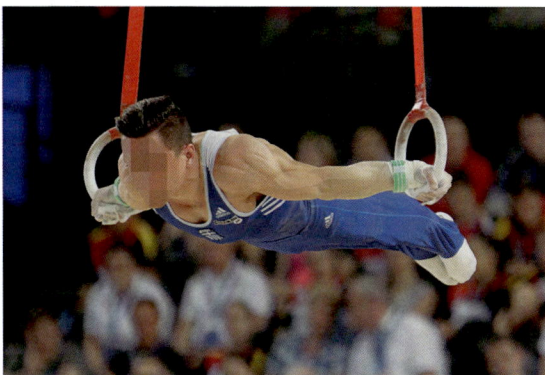

Fig. 3.10 Elite men's artistic gymnastics rings quasi-static strength element (Maltese cross)

frequently associated with chronic shoulder pathology [37]. Men's pommel horse and both men's and women's vaulting performance are associated with chronic wrist injury [37, 38]. In the above events, it is the repetitive impingement (at the dorsal aspect of the radiocarpal joint, for instance) and high forces that are often responsible for the pathology.

3.5 Biomechanical Considerations of Gymnastics Equipment and Matting

Knowledge of the general design and usage parameters of the standard apparatus (equipment) and personal equipment (hand-guards or "grips" as well as wrist supports or "tiger paws") utilized in artistic gymnastics may inform the practitioner about potential injury mechanisms. Any knowledge gap in assumed-versus-actual sport performance parameters in the mind of the clinical practitioner may inadvertently over- or under-load a gymnast recovering from injury and following a return-to-sport protocol [18]. An example of such a scenario has been described wherein which a well-intentioned family-practice physician treating an adolescent female level ten gymnast in the post-acute healing phase of a grade three ankle sprain instructed the gymnast to return to practice and that she was to stay limited in beam, vault, and floor skill training but could return to full uneven bars practice. Enhanced physician knowledge of the requirements for uneven bars performance would have informed the practitioner that the potential loads on the lower extremity during uneven bars training not only include exceptionally high lower extremity forces upon dismount landings but also potentially yield a reinjury of the ankle if the gymnast falls on a Tkatchev ("reverse hecht") release skill – wherein the gymnast's center of mass is displaced nearly 12 feet into the air above the ground. Henceforth, it is advisable to, at minimum, take the opportunity to view practice and competitions for male and female gymnastics at each end of the spectrum of abilities in order to acclimate oneself with potential injury mechanisms and skill terminology.

From an event-by-event perspective, different events in artistic gymnastics vary considerably in their upper body versus lower body strength and power delivery requirements and resultant joint contact stress concentrations. Predominantly upper extremity events include for women the uneven bars and for men the high bar, rings, parallel bars, and pommel horse. A more balanced upper body and lower body contribution scenario exists for both women's and men's floor exercise as well as balance beam for women. Vault requires predominantly lower body strength for both men and women – though the abrupt contact phase with the hands on the vaulting table (required per rules) does lead to a fair number of wrist and other upper extremity maladies in vaulters of both sexes.

While not directly biomechanical, the metabolic considerations vary from event to event considerably as well. In performance of the vault event, the total duration of performance is limited to approximately 5 seconds of predominantly anaerobic metabolism, while in contrast, floor exercise ranges from 60 to 90 seconds, during which aerobic metabolism becomes a contributor to the gymnast's energy system needs.

Matting utilized in training and competition varies greatly between events and, unbeknownst to those outside of the training environment, between men's and women's artistic gymnastics across the board. At present, women's artistic gymnastics requires 12 cm base matting for competition, whereas men's competition requires 20 cm base matting for all events. As such, the force mitigation properties provided via the landing mats in the men's discipline are potentially much greater due to the inherent difference in the *coefficient of restitution* (a shock attenuation parameter) of the different mat sizes.

When considering equipment parameters, note should be made that significant facility-to-facility variability in the specifications, and state of repair, of event-specific equipment, specialty training equipment, flooring, and matting may result in drastically different loading of healthy and injured biological structures during training and competition.

Force transfer, potential (stored) energy, spring coefficients, and coefficients of restitution are factors that a clinician may seek to better understand in an effort to prevent and rehabilitate injury in the gymnast. Specifically, an appreciation for the athlete–equipment interaction wherein the gymnast is "trading" force continuously back and forth with the equipment during nearly all dynamic event performances is an important consideration. For instance, in men's rings, a gymnast may press their body up into an elevated handstand position on the rings. At this point, the center of mass of the athlete may be displaced in excess of 12 feet above the floor surface – resulting in significantly high *potential energy*. As the gymnast swings downward, holding only onto the two rings, through the "bottom" of the skill, the peak kinetic energy must be transferred through the upper extremities and into the ring tower (via the rings and cables) wherein much of that energy is temporarily stored and transferred back into the athlete later in the skill. Uneven bars, high bar, parallel bars, and women's uneven bars all experience similar force transfers during dynamic swinging activities.

In addition to the concepts of force transfer from gymnast to equipment and back again, the concept of *spring coefficients* applies to the vaulting board use, floor exercise performance, and when utilizing specialized training equipment such as trampolines. The spring mechanisms (of which there are a number of variants) act to very briefly store energy from initial contact and return that energy at an opportune time in an effort to propel the athlete forward or vertically (or both). Proper matching ("tuning") of the athlete and skill to the spring mechanisms being utilized help to enhance performance as well as mitigate injury (Fig. 3.11a, b).

Unfortunately, due to time, space, and funding constraints, athlete-specific and skill-specific tuning of spring elements are typically not regularly optimized in training environments at this time [23]. Of special importance on this topic, the use of trampoline training devices poses potentially highly adverse risks when such devices are utilized by more than one performer at a time (and thus against the

Fig. 3.11 (**a–b**) Artistic gymnastics floor exercise apparatus testing methodology in 3D biomechanics laboratory

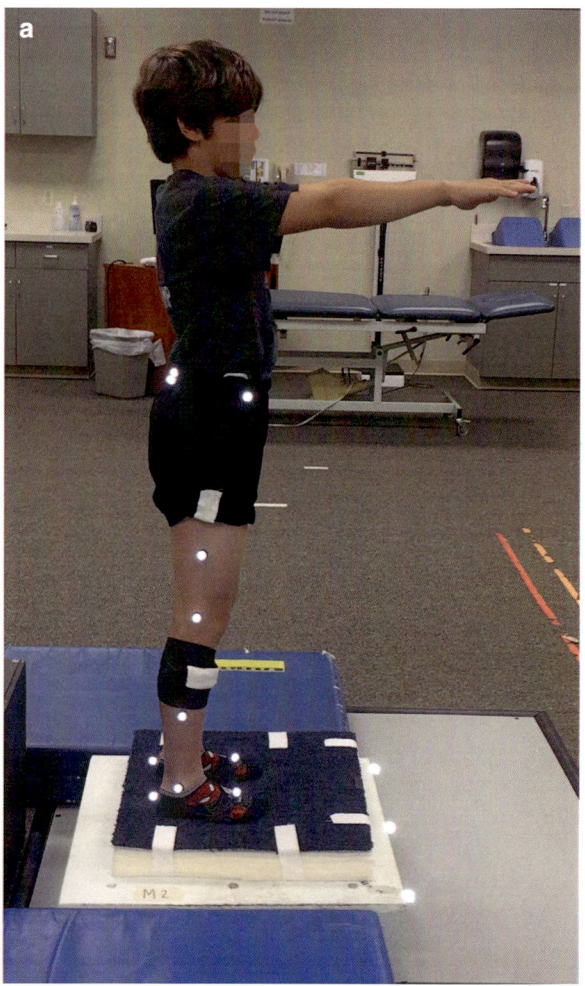

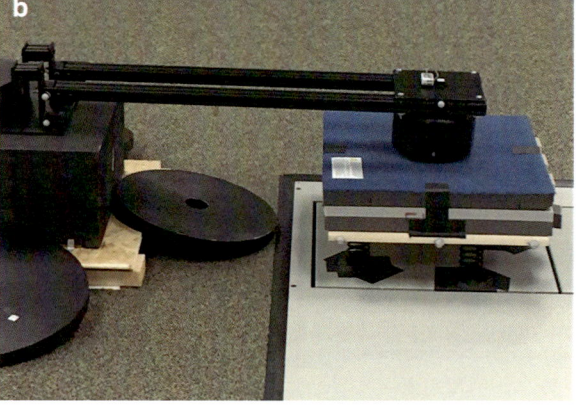

recommendation of the manufacturers and rules of the sport) as excessive force transfers from one performer (exceedingly of concern in the event of a participant size mismatch) to another via stored energy in the series and parallel spring configurations. Catastrophic injury has occurred in the sport as a result, though contemporary evidence demonstrates that this is a far greater concern – and occurs at a vastly higher rate – in "trampoline parks" rather than in gymnastics training facilities. The reason for this facility-type disparity is likely the result of differences in instructor training, usage monitoring, trampoline design parameters, as well as adherence to manufacturer's safety rules between gymnastics training facilities and "trampoline park" facilities.

3.6 Pathomechanical Considerations for High-Perturbation Gymnastics Skills

While few truly static activities are performed in gymnastics, quasi-static activities such as handstand holds, balance scales, and specialized skills on men's rings (Maltese or iron cross, for instance) require exceptional strength, stability, and appropriate joint mobility to be performed technically well and without injury. Without question, those skills that require upper extremity limb positioning overhead, or nearly overhead, while supporting the full weight of the body, are most highly perturbating to the gymnast whether male or female. Because the anatomy of the shoulder complex – in particular the glenohumeral joint – is not the most geometrically stable joint (recall the golf ball on a tee example commonly utilized in anatomy coursework), the soft tissue comprised of the glenoid labrum, joint capsule, glenohumeral ligaments, and muscles of the rotator cuff are taxed heavily as a result. Any dysfunction to one of these static or dynamic stabilizing structures may initiate a cascading paradigm of dysfunction and pain that may precipitate significant injury resulting in loss of performance or requiring surgical intervention.

With respect to the few truly static positions performed regularly in the sport, many of these are combined with excessive single or multiple-joint range of motion skills. For example, a static "bridge" skill (Fig. 3.12) is commonly performed in the sport, even at the most developmental levels. It has been postulated by some in the medical community that excessive lumber hyperextension – especially in prepubescent athletes with preexisting chronically lordotic lumbosacral posture – may increase the rate of occurrence of stress fracture (spondylolysis). Resultantly, many seasoned coaches have embraced utilization of "modification" of these stretches (such as via elevation of the feet upon an extra mat during bridge skill development) and other static holds in order to minimize the potentially adverse effects.

Additionally, and of utmost importance, biomechanical considerations *specific to each athlete* should be made in an effort to "match" skills trained and performed to the individual athlete's range of motion, strength, and power profile in order to minimize risk of injury where possible. For example, the Tkatchev ("reverse hecht"

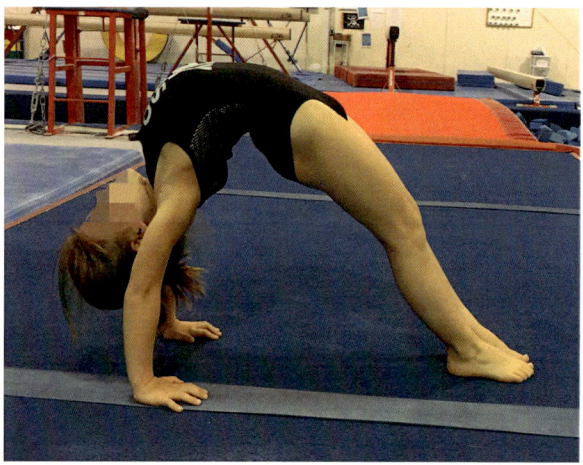

Fig. 3.12 Extensive spine hyperextension required in gymnastics skills such as this bridge (note stress concentration potential via lower thoracic/upper lumbar acute extension angle)

on uneven bars or high bar) release skill places the spine in significant hyperextension *as well as* extensive hip extension and shoulder flexion. Resultantly, if a coach chooses to train this skill longitudinally with an athlete who has reduced mobility at the hips and shoulders, the balance of required extension range of motion will be attempted to be offset by additional extension of the thoracolumbar spine – therein potentially increasing stress concentrations at facet articulations – including the pars interarticularis. This is just one such example of athlete–skill mismatching, as further examples can be seen in nearly every event in gymnastics today.

3.7 Special Clinical Considerations in the Biomechanics of the Gymnast

3.7.1 High Peak (and Chronic) Joint Loading Associated with Training

As well evidenced by the research literature, the ground reaction forces upon "sticking" the landing during vault, bars, or floor exercise performances may exceed 10–14, and possibly as high as 30, times the weight of the body [21]. Such a load during the landing phase of a powerful vault therein approaches or exceeds 10,000 N for a 70 kg gymnast! When this fact is compounded by biomechanical evidence of gymnasts landing with all – or nearly all – of their weight on a single leg in the initial landing phases under suboptimal (asymmetric) performance scenarios, and further compounded by the potential for application of a bending moment at the long bones, the potential for catastrophic joint (ACL rupture) or bone (compound tibial fracture) has been too often realized. Computational modeling (Fig. 3.13) and cadaveric studies have demonstrated that an otherwise healthy long bone such as the tibia can be

Fig. 3.13 Finite-element model of knee utilized in ACL mechanical strain modeling

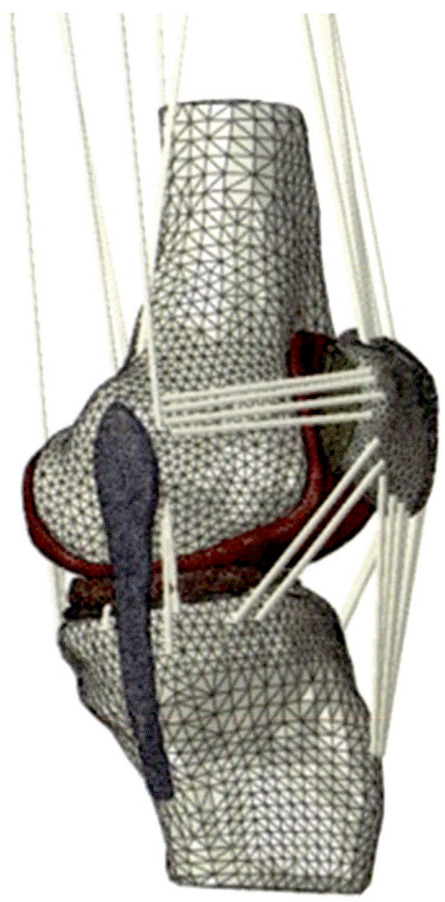

fractured at a load of approximately 4000 N, the ACL ruptured at just over 2000 N [39], and the Achilles tendon at 4000 N [22]. Without a doubt, gymnasts realize forces and moments equivalent or greater than nearly any other athlete.

3.7.2 Extreme Range of Motion and Propensity for Joint Laxity

Whether gymnastics self-selects participants who exhibit hereditarily high levels of laxity or that participation in the sport environment expresses such ranges of motion in participants, the typical gymnast moves his or her body through extensive ranges of motion far beyond that of normal activities of daily living and beyond that required by most other sports. Resultantly, high edge-loading contact forces are experienced at the femoracetabular junction, glenohumeral joint, and many other joints regularly. That FAI is commonly witnessed in the female gymnast is therefore likely not surprising to most medical practitioners. Additionally notable with respect to range of motion is the required chronic hyperextension of the spinal column to ranges exceeding that typically witnessed in other sports. As introduced in Sect. 3.3, chronic bending moments placed upon hard and soft tissues such as those of the spine may lead to injury [1]. Bridging skill performance and other extreme range of motion positions have been implicated in chronic musculoskeletal injury, especially in athletes with less than optimal core strength. It must be mentioned, however, that the extent to which spinal extension skills (such as the backbend or bridge skill, specifically) are linked to injury under controlled training environments has been questioned [40], leaving this specific skill–injury correlation to further longitudinal study.

3.7.3 Footwear (Lack Thereof)

Further compounding the potential risk factors categorized immediately above is the fact that gymnasts typically perform barefoot, making use of orthotics for longitudinal foot posture changes as well as force-mitigating properties typically provided by athletic footwear a moot point. While efforts have been made to provide foot support via taping or specially modified bracing (such as the "X-Brace"), little evidence of long-term consistent injury mitigation via use of such tools in the sport of gymnastics has been demonstrated. Compliance with long-term use of orthotic devices and highly supportive taping methods may also suffer due to the disruption – or perceived disruption by the athlete or coach – to proprioception required by the competitive gymnast.

3.8 Contemporary Research in Gymnastics Biomechanics and Pathomechanics

Contemporary research in the sport of gymnastics with respect to performance enhancement includes recent studies that leverage cutting-edge computer hardware, software, and imaging [5]. Additional efforts include research into performance monitoring [41–43], flexibility [44], strength and power training and testing [45–47], athlete–apparatus interaction [23, 48–52], skill performance optimization [46, 53–65], metabolism [66–68], return-to-sport protocols [18], and gymnastics biomechanics as a whole [36, 69].

Injury prevention biomechanics research in the sport of gymnastics (Fig. 3.14a, b) is now commonplace and may involve 3D motion tracking camera arrays, force platforms, and strain gauge technologies, as well as electromyographic (EMG) approaches in an effort to better understand the mechanisms of injury and optimum performance factors.

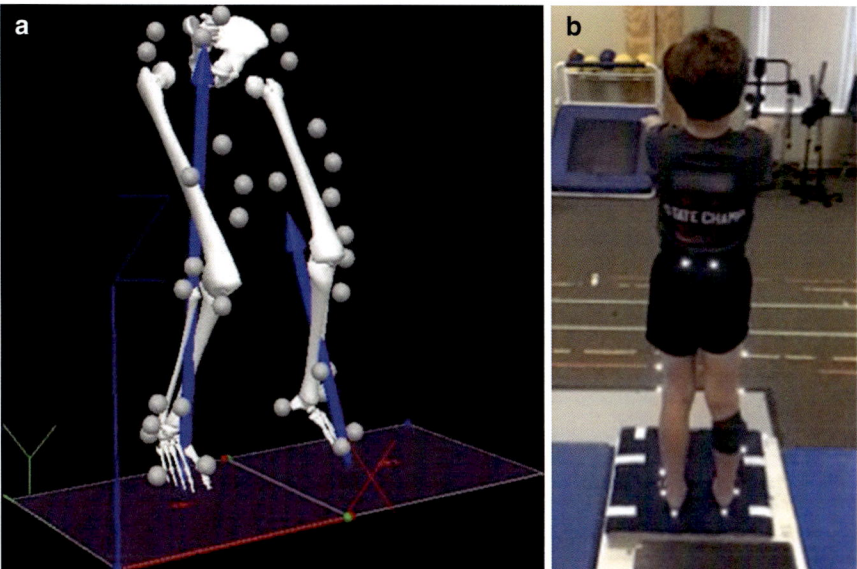

Fig. 3.14 (**a–b**) 3D kinematics laboratory instrumented for gymnast–equipment interaction research

Notable contemporary work includes efforts in the areas of knee injury [20, 21], upper extremity injuries [70, 71], spine injury [40, 72, 73], ankle injuries [74], landing mechanics [21, 30, 75–80] and landing forces [80–82], equipment contact forces [83–86], risk factor stratification/screening [5, 9, 87, 88], bracing [89], and epidemiology [20, 21, 90]. Technological advancements in clinical biomechanical tools for improving risk screening [5, 9, 91, 92] and clinical intervention [76] have also been characterized in modern literature, thereby increasing the availability of evidence-based practice resources available for the care and rehabilitation of the gymnast.

3.9 Conclusion

In conclusion, clinicians are implored to review biomechanical and biological material properties literature as well as familiarize themselves with the typical ranges of motion, forces and joint moments, and training loads experienced across each of the gymnastics disciplines. Mismatched assumptions versus realities of the training and competition environments can, and likely does, lead to delayed healing and/or reinjury in gymnastics athlete patients. It is important to consider the interaction of intrinsic and extrinsic risk factors from a biomechanical perspective as single risk factor injuries (unavoidable acute injury) represent only a portion of the total injuries experienced by the gymnast [9], while complex intrinsic and extrinsic risk factor interactions represent potentially avoidable injuries. From a biomechanical perspective, such injuries may be decreased in magnitude or avoided with more extensive adoption of modern screening and intervention practices. At minimum, enhanced clinician knowledge of the special biomechanical demands and pathomechanics of the sport may improve clinical care outcomes for the injured gymnast.

References

1. Bruggemann GP. Biomechanical and biological limits in artistic gymnastics. ISBS 2005, Beijing, China; 2005.
2. Daly R, Bass S, Finch C. Balancing the risk of injury to gymnasts: how effective are the counter measures? Br J Sports Med. 2001;35:8–20.
3. McGinnis P. Biomechanics of sport and exercise. 3rd ed. Champaign: Human Kinetics; 2013. 442 p.
4. Sands WA, McNeal J. Thinking sensibly about injury prevention and safety. Sci Gymnast J. 2011;3(3):43–58.
5. Sands WA, McNeal J, Stone MH. Thermal imaging and gymnastics injuries: a means of screening and injury identification. Sci Gymnast J. 2011;3(2):5–12.
6. Sands WA, McNeal J. Predicting athlete preparation and performance: a theoretical perspective. J Sport Behav. 2000;23(3):289–310.
7. Sands WA. Injury prevention in women's gymnastics. Sports Med. 2000;30(5):359–73.
8. Sands WA, Shultz BB, Newman AP. Women's gymnastics injuries. A 5-year study. Am J Sports Med. 1993;21(2):271–6.
9. Bradshaw EJ, Hume PA. Biomechanical approaches to identify and quantify injury mechanisms and risk factors in women's artistic gymnastics. Sports Biomech. 2012;11(3):324–41.
10. Quatman CE, Hewett TE. The anterior cruciate ligament injury controversy: is "valgus collapse" a sex-specific mechanism? Br J Sports Med. 2009;43(5):328–35.
11. Bates NA, Nesbitt RJ, Shearn JT, Myer GD, Hewett TE. Knee abduction affects greater magnitude of change in ACL and MCL strains than matched internal tibial rotation in vitro. Clin Orthop Relat Res. 2017;475(10):2385–96.
12. Weber AE, Bedi A, Tibor LM, Zaltz I, Larson CM. The hyperflexible hip: managing hip pain in the dancer and gymnast. Sports Health. 2015;7(4):346–58.
13. Ito K, Minka MA 2nd, Leunig M, Werlen S, Ganz R. Femoroacetabular impingement and the cam-effect. A MRI-based quantitative anatomical study of the femoral head-neck offset. J Bone Joint Surg Br. 2001;83(2):171–6.
14. Amerinatanzi A, Summers R, Ahmadi K, Goel VK, Hewett TE, Nyman E Jr. A novel 3D approach for determination of frontal and coronal plane tibial slopes from MR imaging. Knee. 2017;24(2):207–16.
15. Steffen K, Andersen TE, Krosshaug T, van Mechelen W, Myklebust G, Verhagen EA, et al. ECSS position statement 2009: prevention of acute sports injuries. Eur J Sport Sci. 2010;10(4):223–36.
16. Zadpoor AA, Weinans H. Patient-specific bone modeling and analysis: the role of integration and automation in clinical adoption. J Biomech. 2015;48(5):750–60.
17. Sampath SA, Lewis S, Fosco M, Tigani D. Trabecular orientation in the human femur and tibia and the relationship with lower-limb alignment for patients with osteoarthritis of the knee. J Biomech. 2015;48(6):1214–8.
18. Sweeney EA, Howell DR, James DA, Potter MN, Provance AJ. Returning to sport after gymnastics injuries. Curr Sports Med Rep. 2018;17(11):376–90.
19. Thomas K, Wilson C, Bradshaw E. Fundamental movement assessment of young female gymnasts. XXXI international conference on biomechanics in sports, Taiwan. 2013.

20. Kirialanis P, Malliou P, Beneka A, Giannakopoulos K. Occurrence of acute lower limb injuries in artistic gymnasts in relation to event and exercise phase. Br J Sports Med. 2003;37(2):137–9.
21. Kirialanis P, Dallas G, Di Cagno A, Fiorilli G. Knee injuries at landing and take-off phase in gymnastics. Sci Gymnast J. 2015;7(1):17–25.
22. Piazza C, Pavol M. Achilles tendon forces during a round-off back handspring. Blacksburg, VA: ASB; 2006.
23. Sands WA, Alumbaugh B, McNeal J, Murray S, Stone M. Comparison of floor exercise apparatus spring-types on a gymnastics rearward tumbling take-off. Sci Gymnast J. 2014;6(2):41–51.
24. McNeal JR, Sands WA, Shultz BB. Muscle activation characteristics of tumbling take-offs. Sports Biomech. 2007;6(3):375–90.
25. McNitt-Gray J. Kinetics of the lower extremities during drop landings from three heights. J Biomech. 1993;26(9):1037–46.
26. McNitt-Gray JL, Hester DM, Mathiyakom W, Munkasy BA. Mechanical demand and multi-joint control during landing depend on orientation of the body segments relative to the reaction force. J Biomech. 2001;34(11):1471–82.
27. Panzer V, Bates BT, Mason BR. Lower extremity loads in landings of elite gymnasts. 1987.
28. Beatty KT, McIntosh AS, Frechede B, editors. Variation in landing during gymnastics skills. XXV ISBS symposium, Ouro Preto, Brazil. 2007.
29. Beatty KT, McIntosh AS, Frechede BO, editors. Method for analysing the risk of overuse injury in gymnastics. XXIV ISBS symposium, Salzburg, Austria. 2006.
30. Cuk I, Marinsek M. Landing quality in artistic gymnastics is related to landing symmetry. Biol Sport. 2013;30(1):29–33.
31. Lilley ES, Bradshaw EJ, Rice VJ. Is jumping and landing technique symmetrical in female gymnasts? XXV ISBS symposium, Ouro Preto, Brazil. 2007. p. 345–8.
32. Hewett TE, Myer GD, Ford KR. Anterior cruciate ligament injuries in female athletes: part 1, mechanisms and risk factors. Am J Sports Med. 2006;34(2):299–311.
33. Hewett TE, Myer GD, Ford KR. Decrease in neuromuscular control about the knee with maturation in female athletes. J Bone Joint Surg Am. 2004;86-A(8):1601–8.
34. Hewett TE, Ford KR, Hoogenboom BJ, Myer GD. Understanding and preventing acl injuries: current biomechanical and epidemiologic considerations – update 2010. N Am J Sports Phys Ther. 2010;5(4):234–51.
35. Renstrom P, Ljungqvist A, Arendt E, Beynnon B, Fukubayashi T, Garrett W, et al. Non-contact ACL injuries in female athletes: an International Olympic Committee current concepts statement. Br J Sports Med. 2008;42(6):394–412.
36. Prassas S, Kwon YH, Sands WA. Biomechanical research in artistic gymnastics: a review. Sports Biomech. 2006;5(2):261–91.
37. Wadley GH, Albright J. Women's intercollegiate gymnastics: injury patterns and "permanent" medical disability. Am J Sports Med. 1993;21(2):314–20.
38. Marshall SW, Covassin T, Dick R, Agel J. Descriptive epidemiology of collegiate women's gymnastics injuries: National Collegiate Athletic Association Injury Surveillance System, 1988–1989 through 2003–2004. J Athl Train. 2007;42(2):234–40.
39. Ali N. Predicting risk factors of noncontact anterior cruciate ligament injuries during single-leg landing. Ottawa: University of Ottawa; 2015.
40. Sands WA, McNeal JR, Penitente G, Murray SR, Nassar L, Jemni M, et al. Stretching the spines of gymnasts: a review. Sports Med. 2016;46(3):315–27.
41. Sands WA, Kavanaugh AA, Murray SR, McNeal JR, Jemni M. Modern techniques and technologies applied to training and performance monitoring. Int J Sports Physiol Perform. 2017;12(Suppl 2):S263–S72.
42. Mizuguchi S, Sands WA, Wassinger CA, Lamont HS, Stone MH. A new approach to determining net impulse and identification of its characteristics in countermovement jumping: reliability and validity. Sports Biomech. 2015;14(2):258–72.
43. Bradshaw E, Hume P, Calton M, Aisbett B. Reliability and variability of day-to-day vault training measures in artistic gymnastics. Sports Biomech. 2010;9(2):79–97.

44. Moltubakk MM, Eriksrud O, Paulsen G, Seynnes OR, Bojsen-Moller J. Hamstrings functional properties in athletes with high musculo-skeletal flexibility. Scand J Med Sci Sports. 2016;26(6):659–65.
45. Hall E, Bishop DC, Gee TI. Effect of plyometric training on handspring vault performance and functional power in youth female gymnasts. PLoS One. 2016;11(2):e0148790.
46. Dunlavy J, Sands WA, McNeal J, Stone M, Smith S, Jemni M, et al. Strength performance assessment in a simulated men's gymnastics still rings cross. J Sports Sci Med. 2007;6:93–7.
47. Salonia MA, Chu DA, Cheifetz PM, Freidhoff GC. Upper-body power as measured by medicine-ball throw distance and its relationship to class level among 10-and 11-year-old female participants in club gymnastics. J Strength Cond Res. 2004;18(4):695–702.
48. Sands WA, Kimmel W, McNeal J, Smith S, Penitente G, Murray S, et al. Kinematic and kinetic tumbling take-off comparisons of a spring-floor and an air floor(tm): a pilot study. Sci Gymnast J. 2013;5(3):31–46.
49. Penitente G, Sands WA, McNeal J. Vertical impact force and loading rate on the gymnastics table vault. Port J Sport Sci. 2011;29(11):667–70.
50. Coventry E, Sands WA, Smith SL. Hitting the vault board: implications for vaulting take-off--a preliminary investigation. Sports Biomech. 2006;5(1):63–75.
51. Križaj D, Čuk I. Can miniature accelerometers attached to the gymnastics springboard be used for take-off analysis? Sci Gymnast J. 2015;7(3):69–79.
52. Seeley MK, Bressel E. A comparison of upper-extremity reaction forces between the Yurchenko vault and floor exercise. J Sports Sci Med. 2005;4(2):85–94.
53. Mosscrop E, Penitente G, Sands WA, de Vries JP. A kinematic comparison of backward tucked somersault dismount performed on high bar by elite and non-elite gymnasts. ISSSMC 2013. Br J Sports Med. 47:17.
54. Sands WA, Stone MH, McNeal J, Smith SL, Jemni M, Dunlavy J, et al. A pilot study to measure force development during a simulated maltese cross for gymnastics still rings. XXIV ISBS symposium, Salzburg, Austria. 2006.
55. Potop V, Mihaila JM, Urichianu A. Mathematical modelling of the biomechanical characteristics of the dismounts off uneven bars in women's artistic gymnastics. ICPESK 2015 – 5th international congress on physical education, sport and kinetotherapy, vol. 11. 2016. p. 391–7.
56. Potop V, Manole C, Nistor D, Andreyeva N. Didactic technologies of learning the double back somersault on floor based on the biomechanical analysis of sports technique in women's artistic gymnastics. J Phys Educ Sport. 2015;15(1):120–7.
57. Hiley MJ, Jackson MI, Yeadon MR. Optimal technique for maximal forward rotating vaults in men's gymnastics. Hum Mov Sci. 2015;42:117–31.
58. Hedbavny P, Kalichova M. Optimization of velocity characteristics of the Yurchenko vault. Sci Gymnast J. 2015;7(1):37–49.
59. Yeadon MR, Jackson MI, Hiley MJ. The influence of touchdown conditions and contact phase technique on post-flight height in the straight handspring somersault vault. J Biomech. 2014;47(12):3143–8.
60. Mkaouer B, Jemni M, Amara S, Chaabene H, Padulo J, Tabka Z. Effect of three technical arms swings on the elevation of the center of mass during a standing back somersault. J Hum Kinet. 2014;40:37–48.
61. Mkaouer B, Jemni M, Amara S, Chaabene H, Tabka Z. Kinematic and kinetic analysis of two gymnastics acrobatic series to performing the backward stretched somersault. J Hum Kinet. 2013;37:17–26.
62. Farana R, Jandacka D, Irwin G. Influence of different hand positions on impact forces and elbow loading during the round off in gymnastics: a case study. Sci Gymnast J. 2013;5(2):5–14.
63. Farana R, Jandacka D, Uchytil J, Zahradnik D, Irwin G. Musculoskeletal loading during the round-off in female gymnastics: the effect of hand position. Sports Biomech. 2014;13(2):123–34.
64. Atikovic A. New regression models to evaluate the relationship between biomechanics of gymnastic vault and initial vault difficulty values. J Hum Kinet. 2012;35:119–26.

65. Atiković A, Smajlović N. Relation between vault difficulty values and biomechanical parameters in men's artistic gymnastics. Sci Gymnast J. 2011;3(3):91–105.
66. Jemni M, Sands WA, Friemel F, Stone MH, Cooke CB. Any effect of gymnastics training on upper-body and lower-body aerobic and power components in national and international male gymnasts? J Strength Cond Res. 2006;20(4):899–907.
67. Alves CR, Borelli MT, Paineli Vde S, Azevedo Rde A, Borelli CC, Lancha Junior AH, et al. Development of a specific anaerobic field test for aerobic gymnastics. PLoS One. 2015;10(4):e0123115.
68. Marina M, Rodriguez FA. Physiological demands of young women's competitive gymnastic routines. Biol Sport. 2014;31(3):217–22.
69. Manning ML. Biomechanics of technique selection in women's artistic gymnastics: Cardiff Metropolitan University. 33rd International Conference on Biomechanics in Sports, Poitiers, France, June 29–July 3, 2015. p. 2014.
70. Linderman S. A biomechanical characterization of the gymnastics round-off back handspring first contact and implications for upper extremity orthopedic injury. Boston, MA: Boston University; 2016.
71. McLaren K, Byrd E, Herzog M, Polikandriotis JA, Willimon SC. Impact shoulder angles correlate with impact wrist angles in standing back handsprings in preadolescent and adolescent female gymnasts. Int J Sports Phys Ther. 2015;10(3):341–6.
72. Koyama K, Nakazato K, Min S, Gushiken K, Hatakeda Y, Seo K, et al. Radiological abnormalities and low back pain in gymnasts. Int J Sports Med. 2013;34(3):218–22.
73. Kruse D, Lemmen B. Spine injuries in the sport of gymnastics. Curr Sports Med Rep. 2009;8(1):20–8.
74. Chilvers M, Donahue M, Nassar L, Manoli A 2nd. Foot and ankle injuries in elite female gymnasts. Foot Ankle Int. 2007;28(2):214–8.
75. Slater A, Campbell A, Smith A, Straker L. Greater lower limb flexion in gymnastic landings is associated with reduced landing force: a repeated measures study. Sports Biomech. 2015;14(1):45–56.
76. Nyman E Jr, Armstrong CW. Real-time feedback during drop landing training improves subsequent frontal and sagittal plane knee kinematics. Clin Biomech (Bristol, Avon). 2015;30(9):988–94.
77. Gittoes M, Irwin G. Biomechanical approaches to understanding the potentially injurious demands of gymnastic-style impact landings. Sports Med Arthrosc Rehabil Ther Technol. 2012;4:4.
78. Gittoes MJ, Irwin G, Kerwin DG. Kinematic landing strategy transference in backward rotating gymnastic dismounts. J Appl Biomech. 2013;29(3):253–60.
79. Marinšek M. Basic landing characteristics and their application in artistic gymnastics. Sci Gymnast J. 2010;2(2):59–67.
80. Seegmiller JG, McCaw ST. Ground reaction forces among gymnasts and recreational athletes in drop landings. J Athl Train. 2003;38(4):311–4.
81. Mills C, Pain MT, Yeadon MR. Reducing ground reaction forces in gymnastics' landings may increase internal loading. J Biomech. 2009;42(6):671–8.
82. Burt L, Naughton G, Landeo R. Quantifying impacts during beam and floor training in preadolescent girls from two streams of artistic gymnastics. XXV ISBS symposium, Brazil. 2007.
83. Penitente G, Sands WA. Exploratory investigation of impact loads during the forward handspring vault. J Hum Kinet. 2015;46:59–68.
84. Knoll K, Naundorf F, Bronst A, Wagner R, Brehmer S, Lehmann T. 3 decades of force measurement on vault in gymnastics. XXXII international conference of biomechanics in sports, Johnson City, TN. 2014. p. 610–3.
85. Naundorf F, Brehmer S, Knoll K, Bronst A, Wagner R. Development of the velocity for vault runs in artistic gymnastics for the last decade. ISBS conference 2008, Seoul, Korea. 2008. p. 481–4.
86. Mills C, Yeadon MR, Pain MT. Modifying landing mat material properties may decrease peak contact forces but increase forefoot forces in gymnastics landings. Sports Biomech. 2010;9(3):153–64.

87. Sleeper MD, Kenyon LK, Casey E. Measuring fitness in female gymnasts: the gymnastics functional measurement tool. Int J Sports Phys Ther. 2012;7(2):124–38.
88. Bradshaw E, Thomas K, Moresi M, Greene D, Braybon W, McGillivray K, et al. Biomechanical field test oberservations of gymnasts entering puberty. In: ISBS, editor. XXXII international conference of biomechanics in sports, Johnson City, TN. 2014.
89. Halliday S. Upper extremity vertical ground reaction forces during the back handspring skill in gymnastics: a comparison of various braced vs. unbraced techniques. Ypsilanti: Eastern Michigan University; 2013.
90. Price C. Incidence of injury in relation to limb dominance in Arizona State University Men's and Women's Gymnastics Teams. Arizona State University. 2013.
91. Nyman E Jr. The effects of an OpenNI/Kinect-based biofeedback intervention on kinematics at the knee during drop vertical jump landings: implications for reducing neuromuscular predisposition to non-contact ACL injury risk in the young female athlete. Toledo: The University of Toledo; 2013.
92. Whatman C, Hume P, Hing W. Kinematics during lower extremity functional screening tests in young athletes – are they reliable and valid? Phys Ther Sport. 2013;14(2):87–93.

Chapter 4
Growth and Development in Gymnastics

Lauren Klein Ritchie, Natalie Ronshaugen, and Jennifer Sygo

4.1 Normal Puberty

In order to fully grasp the differences of growth and development in a gymnast, it is crucial to first review normal adolescent growth and development. Puberty is the time in an adolescent's development marked by rapid skeletal and muscular growth along with the development of secondary sex characteristics and reproductive organs. Rapid brain changes occur, along with psychosocial adjustments. Adolescents also develop increased strength and endurance, a key component for success as a gymnast.

Both height and weight significantly increase during puberty. The growth charts compiled by the Centers for Disease Control and Prevention (CDC) depict the normal height and weight trajectory of a child to and through adolescence (Fig. 4.1). A steady, linear incline is noted on the growth chart through young childhood and older childhood, but the pubertal years are marked with a rapid skeletal growth spurt gaining an average of 30.5 cm in boys and 28.5 cm in girls [1].

Lean body mass begins to increase in early puberty. Fat mass increases for females in later puberty [1]. Rapid growth alters the biomechanics of every motion, from walking to handsprings, and increases the risk of both acute and overuse

---

L. K. Ritchie (✉)
University of Colorado School of Medicine, Aurora, CO, USA

Children's Hospital Colorado, Aurora, CO, USA
e-mail: lauren.ritchie@childrenscolorado.org

N. Ronshaugen
Children's Hospital & Medical Center, Omaha, NE, USA

University of Nebraska Medical Center, Omaha, NE, USA
e-mail: nronshaugen@childrensomaha.org

J. Sygo
Cleveland Clinic Canada, Toronto, ON, Canada

Gymnastics Canada – Women's Artistic Program, Gloucester, ON, Canada
e-mail: jsygo@rogers.com

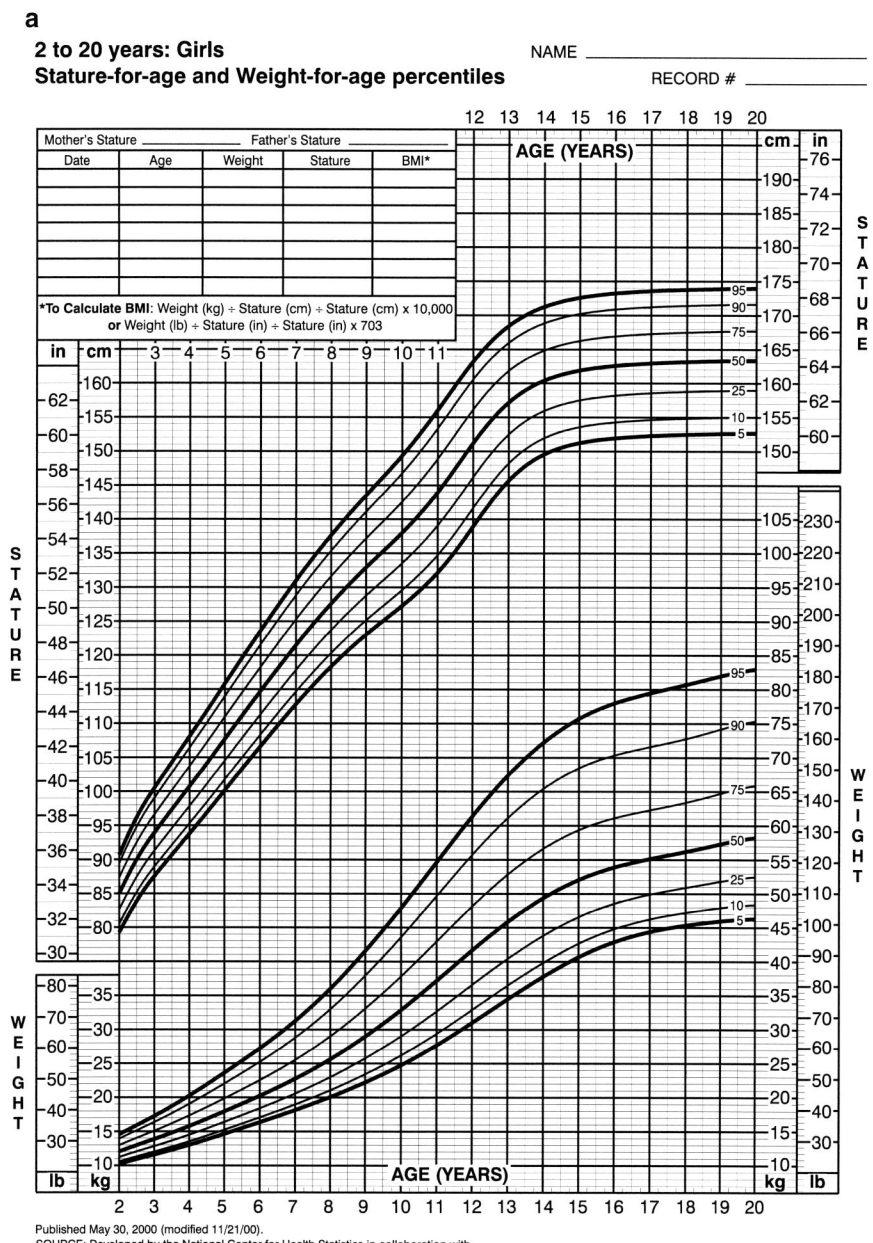

Fig. 4.1 CDC growth charts for females (**a**) and males (**b**)

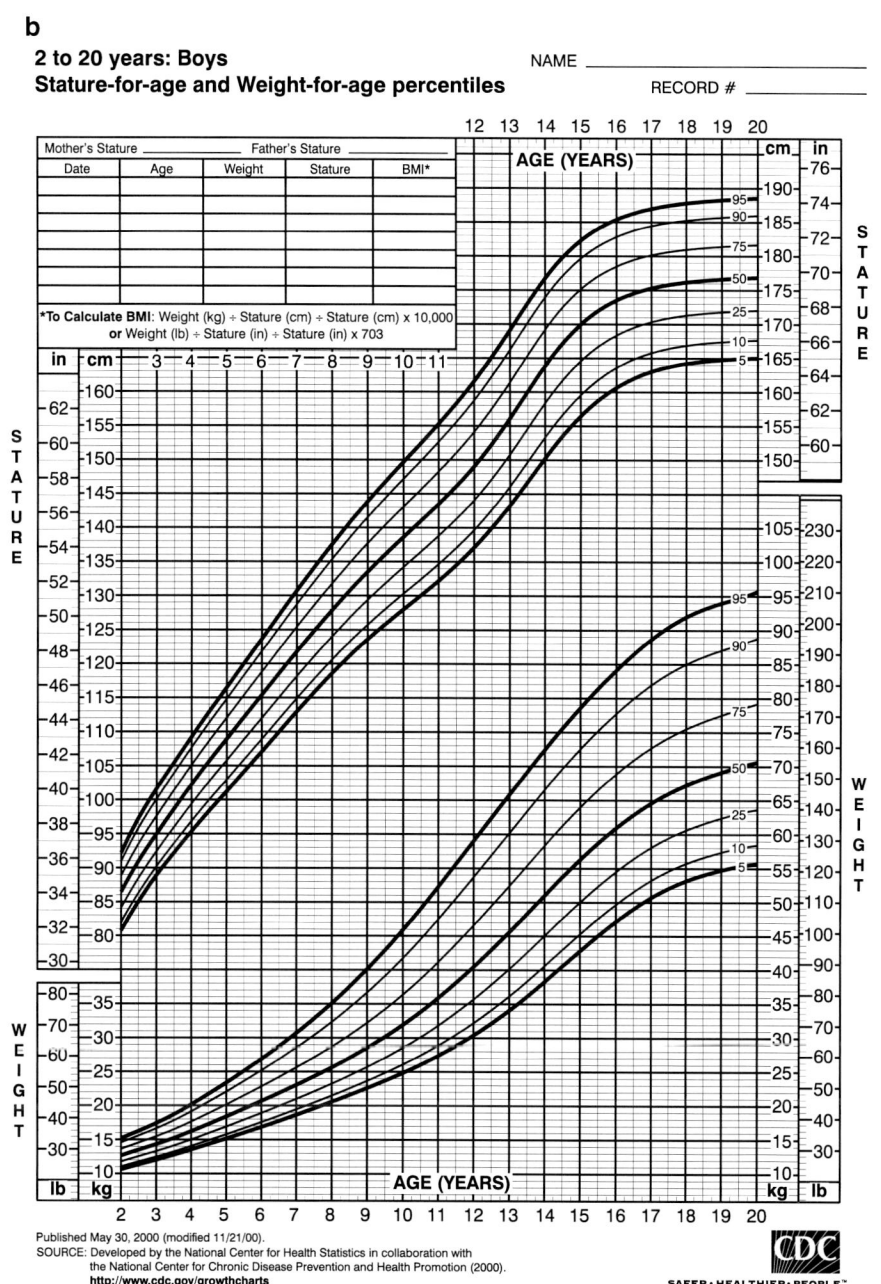

Fig. 4.1 (continued)

injuries for gymnasts, particularly in late puberty for girls [2, 3]. Peak growth velocity is inversely correlated with the age of pubertal onset. Thus, a child with later onset of puberty will have a slower peak growth velocity and may ultimately be shorter than his or her peers [1].

Generally speaking, puberty for girls begins between age 8 and 12 years old. Female pubertal changes typically begin with thelarche, followed by the growth spurt around age 12 years and then pubarche (Fig. 4.2) [4]. Menarche begins at approximately 12 ½ years [5]. Puberty for boys starts between ages 9 and 14 years. Male pubertal changes start with testicular enlargement, followed by pubarche, enlargement of the penis, and then spermarche. Skeletal growth is a later event in male puberty, generally starting around age 14 [6].

Precocious puberty is defined as pubertal changes starting before age 8 years in girls and before age 9 in boys. Delayed puberty is puberty that has not begun by age 13 in girls and age 14 in boys. Primary amenorrhea occurs when menarche has not occurred by age 15 years in girls [4, 7]. Mild delays in puberty are generally thought of as self-limited and benign, and gymnasts who undergo intensive training prior to

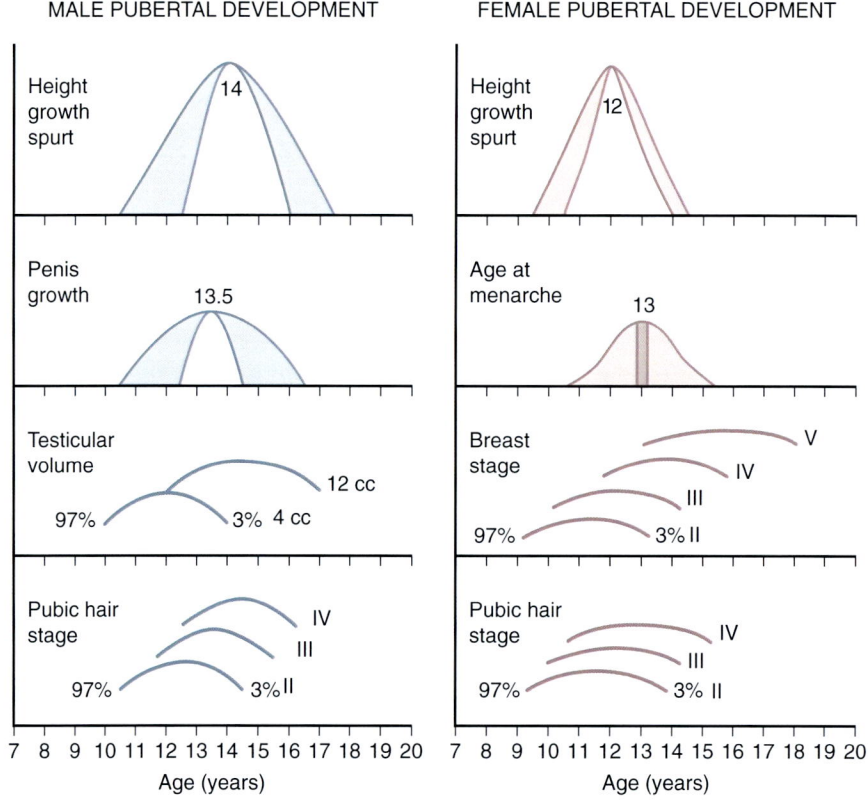

Fig. 4.2 Schematic representing the onset and timing of male and female pubertal development

puberty generally have better bone mineral density than their peers [8]. However, those athletes with significantly delayed puberty or primary amenorrhea are at risk for lower bone mineral density, increased fracture risk, and decreased final adult height [9, 10]. Females who have primary amenorrhea should be evaluated for other components of the Female Athlete Triad (see Chap. 6 for more details).

For both males and females, Tanner staging (Fig. 4.3) is a helpful tool to determine an athlete's stage of development [5, 11]. Initially described in the 1960s, Dr. Tanner outlined the normal progression of pubertal secondary sex characteristics, including penile and testicular growth, pubic hair distribution, and breast development.

A number of genetic and social factors contribute to the age of pubertal onset. These include gender, ethnic background, poverty, diet, activity level, and even nutritional status in-utero and as an infant [12, 13]. It is important to note that national trends show menarche is starting about 4 months to a year earlier than described 30–40 years ago, meaning that puberty may begin as early as 7 years old in girls [14]. These trends coincide with recent data showing increasing BMI levels in adolescents; however, it is unclear if this is the only driver [15, 16]. Despite these trends, many gymnasts have a low weight. A minimum body fat percentage of about 21% required for initiation and maintenance of menses [17]. With this in mind, female gymnasts, especially those who are of a lower weight, may find that their peers are developing more rapidly than they are, even when puberty is progressing normally.

The correlation between weight and puberty is not as linear for boys. Overweight boys have earlier puberty than their normal weight peers; however, as weight continues to increase, obese boys start puberty later than normal and overweight boys [18]. The physiology for this is not well understood currently, but it creates a larger variation of the age of pubertal onset. Thus, low weight male gymnasts may not notice as significant of a difference from their peers in pubertal onset as their female counterparts.

While weight and nutritional deficiencies can certainly contribute to abnormalities in pubertal onset for a gymnast, it is important not to prematurely exclude other health concerns. When evaluating primary amenorrhea, oligomenorrhea, or delayed onset of puberty in a gymnast, a thorough history, physical exam, and sometimes laboratory work-up are necessary to evaluate for other non-nutritional causes. Some of these causes may include thyroid derangements, inflammatory bowel disease, prolactinomas, primary ovarian failure, and genetic syndromes such as Turner Syndrome [19].

4.2 Training, Growth, and Development in Gymnasts

Artistic gymnastics has historically been a sport known to place immense physical and psychological stress on young athlete participants [20, 21]. As seen in other sports, the unique athletic demands give preference to specific body characteristics.

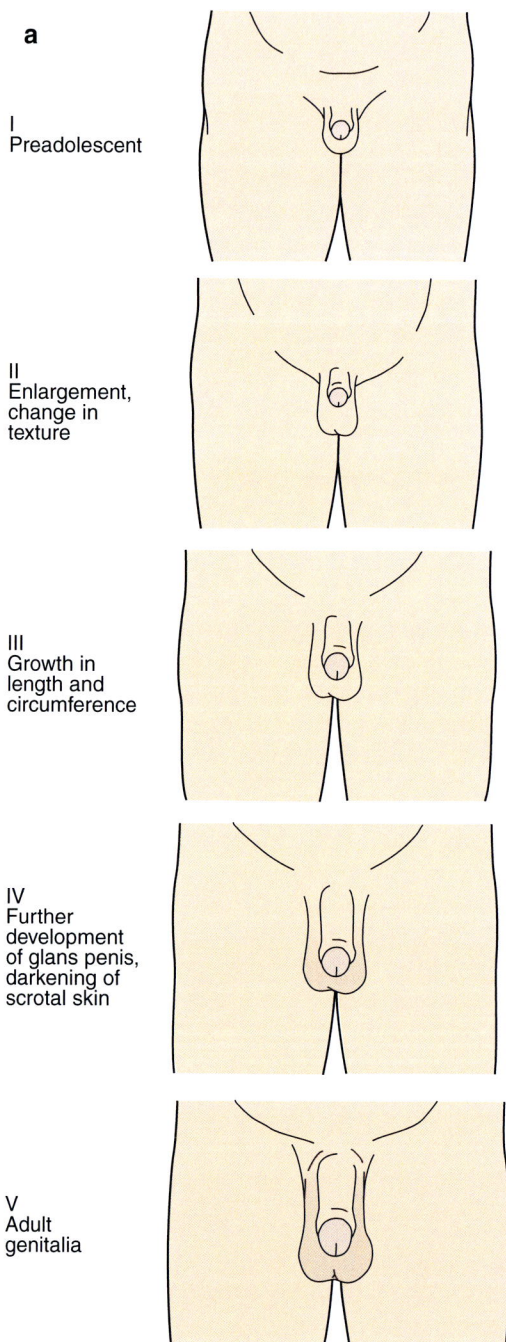

Fig. 4.3 Tanner stages depict the normal male and female development of secondary sex characteristics for male genital development (**a**), male and female pubic hair growth (**b**), and female breast development (**c**)

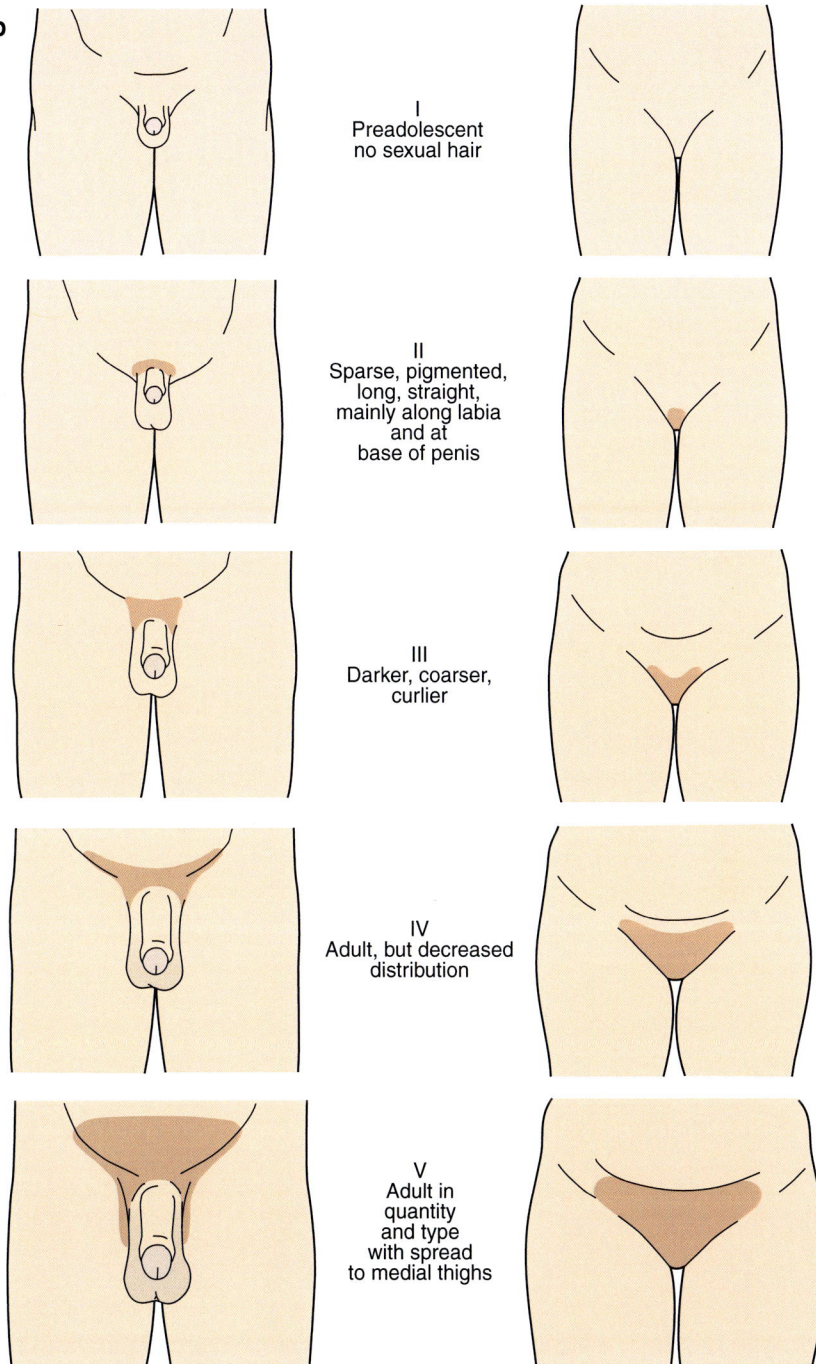

Fig. 4.3 (continued)

Fig. 4.3 (continued)

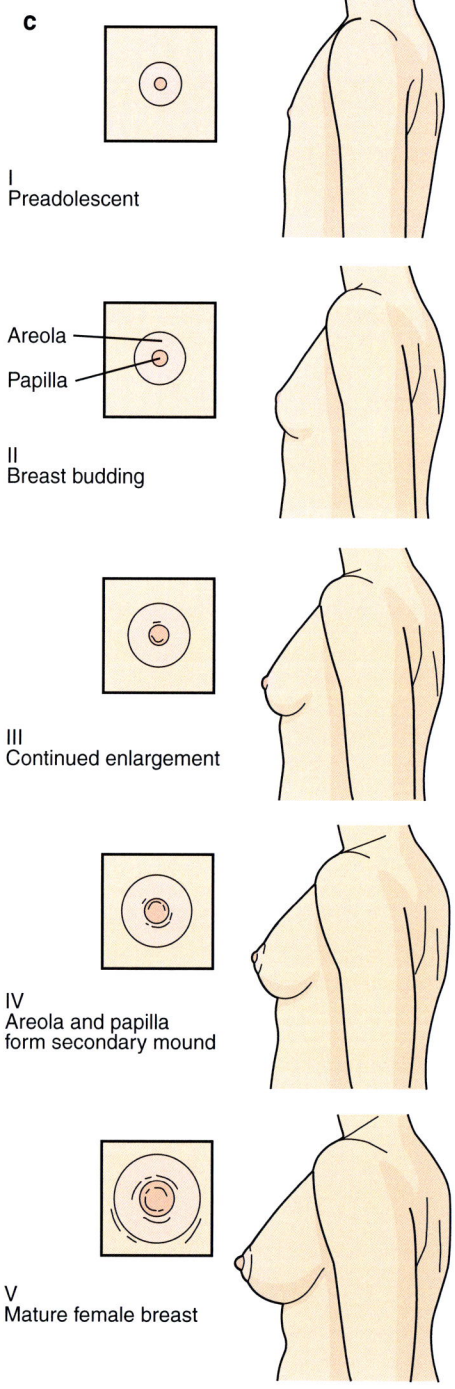

c

I
Preadolescent

Areola
Papilla

II
Breast budding

III
Continued enlargement

IV
Areola and papilla
form secondary mound

V
Mature female breast

The evolution of the sport, with increasingly difficult skills and routines, has favored gymnasts with a prepubescent physique. The optimal somatotype has further been described to include short legs, broad shoulders, and narrow hips [22, 23]. However, growing concerns have surfaced regarding the progressive physical and psychological pressures associated with the sport and their effects on growth and maturation, particularly during adolescence. Based on these concerns, the Federation Internationale de Gymnastique (FIG) raised the age limit for Olympic participation from 15 years of age to 16 years of age in 1997 [20].

Artistic gymnastics is divided into junior Olympic levels (Levels 1–10) and elite. Elite is the top level and allows for a gymnast to compete internationally, including at the Olympics. On average, female gymnasts begin training between 5 and 7 years of age; however, some may start training and competing as young as 3–4 years of age [20, 22]. Although tremendous variability exists, training time and intensity typically increase with increasing age and competitive level. High-level female gymnasts (Levels 9–10) have been reported to practice 4–6 hours daily, 6 days/week, while elite gymnasts typically practice 5–7 hours daily (30–42 hours/week). In addition, most gymnasts train year-round. The amount of time that gymnasts spend training, which occurs largely during the periadolescent years, is in response to the growing demands of the sport and can be compared to gymnasts of the 1970s who reportedly trained approximately 15 hours/week [21, 24, 25]. In contrast, male gymnasts often initiate training and increase the intensity of training at a later age, with maximum training intensity corresponding with the end of puberty [21].

Puberty is a dynamic period of development as evidenced by the rapid changes seen in body size, shape, and composition [23]. Although female gymnasts appear to follow the same pattern of pubertal maturation as the general population, the stages often occur at a later age [20, 22, 25, 26]. This is likely related to the lower height for age, weight for age, and fat mass, in addition to the high level of physical exertion well documented in female gymnasts [21, 25]. These features are thought to modulate hypothalamic activity, limit estrogen production, and correspond with a delayed skeletal age or bone age when compared to chronological age [21, 25]. The onset of puberty is determined by skeletal maturation and occurs at an average bone age of 11 years in females [25]. Therefore, the delayed skeletal age observed in female gymnasts results in a prolonged prepubertal period, shifting the onset of puberty and its subsequent physiological changes including secondary sexual characteristics, growth spurt, and menarche to older ages.

The delays described above have led to female gymnasts being labeled as "late maturers," implying that maturation does typically retain a normal rate of progression throughout puberty (without signs of prolongation or arrest of development) [23, 24, 26, 27]. For example, female gymnasts achieve menarche on average 1 year after reaching peak height velocity as is observed in the general population. Despite normal pubertal progression, there has been evidence of female gymnasts experiencing attenuated growth. This is seen in the form of a "less intense" or lower magnitude pubertal growth spurt, also described as the peak height velocity. Thus, the average peak height velocity among gymnasts is below the mean peak height velocity for adolescents in the United States. Growth attenuation has been appreciated in other sports; however, female gymnasts have statures averaging at the tenth percentile making them the shortest among all female athletes with elite-level gymnasts being at the highest risk for growth faltering [26]. Although elite-level gymnasts make up a very small percentage of all female gymnasts in the United States, reports state that attenuated growth can be seen in gymnasts training a minimum of 18 hours/week [23, 27].

While cause and effect relationships have not been established, it is postulated that the pubertal delay and growth faltering appreciated in female gymnasts are associated with the physical and psychological stresses of the sport [21]. Onset of training and high-intensity training occur earlier in high-level gymnasts resulting in increased prepubertal physical strain when compared to other sports [22, 28]. Furthermore, injuries occur with greater frequency during the period of peak height velocity which is when many gymnasts are increasing their training loads. Thus, gymnasts are more susceptible to lower and upper extremity injuries as well as vertebral injuries [22]. Low body weight reflecting an energy deficit secondary to high-intensity training and restricted caloric intake are likely to be associated with hypothalamic dysregulation and low levels of FSH and LH, decreased serum IGF-1, and ultimately delayed pubertal maturation and reduced growth velocity [20, 27]. Additionally, absence of pubertal rise in estradiol and inability to reach the critical lean mass to body fat ratio can lead to menstrual disturbances [21–23].

Regardless of these associations, researchers pose the question whether the sport causes gymnasts to have delayed puberty or if the sport itself is selective for females with small stature and later pubertal development [26]. Parents of gymnasts, particularly high-level gymnasts, are on average shorter than parents of athletes within other competitive sports and the general population. Female gymnasts are also more likely to have immediate family members, mother or sisters, who report a delay in pubertal maturation [22, 25]. The contribution of these factors is further supported by the fact that prior to initiation of training or high-intensity training, female gymnasts are on average shorter than their peers [26]. This discrepancy is seen in elite gymnasts as young as 2 years of age, demonstrating the importance of monitoring a child's growth from early ages in order to determine individual norms. Although an individual with smaller stature and delayed pubertal maturation may succeed in the realm of competitive gymnastics, additional evaluation should be obtained in any female gymnast if height is less than the fifth percentile or she has fallen across two percentiles on their growth curve [21, 22, 29].

Current literature is heavily weighted toward the effects of the intense physical and psychological stresses on the pubertal maturation of female gymnasts rather than on male gymnasts [25]. While the data are sparse, male gymnasts seem to exhibit unaltered pubertal development compared to their peers. As previously discussed, female gymnasts have a lagging bone age when compared to their chronological age; however, bone age parallels chronological age in male gymnasts. This may be a result of male gymnasts initiating training at later ages and high-intensity training occurring at the end of puberty rather than during the prepubescent years. Moreover, the energy deficit seen in female gymnasts is not often appreciated in male gymnasts secondary to more appropriate intake [21].

Although pubertal development is unaltered in male gymnasts, growth may ultimately be affected. Genetics are thought to be the principal factors influencing the rate of a child's growth and subsequently final adult height; however, genetic predisposition may be modified by unfavorable environmental factors [23]. As previously discussed, female gymnasts are shown to experience an attenuated pubertal growth spurt. However, their growth may continue into later ages (18 years of age) than the average female (15 years of age), and they do often exhibit catch up growth [20]. Catch up growth is seen across many sports and is described as a period of increased growth velocity out of proportion to what is expected based on age. It occurs in the setting of decreased training, for instance during offseason or with injury, or it may occur once an athlete has fully retired from a sport [21, 29]. Despite catch up growth, final adult height was still found to be lower than predicted height based on genetic predisposition in both male and female gymnasts [29]. Although final adult heights were within the standard error of prediction and predicted heights were often based on inaccurate estimates (midparental height), these results raise concern that the growth potential of some male and female gymnasts may truly be impaired [22].

4.3 Body Composition and Anthropometrics

Gymnasts tend to be smaller and lighter than nonathletes and may be leaner than dancers and other athletes [30]. Using dual x-ray absorptiometry (DXA), Deutz et al. [31] reported a mean body fat percentage of 12.36% among elite female gymnasts, while Jonnalagadda et al. [32] reported a similar result of 12.7% ± 2.3%, using skinfold anthropometry. Elite artistic gymnasts have been reported to have lower body fat percentages compared to rhythmic gymnasts (16.6%) and long-distance runners (15.14%) [31]. Intriguingly, at least one study has demonstrated that athletes who have larger and more prolonged energy deficits throughout the day tend to have a higher body fat percentage [31]; this provides further evidence that gymnasts should be encouraged to maintain adequate energy availability, not only over the course of the entire day but also within each part of the day, including the training period.

4.3.1 Weight Changes

At various points in their career, gymnasts may experience a desire to lose weight (mass) and/or body fat (fat mass). While a high strength-to-weight ratio and low body mass may be beneficial for technical success in the sport, intentional weight loss is associated with serious risks to physical and psychological health, as well as performance. Indeed, prolonged periods of intentional or unintentional low energy availability (defined as the amount of energy, or kilocalories, available for basic physiological functioning after factoring in the energy demands of exercise) can lead to menstrual irregularities in female athletes, as well as compromised bone health, impaired immune function, loss of muscle mass, mood changes, and reduced training adaptations in athletes of both genders [33].

The *Handbook of Sports Medicine and Science, Gymnastics* [34], supported by both the International Olympic Committee and the FIG, outline appropriate considerations for managing weight changes in gymnasts. The authors [34] emphasize that coaches should avoid putting pressure on gymnasts to lose weight, and any weight changes should be initiated from the gymnast, not the coach. It was also noted that even lean or light gymnasts may have a desire to lose weight. If a weight loss plan is initiated, it should occur under the guidance of a professional sport dietitian with expertise in the sport, and the focus should be on improving speed and power (i.e., performance) in the gymnast, rather than strictly weight loss. If a weight loss plan is initiated, it should emphasize gradual (0.5 kg/week) weight loss with modest (~200–500 kcal/day) reductions in energy intake to minimize negative effects on health and performance. In female athletes, menstrual irregularities should be avoided, and gymnasts should be monitored both during and after weight loss to ensure both physical health and emotional well-being.

4.4 Nutrition

4.4.1 Energy Needs of Gymnasts

Gymnastics is a largely anaerobic sport characterized by relatively short bursts of intense activity, often involving many or most of the major muscle groups. The energy needs of gymnasts will therefore vary according to the intensity and duration of the training session, the size of the gymnast, and the stage of growth and development. The energy requirements of gymnasts can be subdivided into basal metabolic rate (BMR), activities of daily living (ADL), thermic effect of food (TEF), and the energy expended through training or other physical activity. Additional energy may also be expended to support growth and development. BMR describes the energy required to support basic physiological functioning, including brain and organ function, the autonomic and central nervous system, the endocrine system, and immune system function. ADL encompasses all voluntary movement and activity aside from training, including walking, household activities and personal hygiene, food preparation, and the activities that make up any school or work. TEF describes the energy required to digest and metabolize food.

While a sedentary 16-year-old (160 cm, 55 kg) female's estimated energy requirement to maintain weight is approximately 1700 cal/day [35], gymnasts are expected to have greater requirements due to the energy demands of training, which include not only apparatus-specific activity but also warm up, cool down, conditioning, and any ancillary training, such as dance, pilates, or rehabilitation. The energy requirement of gymnastics training is poorly characterized in the literature, but appears to be lower than the demands of endurance sports, such as running, cycling, or swimming; for example, the total daily energy requirements of competitive female gymnasts has been estimated to be between 2097 ± 144 kcal/day and 2263 ± 199 kcal/day [31]. By comparison, endurance athletes may require 3000–4500 cal/day during intense training [36].

Since gymnastics is a judged, aesthetic sport, gymnasts may, for a variety of reasons, restrict energy intake to control weight. Studies using food diaries have reported mean energy intakes in female gymnasts of 1317 ± 559 kcal/day [31], 1632 ± 533 kcal/day [37], and 1678 ± 543 kcal/day [38]. While this could suggest that female gymnasts tend to follow low-calorie diets, it is also possible that gymnasts, especially female gymnasts, might be prone to underreporting their energy intake, possibly due to pressure to maintain a low body weight. Indeed, Jonnalagadda et al. [32] demonstrated that 61% of the members of the United States' national women's gymnastics team likely underreported their energy intake. Underreporting may be more prevalent among older female gymnasts (aged 15–18 years) versus younger athletes (11–14 years) [38] and in gymnasts with a higher body fat percentage [32].

4.4.2 Macronutrients

Gymnastics training combines static and dynamic movements with a large range of motion, utilizing all major muscle groups. Gymnasts have a high strength-to-weight ratio and engage in numerous activities that can trigger muscle damage. Taken together, this suggests that protein requirements of gymnasts are elevated, not only to support basic physiological functioning but also for muscle repair and recovery and to encourage training adaptations over time. The protein and other macronutrient needs of gymnasts are summarized in Table 4.1. To support optimal muscle protein synthesis and minimize muscle protein breakdown, protein intake should be spread relatively evenly throughout the day, with a target intake of 0.3 g of protein per kilogram body weight per meal and 1.5–2.0 g protein per kilogram body weight per day [39, 40]. For a 55 kg (120 lb) female gymnast, this equals approximately 17 g protein per meal and 80–110 g of protein per day, whereas a 70 kg (154 lb) male gymnast would require approximately 21 g protein per meal and 105–140 g

Table 4.1 Estimated energy and nutrient requirements for weight-stable male and female gymnasts

Gender	Energy (kcal/day)	Protein (g/kg/day)	Carbohydrates (g/kg/day)	Fat (g/kg/day)
Male (postpubertal)	2500–3000	1.5–2.0	5.0–8.0	1.0–1.5
Female (postpubertal)	2200–2500	1.4–2.0	5.0–8.0	1.0–1.5

Recommendations assume gymnasts train ~5 hours/day and have good energy availability

Table 4.2 Protein content of some common foods

Food items	Portion	Protein (g)
Meat/poultry/seafood – various (lean cuts), cooked	85 g (3 oz.)	22–26
Tuna, packed in water, drained.	85 g (1/2 can)	16
Eggs	1 large	6
Milk, cow's (0%, 1%, 2%, 3.25%), chocolate	250 ml (1 cup)	7–8
Yogurt, plain, low fat or skim	170 g (3/4 cup)	9–10
Yogurt, Greek, plain, 0% MF	170 g (3/4 cup)	17
Cottage cheese, 2% MF	125 g (1/2 cup)	12
Cheese, cheddar	30 g (1 oz.)	8
Almonds, roasted	30 g (1 oz.)	6
Peanut butter	30 ml (2 Tbsp.)	7
Lentils, boiled	150 g (3/4 cup)	13
Chick peas, boiled	175 ml (3/4 cup)	11
Quinoa, cooked	125 ml (1/2 cup)	4
Tofu, extra firm	100 g (3.5 oz.)	10

Source: USDA Nutrient Database

protein per day. Examples of protein-containing foods that can be used to meet the target of 15–20 g protein per meal are summarized in Table 4.2.

Relative to endurance athletes, gymnasts tend to engage in more technical and short-burst activities, which, combined with a lower body mass, suggests both absolute and total dietary carbohydrate requirements may be lower than endurance athletes. The carbohydrate requirements of gymnasts are summarized in Table 4.1. Gymnasts engaging in periods of very intense training with a high emphasis on aerobic activities (e.g., conditioning) may have elevated carbohydrate requirements; conversely, carbohydrate needs may decline around competitions when training volumes decrease. To support both satiety and blood glucose control, gymnasts should be encouraged to consume fiber-rich, low-to-moderate glycemic index carbohydrates throughout the day, such as whole fruit, vegetables, and intact grains, while limiting their intake of refined grains and foods high in added sugar.

To maintain stable blood glucose and prevent hunger during training sessions, gymnasts should be encouraged to start training sessions well-fueled, having consumed a mixed meal containing readily digestible carbohydrates, along with lean or low-fat protein foods, 1–4 hours prior to training. Indeed, Batatinha et al. [41] demonstrated that gymnasts with low blood glucose levels may experience greater fatigue and fall from the balance beam more often than those with blood glucose in the optimal range. This suggests that, if necessary, gymnasts be given the opportunity to take a break for a snack during training. This may be especially important if training sessions are long (>4 hours) or if they occur over typical meal times.

The available literature suggests gymnasts tend to consume low-fat diets [38]; however, the emerging trend toward high-fat and low-carbohydrate diets could lead some gymnasts to consume more dietary fat or restrict carbohydrates. Paoli et al.

[42] demonstrated that a very-low-carbohydrate, ketogenic diet resulted in no negative impact on strength and power measures in elite male artistic gymnasts, but importantly, the study did not examine maximum speed or endurance, both of which are vital to gymnastics performance. Since glucose is a critical fuel for brief, maximal intensity sprint activities [43], this suggests that low-carbohydrate diets could impair performance, especially for prolonged high-intensity activities, such as intense conditioning, speed work, and routines with full difficulty. Dietary fat intake can be manipulated to promote satiety and ensure energy balance, but a priority should be placed on nutrient-dense fat sources, such as oily fish, nuts, seeds, avocados, and olive oil, while limiting fats obtained from highly refined, nutrient-poor foods, such as fried foods, processed meats, and commercial pastries. Dietary fat recommendations are listed in Table 4.1.

4.4.3 Micronutrients

While gymnasts should aim to consume a nutrient-dense diet that meets both their energy and macronutrient needs, the available literature suggests gymnasts, especially female gymnasts, may have difficulty meeting their needs for certain key micronutrients, including iron, vitamin D, and calcium.

Iron: Reduced iron stores may occur in gymnasts, especially among female gymnasts. A study assessing iron status in gymnasts and other young athletes [44] demonstrated that mean serum ferritin was 28 ± 18 and 25 ± 10 ng/ml in male and female gymnasts, respectively. While these levels were not different than non-gymnast athletes, gymnasts had, on average, lower levels of serum iron and transferrin saturation than non-gymnast athletes. A study of elite female gymnasts suggested iron intake may be inadequate [38], which may contribute to reduced iron status. To help meet iron needs through diet, gymnasts should be encouraged to consume iron-rich foods, and if necessary, consider iron supplementation. Table 4.3 summarizes key iron-rich foods that gymnasts should include in their diet.

Vitamin D: Vitamin D status is a concern for gymnasts due to the indoor nature of the sport. Even athletes who live and train in warm weather or sunny environments may be prone to vitamin D insufficiency or deficiency, which has important implications for musculoskeletal health and immune system function [47]. For example, a cross-sectional survey of elite Australian gymnasts demonstrated that 15 of 18 athletes had serum vitamin D (25[OH]D) less than 75 nmol/l, and one-third of gymnasts had 25[OH]D less than 50 nmol/l, a threshold consistent with deficiency according to the Institute of Medicine [45]. Since food sources of vitamin D are relatively limited, gymnasts who have difficulty maintaining adequate vitamin status may benefit from routine supplementation or, if appropriate, modest sun exposure (roughly 10 minutes of midday sun exposure to hands, arms, legs, and face). Chapter 6 discusses Vitamin D deficiency in detail.

Table 4.3 Food sources of key nutrients for gymnasts

Food items	Portion	Iron (mg)
Spinach, cooked, boiled, drained	125 ml (1/2 cup)	3.2
Edamame/baby soybeans, frozen, cooked	125 ml (1/2 cup)	1.8
Green peas, cooked, boiled	125 ml (1/2 cup)	1.2
Cereal, dry, various types	30 g (check product label for serving size)	1.1–9.0
Beef, various cuts, cooked	85 g (3 oz.)	1.6–2.4
Chicken, skinless, various cuts, cooked	85 g (3 oz.)	0.9–1.3
Pork, various cuts, cooked	85 g (3 oz.)	0.5–1.2
Tuna, light, canned in water	85 g (3 oz.)	1.4
Pumpkin seeds or squash seeds, roasted	30 g (1 oz.)	0.9
Lentils, cooked, boiled	148 g (3/4 cup)	5.0
Eggs, cooked	2 large	1.76
Hummus	60 g (1/4 cup)	1.5

Iron needs – children 4–8 years: 10 mg/day. Male and female 9–13 years: 8 mg/day. Male 14–18 years: 11 mg/day. Female 14–18 years: 15 mg/day. Male 19+: 8 mg/day. Female 19–50: 18 mg/day

Food items	Portion	Vitamin D (IU)
Milk (3.25%, 2%, 1% skim, chocolate milk)	250 ml (1 cup)	115–124
Soy beverage, fortified with vitamin D	250 ml (1 cup)	119
Eggs, cooked	2 large	82
Salmon, sockeye, cooked	85 g (3 oz.)	570
Trout, rainbow, cooked	85 g (3 oz.)	645
Tuna, light canned in water	85 g (3 oz.)	40
Cod liver oil	5 ml (1 tsp.)	450

Vitamin D needs – male and female, 4–50 years: 600 IU/day

Food items	Portion	Calcium (mg)
Spinach, fresh or frozen, cooked	125 ml (1/2 cup)	122
Kale, cooked, boiled, drained	125 ml (1/2 cup)	88
Collard greens, fresh or frozen, cooked	125 ml (1/2 cup)	134
Soy beverage, fortified with calcium	250 ml (1 cup)	301
Milk, 3.25%, 2%, 1% skim, chocolate milk	250 ml (1 cup)	272–305
Yogurt, plain, low fat or skim	170 g (6 oz.)	311–338
Cheese, various (cheddar, Gouda, Swiss, mozzarella)	30 g (1 oz.)	198–252
Yogurt, Greek, plain, nonfat	170 g (6 oz.)	187
Cottage cheese	125 g (1/2 cup)	125
Almonds	23 whole (1 oz.)	76

Calcium needs – children 4–8 years: 1000 mg/day. Male and female 9–18 years: 1300 mg/day. Male and female 19–50 years: 1000 mg/day

Source: Dietary Reference Intakes [45, 46]

Calcium: Calcium, along with Vitamin D, is necessary for the maintenance of optimal bone health, which is particularly important during the adolescent years when peak bone accrual occurs. Several studies suggest that gymnasts have difficulty meeting calcium needs through diet. Lovell et al. [48] found that 13 of 18 elite female gymnasts did not meet their age-related calcium requirements. Similar results have been observed in prepubescent female gymnasts [30] and elite members of the United States' women's national gymnastics team [38]. To help meet calcium requirements, gymnasts should be encouraged to consume calcium-rich foods, and if necessary, make up any difference with supplements to meet the Dietary Reference Intake (DRI) for their age. Table 4.3 outlines some common food sources of calcium.

References

1. Soliman AT, De Sanctis V, Elalaily R, Bedair S. Advances in pubertal growth and factors influencing it: can we increase pubertal growth? Indian J Endocrinol Metab. 2014;18:S53–62.
2. Baxter-Jones A, Maffulli N, Helms P. Low injury rates in elite athletes. Arch Dis Child. 1993;68(1):130–2.
3. Hawkins D, Metheny J. Overuse injuries in youth sports: biomechanical considerations. Med Sci Sports Exerc. 2001;33(10):1701–7.
4. Deligeoroglou E, Tsimaris P. Menstrual disturbances in puberty. Best Pract Res Clin Obstet Gynaecol. 2010;24(2):157–71.
5. Marshall WA, Tanner JM. Variations in pattern of pubertal changes in girls. Arch Dis Child. 1969;44(235):291–303.
6. Marshall WA, Tanner JM. Variations in the pattern of pubertal changes in boys. Arch Dis Child. 1970;45(239):13–23.
7. Johnson TR, Moore WM, Jeffries JE. Adolescent developmental stages. In: Children are different: developmental physiology. 2nd ed. Columbus: Ross Laboratories a Division of Abbott Laboratories; 1978. p. 25–9.
8. Bass S, Pearce G, Bradney M, Hendrich E, Delmas PD, Harding A, Seeman E. Exercise before puberty may confer residual benefits in bone density in adulthood: studies in active prepubertal and retired female gymnasts. J Bone Miner Res. 1998;13:500–7.
9. Yingling VR, Xiang Y, Raphan T, Schaffler MB, Koser K, Malique R. The effect of a short-term delay of puberty on trabecular bone mass and structure in female rats: a texture-based and histomorphometric analysis. Bone. 2007;40(2):419–24.
10. Zhu J, Chan YM. Adult consequences of self-limited delayed puberty. Pediatrics. 2017;139(6):e20163177.
11. Chemaitilly W, Escobar O, Witchel SF. Endocrinology. In: Zitelli BJ, McIntire SC, Nowalk AJ, editors. Zitelli and Davis' atlas of pediatric physical diagnosis. 6th ed. Philadelphia: Elsevier Saunders; 2012. p. 373–5.
12. Qamra SR, Mehta S, Deodhar SD. A mixed-longitudinal study on the pattern of pubertal growth: relationship to socioeconomic status and caloric-intake--IV. Indian Pediatr. 1991;28(2):147–56.
13. Proos L, Gustafsson J. Is early puberty triggered by catch-up growth following undernutrition? Int J Environ Res Public Health. 2012;9(5):1791–809.

14. Herman-Giddens ME, Slora EJ, Wasserman RC, Bourdony CJ, Bhapkar MV, Koch GG, et al. Secondary sexual characteristics and menses in young girls seen in office practice: a study from the Pediatric Research in Office Settings network. Pediatrics. 1997;99(4):505–12.
15. Kaplowitz PB, Oberfield SE. Reexamination of the age limit for defining when puberty is precocious in girls in the United States: implications for evaluation and treatment. Drug and Therapeutics and Executive Committees of the Lawson Wilkins Pediatric Endocrine Society. Pediatrics. 1999;104(4 Pt 1):936–41.
16. Biro FM, Greenspan LC, Galvez MP. Puberty in girls of the 21st century. J Pediatr Adolesc Gynecol. 2012;25(5):289–94.
17. Tokatly Latzer I, Kidron-Levy H, Stein D, Levy AE, Yosef G, Ziv-Baran T, et al. Predicting menstrual recovery in adolescents with anorexia nervosa using body fat percent estimated by bioimpedance analysis. J Adolesc Health. 2019;64(4):454–60.
18. Lee JM, Wasserman R, Kaciroti N, Gebremariam A, Steffes J, Dowshen S, et al. Timing of puberty in overweight versus obese boys. Pediatrics. 2016;137(2):e20150164.
19. Fenichel P. Delayed puberty. Endocr Dev. 2012;22:138–59.
20. Georgopoulos NA, Theodoropoulou A, Roupas NA, Rottstein L, Tsekouras A, Mylonas P, et al. Growth velocity and final height in elite female rhythmic and artistic gymnasts. Hormones (Athens). 2012;11(1):61–9.
21. Weimann E, Witzel C, Schwidergall S, Bohles HJ. Peripubertal perturbations in elite gymnasts caused by sport specific training regimes and inadequate nutritional intake. Int J Sports Med. 2000;21(3):210–5.
22. Caine D, Lewis R, O'Connor P, Howe W, Bass S. Does gymnastics training inhibit growth of females? Clin J Sport Med. 2001;11(4):260–70.
23. Georgopoulos NA, Roupas ND, Theodoropoulou A, Tsekouras A, Vagenakis AG, Markou KB. The influence of intensive physical training on growth and pubertal development in athletes. Ann N Y Acad Sci. 2010;1205:39–44.
24. Georgopoulos NA, Theodoropoulou A, Leglise M, Vagenakis AG, Markou KB. Growth and skeletal maturation in male and female artistic gymnasts. J Clin Endocrinol Metab. 2004;89(9):4377–82.
25. Malina RM, Baxter-Jones AD, Armstrong N, Beunen GP, Caine D, Daly RM, et al. Role of intensive training in the growth and maturation of artistic gymnasts. Sports Med. 2013;43(9):783–802.
26. Thomas M, Claessens AL, Leferve J, Philippaerts R, Beunen GP, Malina RM. Adolescent growth spurts in female gymnasts. J Pediatr. 2005;146(2):239–44.
27. Daly RM, Caine D, Bass SL, Pieter W, Broekhoff J. Growth of highly versus moderately trained competitive female artistic gymnasts. Med Sci Sports Exerc. 2005;37(6):1053–60.
28. Theodoropoulou A, Markou KB, Vagenakis GA, Benardot D, Leglise M, Kourounis G, et al. Delayed but normally progressed puberty is more pronounced in artistic compared with rhythmic elite gymnasts due to the intensity of training. J Clin Endocrinol Metab. 2005;90(11):6022–7.
29. Bass S, Bradney M, Pearce G, Hendrich E, Inge K, Stuckey S, et al. Short stature and delayed puberty in gymnasts: influence of selection bias on leg length and the duration of training on trunk length. J Pediatr. 2000;136(2):149–55.
30. Soric M, Misigoj-Durakovic M, Pedisic Z. Dietary intake and body composition of prepubescent female aesthetic athletes. Int J Sport Nutr Exerc Metab. 2008;18(3):343–54.
31. Deutz RC, Benardot D, Martin DE, Cody MM. Relationship between energy deficits and body composition in elite female gymnasts and runners. Med Sci Sports Exerc. 2000;32(3):659–68.
32. Jonnalagadda SS, Benardot D, Dill MN. Assessment of under-reporting of energy intake by elite female gymnast. Int J Sport Nutr Exerc Metab. 2000;10(3):315–25.
33. Mountjoy M, Sundgot-Borgen JK, Burke LM, Ackerman KE, Blauwet C, Constantini N, et al. IOC consensus statement on relative energy deficiency in sport (RED-S): 2018 update. Br J Sports Med. 2018;52(11):687–97.

34. Sundgot-Borgen J, Garthe I, Meyer N. Energy needs and weight management for gymnasts. In: Caine DJ, Russel K, Lim L, editors. Handbook of sports medicine and science, gymnastics. Hoboken: Wiley-Blackwell; 2013.
35. Harris JA, Benedict FG. A biometric study of human basal metabolism. Proc Natl Acad Sci U S A. 1918;4(12):370–3.
36. Stellingwerff T, Boit MK, Res PT, International Association of Athletics Federations. Nutritional strategies to optimize training and racing in middle-distance athletes. J Sports Sci. 2007;25 Suppl 1:S17–28.
37. Fogelholm GM, Kukkonen-Harjula TK, Taipale SA, Sievanen HT, Oja P, Vuori IM. Resting metabolic rate and energy intake in female gymnasts, figure-skaters and soccer players. Int J Sports Med. 1995;16(8):551–6.
38. Jonnalagadda SS, Bernadot D, Nelson M. Energy and nutrient intakes of the United States National Women's Artistic Gymnastics Team. Int J Sport Nutr. 1998;8(4):331–44.
39. Areta JL, Burke LM, Ross ML, Camera DM, West DW, Broad EM, et al. Timing and distribution of protein ingestion during prolonged recovery from resistance exercise alters myofibrillar protein synthesis. J Physiol. 2013;591(9):2319–31.
40. Moore DR, Areta J, Coffey VG, Stellingwerff T, Phillips SM, Burke LM, et al. Daytime pattern of post-exercise protein intake affects whole-body protein turnover in resistance-trained males. Nutr Metab (Lond). 2012;9(1):91.
41. Batatinha HA, da Costa CE, de Franca E, Dias IR, Ladeira AP, Rodrigues B, et al. Carbohydrate use and reduction in number of balance beam falls: implications for mental and physical fatigue. J Int Soc Sports Nutr. 2013;10:32.
42. Paoli A, Grimaldi K, D'Agostino D, Cenci L, Moro T, Bianco A, et al. Ketogenic diet does not affect strength performance in elite artistic gymnasts. J Int Soc Sports Nutr. 2012;9(1):34.
43. Parolin ML, Chesley A, Matsos MP, Spriet LL, Jones NL, Heigenhauser GJ. Regulation of skeletal muscle glycogen phosphorylase and PDH during maximal intermittent exercise. Am J Phys. 1999;277(5):E890–900.
44. Constantini NW, Eliakim A, Zigel L, Yaaron M, Falk B. Iron status of highly active adolescents: evidence of depleted iron stores in gymnasts. Int J Sport Nutr Exerc Metab. 2000;10(1):62–70.
45. Institute of Medicine. Dietary reference intakes for calcium and vitamin D. Washington, DC: National Academy Press; 2010.
46. Institute of Medicine. Dietary reference intakes for vitamin A, vitamin K, arsenic, boron, chromium, copper, iodine, iron, manganese, molybdenum, nickel, silicon, vanadium, and zinc. Washington, DC: National Academies Press; 2001.
47. Owens DJ, Allison R, Close GL. Vitamin D and the athlete: current perspectives and new challenges. Sports Med. 2018;48(Suppl 1):3–16.
48. Lovell G. Vitamin D status of females in an elite gymnastics program. Clin J Sport Med. 2008;18(2):159–61.

Chapter 5
Psychological Aspects of Injury in Gymnastics

Jamie L. Shapiro, Michelle L. Bartlett, and Leah E. Lomonte

5.1 Introduction

While many sports medicine professionals (e.g., medical doctors, physical therapists, athletic trainers, chiropractors, massage therapists) focus on the physical aspects of injury recovery, the psychological effects of sport injury and impact on recovery also warrant attention by medical providers. Psychological factors can increase or decrease the risk of injury occurring, can impact an athlete's emotional and behavioral response to injury, and can affect the recovery process. Psychological interventions, such as mental skills interventions, can both prevent injury and enhance injury rehabilitation and return to sport. When emotional disturbances and clinical issues (e.g., major depression, anxiety, eating disorders, substance abuse, trauma) are present, sports medicine professionals should refer athletes to a qualified mental health professional. This chapter addresses (a) psychological and sociocultural antecedents of injury; (b) psychological responses to injury; (c) psychological interventions during rehabilitation; and (d) psychological aspects of returning to gymnastics following injury. The referral process to mental health professionals and multidisciplinary treatment of the injured athlete will also be discussed.

J. L. Shapiro (✉) · L. E. Lomonte
University of Denver, Denver, CO, USA
e-mail: Jamie.Shapiro@du.edu; leah.lomonte@du.edu

M. L. Bartlett
West Texas A&M University, Canyon, TX, USA
e-mail: mbartlett@wtamu.edu

© Springer Nature Switzerland AG 2020
E. Sweeney (ed.), *Gymnastics Medicine*,
https://doi.org/10.1007/978-3-030-26288-4_5

5.2 Psychological and Sociocultural Antecedents of Sport Injury

Because of the physical demands of gymnastics, the sport is "chalk-full" of injuries, with an annual estimated injury rate of 198–364% (i.e., 1.98–3.64 injuries per person per year) for competitive gymnasts [1]. There are many potential causes of injuries in gymnastics. As outlined in Ray and Wiese-Bjornstal [2], there may be physical causes of injury, such as an increase in training load and subsequent load on the body, musculoskeletal imbalances, being under-recovered, or continuing to overwork a minor injury to the point of it becoming a major injury. There are also environmental factors such as damaged equipment, faulty apparatus settings, humidity, or even having to compete on unfamiliar equipment that can contribute to injuries. However, there are two other categories of antecedents of injury that are less acknowledged by coaches, athletes, and sports medicine professionals but may be even more impactful than the physical or environmental causes. These are the psychological and sociocultural antecedents of injury. Unfortunately, psychological and sociocultural factors are rarely accounted for in sport injury prevention guidelines [3]. Therefore, it is important that sports medicine professionals are knowledgeable of these risk factors so that they may take them into account for injury or re-injury prevention.

5.2.1 Psychological Antecedents of Injury

There is ample evidence to demonstrate that athletes' psychological states can contribute to injury risk. For instance, athletes who have had a previous serious injury are 4.6 to 176 times more likely to succumb to another injury [4], and it may not even be the same injury. While some may think this is due to an inherent physical weakness, it actually may have more to do with psychological reasons. This can be due to a psychological factor of concentration, where the athlete is distracted by thoughts of protecting an injured area or avoiding an injury while *not* concentrating on relevant performance factors, like how close to the end of the beam she is or that the vaulting table is set too low. Another major psychological factor that can account for increased injury risk is psychological stress, defined as the (usually unpleasant) nonspecific response of the body to any demand placed on it [5].

5.2.1.1 The Stress and Injury Model

One model that suggests psychological factors are antecedents to sport injury is Andersen and Williams' [6] (and then later revised by Williams and Andersen in 1998 [7]) *stress and injury model* (Fig. 5.1). Introduced over 30 years ago, it still remains the most dominant model to explain the connection between psychological factors and injury risk, prevention, and incidence [3]. The model was developed in the late 1980s to streamline much of the previous research that was done in the 1960s and 1970s highlighting that athletes under psychological stress were significantly more likely to sustain acute injuries while performing, and that the influence of psychological variables on injury incidence is primarily through stress (i.e., distress) [7].

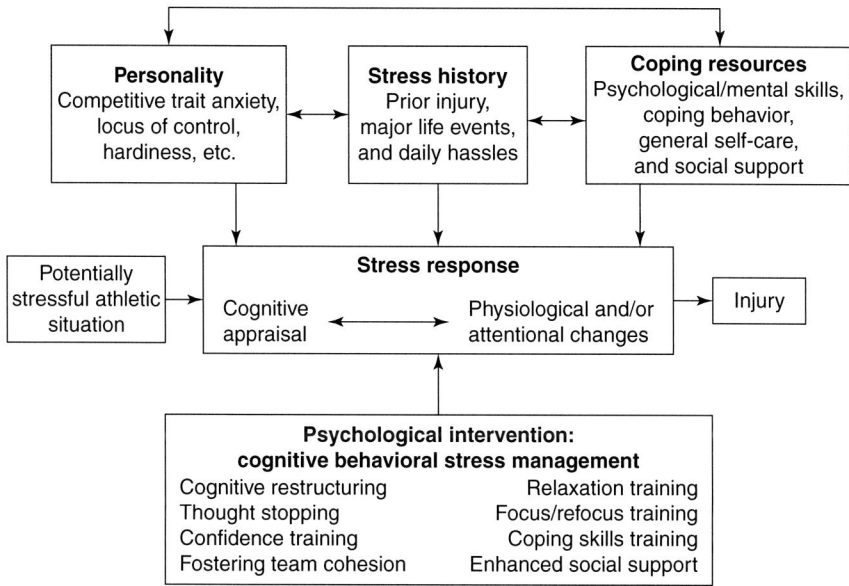

Fig. 5.1 The stress and injury model. (Williams and Andersen [7]. Appaneal and Habif [2]. Reprinted with permission of the publisher [Taylor & Francis Ltd., http://www.tandfonline.com]. Permission conveyed through Copyright Clearance Center, Inc.)

Williams and Andersen's [7] model stipulates that four broad categories – personality, history of stressors, coping resources, and cognitive interventions (stress management skills) – serve as moderators to the central component of the stress and injury model, the stress response process, which in turn influence risk of injury. The stress response process is bidirectional and two-fold: (1) the occurring cognitive appraisal, and (2) the subsequent effects of that appraisal on attention/concentration and on physiological activation levels, or the effects of the changes in attention/concentration and physiological activations on one's cognitive appraisal.

Cognitive appraisal is a process in which people evaluate the environmental/situational demand being placed on them by sizing up that demand in terms of threat, harm, and consequence (primary appraisal), and then whether or not they possess sufficient resources to meet that demand (secondary appraisal) [3, 8]. If an athlete thinks that an event (e.g., an important gymnastics meet) is threatening and with severe consequences (e.g., "If I don't stick these routines then I will not make the Olympic team and I will lose my endorsements"), and that they do not have the resources to meet this demand ("I don't have enough coaching support to perform well here"), then there will be a subsequent change in the athlete's attentional field (narrowing; i.e., "tunnel vision") and potentially delayed decision-making with an increase in physiological activation. This physiological activation may include increased muscle tension, increased sweating, and decreased coordination. Both the inability to pay attention to performance relevant cues and the aforementioned bodily changes make optimal performance difficult and greatly increase the risk of an injury occurring.

5.2.1.2 Moderators of the Stress Response Process in the Stress and Injury Model

A moderator is a variable that changes the strength and form of a relation between two variables [9]. In the stress and injury model, the relationship between stress and injury can be impacted positively or negatively by athletes' personalities, their history of stressors, their coping resources, and the extent to which they have had previous experience with learning psychological/stress management interventions.

Personality Personality is composed of the relatively stable characteristics and traits that people uniquely possess that influence behavior. Andersen and Williams [6] proposed that certain positive personality traits, such as hardiness (e.g., committing to tasks and having purpose in life, having a sense of control, and viewing stressful life events as challenges and opportunities) and "positive states of mind," can buffer the stress response process and help lower injury risk. Negative or disadvantageous traits, such as trait anxiety, can exacerbate injury risk. It should be noted, however, that an overall "injury-prone" personality type has not been found or documented [10].

Andersen and Williams [6] offered six different personality characteristics as potentially having an effect on the stress-injury relationship: (1) hardiness; (2) sense of coherence (a belief that the world is predictable and meaningful); (3) sensation seeking (desiring stimulation); (4) locus of control (one's perspective of whether one is generally in control of his/her own fate or not); (5) trait anxiety (the extent to which an individual is over-activated/worried on a general basis); and (6) achievement motivation (a drive to reach one's goals and experience the success of doing so). In 1998, Williams and Andersen [7] noted that items 1, 2, and 6 had not been studied and the others had mixed results regarding their relationships to injury. Eleven years later, however, Appaneal et al. [11] found in an analysis of over 45 studies from 1986 to 2009, on over 20 different aspects of personality, that 69% of studies showed a relationship between personality and injury. The most commonly studied personality variables were trait anxiety, locus of control, and mood.

Anxiety Anxiety is one of the most frequently studied personality traits in the antecedents of injury literature, and more specifically, competitive anxiety [3]. Competitive anxiety is defined as a tendency to perceive a competitive situation as threatening and respond with inappropriately heightened activation levels, fear, and/or tension [12]. Of all the personality variables, it has shown the most consistent association with sport injury [10]. Since the aforementioned definition of competitive anxiety looks very similar to what occurs in the stress response process, it would make sense that an athlete with competitive anxiety would have a more drastic stress response to competition than an athlete who is generally not anxious, and thus face a higher likelihood of injury during competition. Even further, athletes who not only have high anxiety, but also perceive that their anxiety is detrimental to performance, may be at highest risk for injury [7].

Locus of Control Locus of control is the perspective of who or what controls what happens to oneself. If gymnasts have an internal locus of control, they would generally feel like they mostly control the events and outcomes in their lives. If they have an external locus of control, this means they generally feel like something outside of their control such as luck, a higher power, or the universe makes things happen to them. Much less research has been conducted in this area than with anxiety, but according to two studies, athletes with a higher internal locus of control had a higher number of injuries than those with an external locus of control [3].

Mood Mood is the most common mental and/or emotional state to be examined in conjunction with sport injury. Athletes who report negative mood states or more total mood disturbance are more likely to become injured [3]. It is important to note the bi-directionality of the arrow between personality and history of stressors in the stress and injury model (added to the revised model in 1998) when examining mood. Negative mood may be associated with an increase in stressors and not necessarily something that is stable and dispositional within the athlete like trait/competitive anxiety and locus of control.

History of Stressors Of the three moderating variables found in the boxes above the stress-response in the stress and injury model, history of stressors continues to be the most heavily researched, with the Appaneal et al. [11] review indicating nearly 80 percent of studies supporting a relationship between amount and type of stressors and injury occurrence. In a small sample of artistic gymnasts, total stress, negative stress, and positive stress were all associated with injury occurrence [13]. Williams and Andersen [6, 7] categorized stressors into three groups: major life events, or life stress, daily hassles, and previous injury history.

Major Life Events Major life events are significant life and/or sport events that require a significant allocation of resources (e.g., emotion, energy, time, etc.). Such events include death of a loved one, moving/relocating to a new place, the breakup of a relationship, or a new coach. Passer and Seese [14] determined that differentiating between perceptions of life events as being positive or negative was important in influencing injury risk. For example, getting a new coach can be perceived as a positive or negative event. Each can increase allostatic load and injury susceptibility, but the life events that athletes perceive as negative make a greater impact on injury risk.

Daily Hassles While major life events may have a more drastic impact on injury susceptibility, daily hassles can also compound life events to increase injury risk. Daily hassles are defined by Williams and Andersen [7] as minor daily problems, irritations, and/or changes, such as car problems, late payments on bills, or struggling to learn a new skill at practice. It may be that major life events impact injury risk because of all the daily hassles that usually accompany them. From the previous example of a major life event, a new coach may institute a change of practice times, change an athlete's position in the lineup, or require additional training sessions compared to the previous coach. All of these things are changes that an athlete must spend additional energy on adapting to, hence, increasing daily hassles.

Previous Injury While less studied than major life events and daily hassles, an athlete's history of previous injury may impact the risk of injury. Brewer and Redmond [10] offered potential explanations for this as incompletely rehabilitating the previous injury, negative interpretations of current injury (e.g., "I must be weak if I keep getting injured"), and resulting negative mood from such interpretations (again highlighting the bi-directionality of the arrow between personality and history of stressors in the model) and/or distraction from sport relevant cues from worrying about re-injury.

Coping Resources and Psychological Interventions Coping resources include resources that athletes may possess to help them deal with stress, thus decreasing the impact of the stress response and risk of injury. Additionally, athletes who have low coping resources will, according to the model, have a much worse stress response and higher risk of injury. Examples of coping resources include self-care activities (e.g., getting an appropriate amount of sleep, eating a nutritious diet, staying hydrated), psychosocial resources (e.g., social support), possessing cognitive-behavioral coping skills (e.g., stress management skills, relaxation skills), and ability to modify intrapersonal communication (e.g., changing one's self-talk, reframing thoughts, cognitive restructuring). In the stress and injury model, behavioral coping skills are in the *Psychological Interventions* box, below the *Stress Response* box. The model postulates that athletes who possess such skills will be better able to manage stress, since they have had training in doing so, and will be less likely to get injured. Perna et al. [15] affirmed this when they found that athletes exposed to a short psychological intervention-based stress management program had a significant reduction in the number of injury and illness days compared with a control group. Kolt et al. [1] saw similar (but nonsignificant) trends in their study of gymnasts undergoing a stress management program. These particular psychological interventions will be discussed in depth in Sect. 5.5.

Social support, or having relationships with others who are caring both in and out of the sport environment, has been the most researched aspect of coping resources in the stress-injury relationship. The stress and injury model proposes that social support both buffers the effect of stressful life events and also directly lessens an athlete's stress response [10]. Williams and Andersen [7] summarized that high social support seems to buffer the effects of stressful life events, thereby reducing injury, while low social support makes the harmful effects of life stress worse, thus increasing injury vulnerability significantly. Sports medicine professionals are in a position to provide several sources of social support to athletes, as will be discussed in Sect. 5.5.

Overall, if sports medicine professionals are able to identify athletes who are at high risk for injury and connect them with the appropriate resources, then they can optimize the chances of injury prevention. The stress and injury model provides a useful guide for such prevention. Gymnasts who have maladaptive personality traits, such as high trait anxiety and negative mood, significant life stress, and low coping resources are most likely to become injured.

5.2.2 Sociocultural Antecedents of Injury

The culture of sport may itself contribute to injury. Hughes and Coakley [16] identified the "sport ethic" which describes the culture of competitive sport as one that encourages athletes to take undue physical risks in pursuit of performance, making personal sacrifices for "The Game," striving for distinction among other athletes, playing through pain, and not accepting any limits.

This sport ethic is ever present in the socialization of young athletes into their sport. A young gymnast may learn that to be accepted by her team and her coach that she must not cry when injured, she must view pain as just part of gymnastics, and that she is expected to practice when hurt. These attitudes are also reflected in the types of slogans we see plastered in locker rooms and on team gear like "no pain, no gain," "pain is temporary, pride is forever," and "whatever it takes." Whereas outside of the sport culture a person would not, for example, walk on a sprained ankle, the culture of sport may encourage an athlete to do just the opposite of that – tape it up and get to practice. Altogether, these cultural forces increase an athlete's risk of injury.

Coaches may inadvertently (or purposely) foster this culture of risk-taking by ignoring or making fun of gymnasts who report an injury, who take time off to recover from an injury, and/or by giving accolades to gymnasts who compete when hurt. Media and fans similarly contribute by glorifying gymnasts who perform while injured. One prominent example is when gymnast Kerri Strug vaulted with an injured ankle in the 1996 Olympics to help Team USA win the gold medal. While this event is considered one of the most iconic sports moments in history [17], it can set an example for other athletes that it is acceptable to compete while injured to win at any cost. It is important for sports medicine professionals to be aware of the impact that the sport ethic culture may have on gymnasts and not be a contributor to the sociocultural antecedents of sport injury.

5.3 Psychological Response to Sport Injury

After an injury occurs, an athlete may experience a wide range of emotional and behavioral responses. For instance, athletes may experience frustration, anger, negative mood, anxiety, confusion, helplessness, loss of athletic identity, and feelings of isolation from their team [10, 18, 19]. An athlete could also feel a sense of relief to get some time off of practice if she or he feels burned out. Some athletes may be very motivated for physical therapy and demonstrate high compliance and adherence to the rehabilitation protocol, while others may not feel motivated to put a large amount of effort into rehabilitation. The general trend in the literature is that injured athletes experience negative emotions following injury that decrease over time, while adaptive or positive emotions tend to increase as time progresses; however, spikes in negative emotions can occur throughout the rehabilitation process [10, 20, 21]. The trajectory following injury can be full of ups and downs, and this should be normalized by medical providers. However, researchers have found that a minority of athletes (5–27%) experience clinical levels of psychological distress following injury [18, 20], and these athletes should be referred to a mental health professional (see Sect. 5.4 for information about the referral process). On the other hand, many athletes can be quite resilient after injury [21], and some researchers have found that athletes may experience positive or adaptive emotions and outcomes following injury [10, 22]. For example, after injury, some athletes have reported personal growth, gaining a new perspective on sport and life, learning new psychological skills, feeling more mentally tough, learning more about the technical aspects of the sport, gaining physical strength from physical therapy, developing interests outside of sport, expanding their social network, and developing empathy for others [22, 23]. Such responses may be considered *stress-related growth*, which is defined as positive changes in individuals following a stressful event (such as injury) that result in a higher level of functioning than prior to the event [24]. Clearly, the manner in which an athlete responds to an injury is very individualized and depends on numerous factors, which have been conceptualized using several models. It is important for sports medicine professionals caring for gymnasts to be familiar with these models to aid in the holistic recovery of the injured athlete.

5.3.1 Models of Psychological Response to Injury

Since injury could be considered as a loss of an aspect of the self, *grief-response models*, or *stage models*, have been applied to sport injury [18, 19]. One of the most popular grief-response models is the Kubler-Ross [25] model, which proposed that in response to a loss, one would sequentially progress through the stages of denial, anger, bargaining, depression, and acceptance. For a gymnast who experienced a severe knee injury, she might minimize the severity of the injury and believe she will be back in a few weeks (denial), then feel upset and frustrated when she learns that the rehabilitation will take 6 months (anger). Next, she might plea with a higher power to speed up her recovery if she goes to physical therapy every day (bargaining), then she could experience sadness and negative mood when she sees her teammates compete without her (depression), and finally she might realize that she will be back on the team next season and will make the most of her time on the sidelines by conditioning, learning what the judges are looking for, and supporting her teammates (acceptance). Although this model could be useful for sports medicine professionals to normalize the progression of emotional responses with their athletes, support for this model has not been strong in the sport injury literature [10, 26], especially because it does not take into account individual variability in response to an injury or personal or situational variables that are specific to an individual.

A model that does take into account individual variability and numerous personal and situational variables is the *integrated model of psychological response to the sport injury and rehabilitation process* (Fig. 5.2) [27]. Pre-injury variables from the stress and injury model (discussed in Sect. 5.2.1.1) [6] such as stress, personality, coping skills, and interventions interact with post-injury variables (personal and situational factors) to determine athletes' cognitive, emotional, and behavioral responses to injury. According to this model, following injury, an athlete appraises the injury (cognitive appraisal) in terms of what the injury means to him or her (primary appraisal) and if she or he believes that she or he has the resources to cope with the injury (secondary appraisal). The cognitive appraisal is influenced by personal factors (e.g., demographics, injury severity, personality, athletic identity, and coping skills) and situational factors (e.g., level of sport, time of the season, social support, and rehabilitation facilities). Cognitive appraisal of the injury then affects emotional (e.g., fear, tension, anger, depression, frustration, attitude) and behavioral (e.g., adherence, effort in rehabilitation, use of mental skills, use of social support) responses to injury. According to this model, cognitive appraisals, emotional responses, and behavioral responses reciprocally influence each other, and these responses influence physical and psychological recovery outcomes. Researchers have not found support for the model as a whole, but have supported elements of the model [19]. Practically speaking, this model would help explain why one gymnast who has an athletic trainer avail-

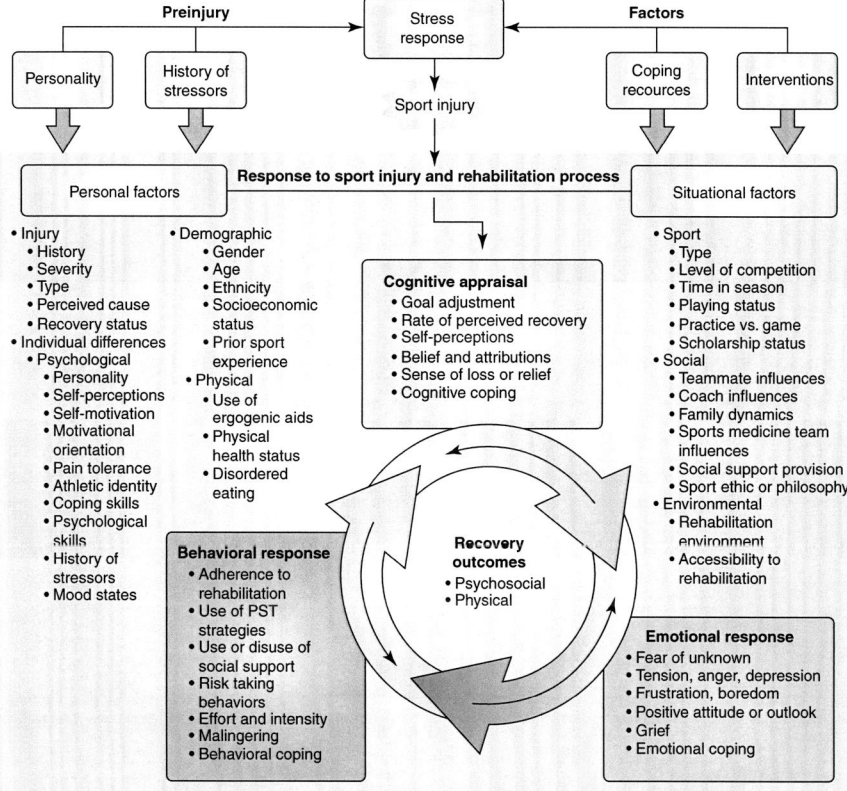

Fig. 5.2 Integrated model of psychological response to the sport injury and rehabilitation process. (Wiese-Bjornstal et al. [27]. Reprinted with permission of the publisher [Taylor & Francis Ltd., http://www.tandfonline.com]. Specific design republished with permission of the publisher [Human Kinetics, Inc.], from Brewer and Redmond [10]. Permission conveyed through Copyright Clearance Center, Inc.)

able at practice, has great relationships with her coach and teammates, is attending physical therapy multiple times per week, and is confident that she will return this competitive season has more positive rehabilitation outcomes than a gymnast who lacks financial resources for physical therapy, does not get along with her coach, is in the last year of her sport, and is experiencing depression about the injury. In order to maximize rehabilitation effectiveness, sports medicine professionals should pay attention to various personal and situational factors that influence how gymnasts appraise their injury, how that appraisal impacts emotional and behavioral responses, and then intervene when appropriate (e.g., helping the gymnast implement mental skills and creating a positive motivational climate in the rehabilitation setting).

Another model of psychological response to sport injury is the *biopsychosocial approach to sport injury rehabilitation* [28]. The model has seven interacting components (Fig. 5.3): injury characteristics, sociodemographic factors, biological factors

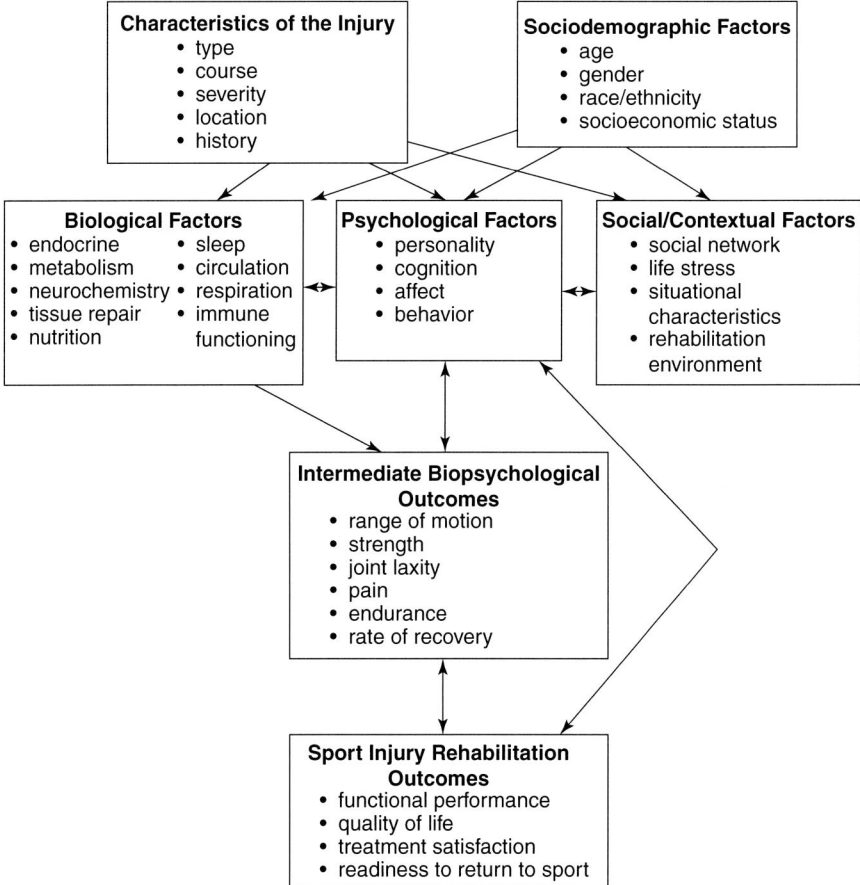

Fig. 5.3 A biopsychosocial approach to sport injury rehabilitation. (Republished with permission of the publisher [Fitness Information Technology Inc.], from Brewer et al. [28]. Permission conveyed through Copyright Clearance Center, Inc.)

(e.g., nutrition, sleep, immune function), psychological factors (e.g., personality, affect, cognition), social/contextual factors (e.g., social network, life stress, rehabilitation environment), intermediate biopsychological outcomes (e.g., range of motion, strength, pain, recovery rate), and sport injury rehabilitation outcomes (e.g., treatment satisfaction, readiness to return to sport, functional performance). Similar to the integrated model, the model is quite complex and has not been tested as a whole, but there is support for various elements of the model [19]. Sports medicine professionals can apply this model with gymnasts by realizing that physical markers of the rehabilitation process are affected by a host of personal, situational, biological, and psychological factors, and they could assess how these factors are impacting rehabilitation outcomes. For example, if a gymnast's strength and range of motion are not improving, the sports medicine professional can ask about her sleep, nutrition, stress level, and social support and make recommendations about those areas if appropriate or connect her to relevant resources, such as a mental health professional.

5.4 Multidisciplinary Team in Treatment and the Referral Process

The ideal treatment of injured athletes would include a multidisciplinary team available to athletes during injury recovery and rehabilitation. The primary rehabilitation team would include sports medicine professionals who work most closely with the injured athlete (e.g., sports medicine physicians, surgeons, athletic trainers, physical therapists), while a secondary rehabilitation team might include sports nutritionists, strength and conditioning coaches, athletic coaches, teammates, family/friends, sport psychologists, psychiatrists, clinical/counseling psychologists, chiropractors, massage therapists, biomechanists, and exercise physiologists [29]. Depending on the gymnast's injury and rehabilitation process, different members of the rehabilitation teams may or may not interact or collaborate, but it is important that sports medicine professionals build networks of other medical and allied health professionals to address both the physical and psychological aspects of injury recovery. Also, various settings and levels of gymnasts may have differing amounts of access to such rehabilitation teams. For instance, collegiate or elite gymnasts may have more resources than club gymnasts. Regardless of the resources, sports medicine professionals are in a prime position to assist injured gymnasts with the psychological aspects of recovery, either directly by incorporating mental skills into rehabilitation, or indirectly by providing referrals to mental health or sport psychology professionals.

Since the late 1980s, researchers have been suggesting that sports medicine professionals who have regular contact with athletes are optimally positioned to inform, educate, and attend to injured athletes' psychological needs as well as physical needs [30]. In order to effectively account for psychological factors in the prevention and treatment of sport injuries, it is vital that all members of the sports medicine team are knowledgeable in both the identification of and treatment of nonclinical psychological issues. While there is nothing inherently unethical about any member of the sports medicine team administering basic psychological interventions (e.g., goal-setting, imagery, relaxation training, etc.), more clinically based psychological issues, such as eating disorders, clinical depression/anxiety, sexual assault, and drug abuse, require treatment by a qualified mental health professional. As a sports medicine professional, it is important to have the skills to identify such issues in a timely manner and refer appropriately.

Sports medicine professionals might provide a referral to a sport psychologist or certified mental performance consultant (CMPC) [31] to provide mental training for enhancing the mental aspects of rehabilitation and return to sport, but it is essential to refer an athlete with clinical levels of psychological distress to a mental health professional (e.g., clinical [sport] psychologist, psychiatrist, counselor/therapist). The referral process to a mental health professional consists of the following steps [10, 32]: (1) *Assessment* of the gymnast's psychological response to injury by listening and observing the gymnast; (2) *Consultation* with a mental health professional to confidentially discuss the gymnast's psychological symptoms. The mental health professional might recommend immediate referral, additional assessment, or a trial intervention; (3) *Trial intervention* includes basic mental skills interventions to help the athlete with coping skills. If the intervention works, no further action is necessary, but if it does not, additional consultation or the referral would occur next; (4) *Referral* to a mental health professional can be done by expressing concern to the gymnast in a caring manner, explaining the rationale for the referral, allowing the gymnast and/or her parents (if a minor) to ask questions, and connecting the gymnast with the mental health professional. If possible, the sports medicine professional can help schedule the appointment or introduce the gymnast to the mental health professional; (5) *Follow-up* should take place with the mental health professional (while respecting the gymnast's confidentiality if she did not sign a release of information) and with the gymnast. The sports medicine professional should continue to monitor psychological symptoms.

Particular emphasis regarding the need to be knowledgeable and comfortable in the referral process coincides with the unfortunate presence of sexual abuse in sports, particularly in gymnastics. Many documented cases exist in which prominent coaches and/or athletic staff were sexually abusing the athletes under their authority (e.g., Dr. Larry Nassar who was a medical provider for USA Gymnastics and the Michigan State University Athletic Department) [33]. Sadly, numerous sports medicine professionals neglected to refer these athletes who were sometimes clearly (or subtly) suffering from emotional trauma as a result of the abuse. Interestingly, while teachers and health professionals, such as the sports medicine professional, are mandated reporters for child abuse, coaches presently do not have this requirement in all states. There is also not a standard education that coaches receive about identification of abuse and protocol on how to assist athletes. Therefore, the sports medicine professional may be the only person that the gymnasts interact with that would have such trauma identification skills and referral knowledge that could intervene and help them.

Trauma is defined as an event that confronts individuals with an acute or overwhelming threat [34] that exceeds their ability to cope [35]. An athlete experiencing sexual abuse or assault could certainly fit this definition. It is important to note that it is not typical of sports medicine professional training and education to be trained on the identification of trauma and certainly not in the treatment of trauma. In fact, even for a licensed mental health professional, expertise in treating trauma is usually an advanced specialization requiring additional training. This illustrates the importance of not only being able to make a referral, but also making sure the athlete is referred to an appropriately qualified professional.

Because of a sport culture that encourages conformity and the withholding of emotions, it is important to be mindful that athletes, especially gymnasts, may also struggle in ways that do not mimic traditional clinical features. While not meant to be comprehensive, below are signs that may indicate that an athlete is experiencing trauma [36]:

- Negative affect (emotional state)
- Decreased interest in activities
- Feeling isolated
- Difficulty experiencing positive affect (emotional state)
- Irritability or aggression
- Risky or destructive behavior
- Hypervigilance
- Heightened startle reaction
- Difficulty concentrating
- Difficulty sleeping

For trauma over a long duration, athletes may also experience the following changes to various aspects of their lives (originally described by Herman in 1992) [37, p. 109]:

- Emotional Regulation. May include persistent sadness, suicidal thoughts, and explosive or inhibited anger.
- Consciousness. Includes forgetting or reliving traumatic events, or having episodes in which one feels detached from one's mental processes or body (dissociation).
- Self-Perception. May include helplessness, shame, guilt, stigma, and a sense of being completely different from other human beings.
- Distorted Perceptions of the Perpetrator. Examples include attributing total power to the perpetrator, becoming preoccupied with the relationship to the perpetrator, or having thoughts of revenge.
- Relations with Others. Examples include isolation, distrust, or a repeated search for a rescuer.
- One's System of Meanings. May include a loss of sustaining faith or a sense of hopelessness and despair.

Again, it is critical that sports medicine professionals and all athletic staff can identify athletes who need a referral and take the recommended steps presented here to put the athlete in contact with the appropriate professional to whom the referral should be made. It is also essential that if child abuse or neglect of any kind (physical, sexual, verbal, emotional) is suspected, that the appropriate authorities are contacted and a full report is made with child protective services. Sports medicine professionals must become familiar with state laws regarding the mandatory reporting of the abuse of a minor, which can be found at this link: https://www.childwelfare.gov/topics/systemwide/laws-policies/state/ [38].

Since the majority of athletes recovering from an injury do not report clinical levels of psychological distress [20], and a sports medicine professional would likely interface with athletes more frequently than a sport psychology professional, therein lies a need for the preparation of sports medicine professionals to address a basic nonclinical counseling component in sports medicine in order to enhance athletes' psychological recovery of injury. Sports medicine professionals report that despite an interest in gaining the knowledge necessary to incorporate psychological skills in rehabilitation, there are few opportunities and trainings accessible to develop that knowledge [39–41]. Sports medicine professionals are already required to "wear many hats," fulfilling roles that may not necessarily be neatly within their job description. As suggested by Bartlett [42], integrating sport psychology professionals into the sport injury treatment team would be an optimal option to bridge this gap between need and resource. While athletes may primarily see the role of the sports medicine professional as attending to the physical aspect of the injury, there is also a need for them to implement subtle psychosocial interventions to optimally facilitate injured athlete recovery and a smooth return to sport [30], especially when a sport psychologist is not a member of the sports medicine team or available as a referral source. The subsequent section of this text provides an overview of nonclinical sport psychology interventions (i.e., mental skills interventions) that members of the sports medicine team can apply with their athletes.

5.5 Psychological Interventions During Rehabilitation

As mentioned earlier, a CMPC is trained to teach mental skills to athletes, including injured athletes. However, it is important for sports medicine professionals to consider how they might integrate some psychological interventions into appointments with patients and rehabilitation sessions.

5.5.1 Social Support

Social support provides athletes with a sense of being cared for, belonging to a network, and having access to resources in times of need, such as during an injury [43, 44]. Types of social support include [43–45] (1) *emotional support*, which can consist of (a) esteem support (enhancing athletes' self-confidence or self-esteem through delivering positive feedback), (b) listening support (actively listening nonjudgmentally), (c) emotional support (showing care, empathy, and encouragement), (d) emotional challenge support (challenging individuals' attitudes toward rehabilitation and obstacles), and (e) shared social reality (validating athletes' perspectives); (2) *technical support*, including technical appreciation (reinforcing effort, intensity, and achievements in rehabilitation) and technical challenge (encouraging athletes to challenge themselves and do more in rehabilitation); (3) *informational support*, which includes providing information, advice, and guidance about the injury and rehabilitation; and (4) *tangible support*, which is providing concrete assistance, such as transportation or help with daily living tasks.

Sports medicine professionals should assess the types of support that gymnasts are receiving from coaches, teammates, family, and friends to make sure they are getting the support and assistance they need. They can also provide support themselves. For example, a sports medicine doctor may provide informational support by informing the gymnast about each step of surgery and the recovery process. An athletic trainer could provide technical challenge support by creating a contest for a gymnast to safely add more weight to the leg press exercise each week. A physical therapist could provide emotional support by listening attentively to the gymnast's struggles with rehabilitation and normalizing feelings of frustration, yet encouraging her that despite obstacles, progress is being made overall. Sports medicine professionals might also organize injury support groups or performance enhancement groups for injured athletes to enhance various types of social support among injured athletes, including shared social reality [46, 47]. Providing social support to injured athletes will help build trust and rapport with them, and the athletes will likely be more receptive to rehabilitation protocols and utilizing other mental skills in rehabilitation that are recommended below. In addition, as mentioned in Sect. 5.2.1.2, having social support can lower the athlete's risk of re-injury during rehabilitation or future injury once returned to sport.

5.5.2   Goal Setting

Athletes are likely to be familiar with goal setting in their sport, so it would be a natural transfer to include goal setting during injury recovery. Goals are aims or objectives of an action [48]. Researchers have found that goal setting improves injury outcomes, such as performance on rehabilitation tasks [49], self-efficacy (confidence) for rehabilitation [50], and adherence to rehabilitation [50].

There are different content domains that goals could be set for during injury recovery, including physical rehabilitation goals (e.g., range of motion, strength), psychological goals (e.g., confidence, motivation, focus), sport performance goals (e.g., sport-specific technique and skills), and lifestyle goals (e.g., nutrition, sleep, relationships) [44, 51]. Types of goals include outcome, performance, or process goals [52]. Outcome goals focus on the end result, such as a gymnast wanting to fully return to gymnastics 8 months post-ACL surgery. Performance goals focus on measurable standards compared to one's own performance, such as a gymnast who wants to increase weight and repetitions on squats. Process goals refer to the specific action steps one must take to perform (i.e., HOW they can accomplish performance and outcome goals), such as the gymnast having proper form on her squat.

Sports medicine professionals can easily incorporate goal setting into the rehabilitation process by collaboratively setting various types of goals with the gymnast. Getting the gymnast's input is important for fostering commitment [51]. To set effective goals for recovery, gymnasts should set SMARTER goals [44, 51, 52]:

- *S*pecific – precise aim to be achieved (versus general, vague goals)
- *M*easurable – quantifiable
- *A*djustable – flexible, especially since injury recovery can have peaks, valleys, and plateaus
- *R*ealistic – not too easy, but not too difficult
- *T*ime-based – include target dates or date ranges
- *E*valuated – periodically reviewed and adjusted as needed
- *R*ecorded – written down

Gymnasts should also set long-term, short-term, and daily goals for rehabilitation that should link together as a "goal ladder" – daily goals should help accomplish short-term goals, which help accomplish long-term goals. The daily goals are especially important for lengthy rehabilitation to help the gymnast stay motivated and focused during rehabilitation.

5.5.3 Relaxation

Relaxation training is an important tool for injury rehabilitation because it can help alleviate stress, anxiety, muscle tension, and pain, which are both physiological and psychological responses [10, 53]. Cupal and Brewer [54] found that a relaxation and imagery intervention produced greater muscle strength and lower levels of re-injury anxiety and pain compared to placebo and control groups following knee surgery. Relaxation techniques that may be useful for injured athletes include diaphragmatic breathing, progressive muscle relaxation, and passive relaxation [44, 55].

For *diaphragmatic breathing*, an athlete would begin the inhalation of a deep breath by pushing out the abdomen (diaphragm), then filling the rib cage, and then filling the upper part of the lungs by raising the chest and shoulders [52]. The exhalation would proceed in the opposite order and would be longer than the inhale (for instance, count for four on the inhale and six on the exhale, also known as ratio breathing). Gymnasts could practice diaphragmatic breathing during a painful procedure during injury rehabilitation such as scar tissue mobilization. *Progressive muscle relaxation* (PMR) [56] consists of tension and relaxation cycles throughout the body. For instance, a gymnast would tense her right hand for about 5 seconds, and release the tension (relax) for about 20 seconds and repeat this for every muscle group. Injured athletes may need to avoid tensing the injured part of their body. Gymnasts might practice PMR during a stimulation treatment in rehabilitation or after a rehabilitation session at home. *Passive relaxation* is when athletes would do a body scan and release tension throughout every muscle in their body, for instance, they could imagine the tension draining out of the bottom of their feet [44]. Gymnasts could do this while they are icing or heating parts of their body or before they go to sleep. Many relaxation scripts and audio recordings can be found online and even in smartphone applications, such as "Calm" and "Headspace."

5.5.4 Self-Talk

Self-talk is an individual's thought(s) that she or he says aloud or internally and privately [57]. Types of self-talk include positive or motivational self-talk, negative or critical self-talk, and instructional self-talk [52]. During injury recovery, helping athletes have a productive (positive or neutral) mindset is important considering the negative psychological responses that athletes could experience. Researchers have found that for injured athletes, self-talk interventions improved strength [58] and balance [59] and, along with relaxation, contributed to reductions in re-injury anxiety [60] and negative mood [61].

Sports medicine professionals can assess and monitor gymnasts' self-talk by asking what they are thinking during rehabilitation. If self-talk is unproductive for the gymnast, the cognitive restructuring (reframing) or thought stopping technique can be implemented [45, 52]. The thought-stopping technique consists of (1) helping the athlete recognize her unproductive self-talk, (2) insert a thought-stopping cue (e.g., saying "STOP" to herself), and (3) reframing the unproductive self-talk to productive self-talk. For example, a gymnast who says, "I can't imagine ever doing a back handspring on beam after my shoulder injury" can reframe her self-talk to, "I know it's a few months off, but if I do my physical therapy exercises each day and do my progressions on beam, I know that I can get my back handspring on beam back eventually." Self-talk, specifically instructional self-talk or cue words, can also be used to help injured athletes focus and concentrate during rehabilitation and return to sport [44]. For example, a gymnast could say, "push off your feet," as she does a squat jump exercise during rehabilitation.

5.5.5 Imagery

Imagery is the creation or re-creation of an experience in the mind, also known as mental practice. For injured athletes, imagery can be beneficial for maintaining (or possibly improving) athletic performance while the athlete cannot physically practice due to injury [10, 62]. As mentioned in the relaxation section, a study incorporating relaxation and imagery resulted in lower pain and re-injury anxiety and greater knee strength after ACL surgery [54]. Numerous other benefits of imagery for injured athletes have been reported in the literature, including quicker recovery time [63], better ability to cope with injury [64], increased motivation and adherence to rehabilitation [65], emotion management associated with injury and rehabilitation [65], and increasing confidence for return to sport following injury [62].

There are four types of imagery that have been described in relation to injury recovery [42, 62, 66]: (1) *healing imagery*, in which athletes imagine the body mending the injured area; (2) *pain management imagery*, which might include (a) soothing imagery, in which athletes picture themselves in a pleasant setting or (b) pain acknowledgment imagery, where athletes assign physical properties such as color, shape, size, or sounds to their injury pain; (3) *rehabilitation imagery*, during which athletes imagine themselves performing rehabilitation exercises; and (4) *performance imagery*, in which athletes picture themselves practicing or competing in sport. For example, during a physical therapy session, a gymnast could practice healing imagery while receiving a stimulation treatment, rehabilitation imagery right before she's about to do a lunge, soothing imagery while she's in the ice bath, and sport-specific imagery at home before she goes to bed. A key to effective imagery is to use all the senses (sight, sound, smell, taste, touch, and the kinesthetic sense [sensation of body position and movement]). Starting an imagery session with relaxation is helpful as well [44, 52, 62].

5.5.6 Mindfulness

An ancient Buddhist practice, mindfulness can be defined as "paying attention in a particular way: on purpose, in the present moment, and nonjudgmentally" [67, p. 4]. Mindfulness meditation can be practiced in a number of forms and settings, including sitting, lying down, walking, and while eating. While the type of meditation can change, the intention is always the same: the generation of awareness and acceptance of all present-moment thoughts, emotions, and bodily sensations without the infusion of interpretation, meaning, or judgment [67]. Mindfulness practice influences sport-specific coping through attentional control and emotion regulation [68–70].

The attentional control component of mindfulness practice enhances gymnasts' awareness of where their attention is wandering from moment-to-moment and influences pain tolerance. Awareness of attention allows for control of attention. Gymnasts learn to recognize when their attention has wandered to performance inhibiting thoughts, emotions, and sensations and to nonjudgmentally bring their attention back to goal-directed behaviors, including rehabilitation techniques, physical conditioning exercises, and fueling their bodies with proper nutrition [68]. Attentional control also influences pain tolerance. A study of injured athletes suggested that Mindfulness Based Stress Reduction (MBSR), a group program consisting of eight weekly classes incorporating guided mindfulness meditation, informational presentations, discussions, and homework assignments, increased pain tolerance [70]. Cultivating a present-moment focus increases one's ability to notice each experience as it arises and to let it pass by without clutching onto it [71]. Injured athletes learn how to acknowledge the pain when it comes, but also how to let it go, decreasing their attention and sensitivity to the pain [70].

The emotion regulation component of mindfulness practice emphasizes the acceptance of all experiences, both the good and bad, without passing judgment. *Reperceiving* is a term coined by Shapiro and colleagues [71] that characterizes a shift in perspective, allowing individuals to view moment-to-moment experiences as objective information, rather than emotionally charged descriptors. This process of reperceiving influences the pain catastrophizing process. The gymnasts no longer view the pain as a threat they are unable to cope with, but simply as information regarding the intensity of the injury and phase of rehabilitation [72].

Heightened attentional control and emotion regulation also interrupt the rumination process, bringing the repetitive cycle of negative thoughts surrounding the injury to a halt [69]. Diminished rumination frees up attentional capacity that the gymnasts can direct toward productive, goal-oriented thoughts and behaviors, as they are no longer using up their mental energy on negativity [69]. Mohammed and colleagues [70] also found that mindfulness practice improves the psychological well-being of injured athletes, as they recorded a decrease in depression, anxiety, fatigue, and confusion after the athletes engaged in MBSR.

Because most gymnasts do not have much free time in their schedules between school and practice, implementing a daily mindfulness exercise into their rehabilitation program can be an effective way to expose athletes to the benefits of mindfulness without adding an extra responsibility to their already hectic schedules. Having the injured athletes begin and end each rehabilitation session with a brief mindful breathing exercise or body scan can help the athletes get in touch with the present moment and reap the physical, psychological, and emotional benefits of a mindful rehabilitation session. Mindfulness audio recordings can also be found online and in smartphone applications listed above in the relaxation section.

5.6 Psychological Aspects of Returning to Gymnastics Following Injury

Once injury rehabilitation has been successfully completed, it is time for the gymnasts to return to training and competition. This return to gymnastics can be an emotionally tumultuous time for the athletes, as the excitement of being cleared to train is often accompanied by the fear of returning to many unknown factors. Because of the complexities involved in the return to sport phase of rehabilitation, physical readiness and psychological readiness to return to gymnastics do not always coincide [73].

Many of the psychological challenges that athletes encounter upon their return to sport are related to their perceptions of three basic psychological needs – *competence, autonomy,* and *relatedness* [74]. *Competence* refers to the need for athletes to believe they are capable of succeeding in a particular task; competency concerns related to injury primarily consist of fear of re-injury and uncertainty regarding their ability to perform at pre-injury levels [74]. For example, a gymnast who suffered an

Achilles tendon tear on a double backflip on the floor exercise may be hesitant to tumble on the floor or punch the vault springboard upon her return for fear of re-tearing her Achilles tendon. A gymnast who underwent surgery to repair a torn labrum in her shoulder may worry that she will not regain all of her release moves on the uneven bars.

The fear of re-injury can manifest in many forms, including heavy taping of the injured body part, being hesitant and withholding effort, particularly in injury-provoking situations, and even avoiding the return to sport altogether [74]. A gymnast who broke her ankle on a beam flight series may consistently tape her ankle long after it has healed, while a gymnast who tore her ACL on a front twisting double full on floor may avoid training that skill again.

The uncertainty surrounding returning to pre-injury performance standards largely stems from the extended absence from training, loss of strength and physical conditioning, and subsequent difficulty regaining skills and routines [75]. These concerns include the fear of not meeting others' expectations; letting down teammates, coaches, and family; performing poorly; and failing to meet personal goals and expectations. These concerns are largely expressed through frustration and lack of confidence [74]. A gymnast who consistently falls during balance beam routines her first season back after ankle surgery may become frustrated and lose confidence in her ability to perform her beam routine successfully, resulting in more falls and even more frustration. After 3 years away from the competition arena due to multiple ACL reconstruction surgeries, a gymnast may fear falling on her uneven bars routine and letting down her teammates and coaches, who have spent time and energy guiding her through her recoveries.

The psychological need of *autonomy* refers to the need for athletes to have agency or control over their choices and actions; a common concern related to autonomy after injury includes returning to the sport before one is physically or psychologically prepared to do so. The premature return is often due to external pressures from coaches, the "sport ethic" discussed in Sect. 5.2.2, and the athletes' athletic identity [74]. These external pressures can have detrimental consequences to the health and well-being of the athletes, including increased anxiety and tension, decreased motivation, guarding of the injured body part, and inappropriate focus on the injured body part rather than on performance-relevant cues, all of which contribute to an increased risk of another injury occurring [74]. Feeling pressured to compete by her coaches, a gymnast still crippled with fear of re-injuring her newly healed hand may ignore her beam flight series cues, resulting in her missing her feet on the landing and re-injuring her hand. A gymnast who believes her identity to be rooted in gymnastics may begin tumbling before she has finished her knee rehabilitation, increasing her chance of re-injury.

Finally, the psychological need of *relatedness* recognizes the athlete's need to feel a sense of belonging and connectedness to others; during injury, a potential relatedness concern would be if the athlete perceived alienation or isolation from teammates or coaches throughout the injury rehabilitation process [74]. Because they are not training or competing, the communication and interaction between the injured gymnasts and their coaches decreases dramatically and can result in a perceived lack of attention. This sense of isolation is exacerbated when the team travels out of town for competitions and leaves the injured gymnasts at home. The perceived lack of social support from their teammates and coaches can leave injured athletes feeling like they have no one to help them navigate the physical, psychological, and emotional challenges of returning to sport [74]. As an example, a gymnast recovering from a concussion who felt invisible to her coach throughout her rehabilitation may not feel comfortable asking for a spot on her uneven bar release move, increasing her fear of the skill.

These competency, autonomy, and relatedness concerns act as psychological barriers to athletes' successful return to sport. It is important that psychological rehabilitation is emphasized along with the physical rehabilitation. A study of athletes across sports, including soccer, rugby, gymnastics, and martial arts, defined *psychological readiness* as confidence in returning to sport, having realistic expectations of one's performance capabilities, and the motivation to regain previous performance standards [76]. Many of the same psychological interventions utilized during the rehabilitation process can also facilitate the athletes' return to sport; imagery, goal setting, and social support are important strategies in easing athletes' fears and enhancing their confidence when returning to training and competition [74, 76].

Through imagery training, injured athletes can prepare for their return to the gym by creating a vivid mental picture of their skills and routines, the gym or arena they will be training and competing in, and the emotions that are present at the time of the performance [30]. Performance imagery provides the opportunity for gymnasts to mentally rehearse the visual, kinesthetic, and other relevant sensory experiences of specific skills and routines, helping gymnasts to practice their skills and routines when not physically able to practice, reduce the fear of re-injury, and enhance perceptions of confidence and competence regarding their ability to return to gymnastics [66, 74].

Achieving return-to-sport goals further enhances athletes' perceptions of autonomy and competence. Setting and achieving process, performance, and outcome goals allows the gymnasts to feel in control of their performance, signals that they are "strong and fit," and increases their motivation to adhere to their continued rehabilitation and reintroduction to training and competition [75, p. 470, 76].

Social support is one of the most important contributors to athletes' return to sport. Informational support provided by medical professionals provides athletes the information they need to trust in their rehabilitation and newly healed body part, while the emotional support gymnasts receive through reassurance, positive feedback, encouragement, and praise from coaches and teammates communicates to the gymnasts that those around them believe in their ability to make a full recovery and perform well once they return to sport [74–76].

While there are many challenges that accompany the return to sport following an injury, there is also a degree of anticipation and excitement. Even amidst the fear, athletes return to sport because it offers the opportunity to achieve personal goals, maintain their fitness, preserve their athletic identity, pursue lifelong friendships with their teammates and coaches, and ultimately for the passion and love they feel for the sport [77]. Walking back into the gym after suffering an injury is fear-provoking, as there are many unknowns. By incorporating a holistic recovery approach that emphasizes the gymnasts' physical, psychological, and emotional health throughout the rehabilitation and return to sport processes, the athletes are equipped to effectively manage their uncertainty and fear, freeing them to experience the joy of gymnastics.

5.7 Conclusion

While the physical aspects of sport injury have been the primary focus of medical professionals, there is a growing need to expand professionals' understanding of the sport injury rehabilitation and recovery process to include the psychological and sociocultural influences. Present throughout the entirety of the injury process, psychological factors contribute to both an athlete's risk of injury and to the effectiveness of the rehabilitation process [7]. Key psychological and sociocultural antecedents of injury include personality, history of stressors, coping resources, psychological interventions, and the "sport ethic," which glorifies playing through pain and making sacrifices for "The Game" [7, 16]. After an injury has been sustained, it is common for athletes to experience a rollercoaster of emotions, including frustration, anxiety, confusion, isolation from teammates, loss of athletic identity, relief, fear of re-injury, and uncertainty regarding their ability to perform at pre-injury levels [10, 18, 19, 74]. Psychological interventions implemented during the rehabilitation and return to sport processes can help athletes manage the psychological and emotional distress that accompanies injury, and include social support, goal setting, relaxation, self-talk, imagery, and mindfulness. Due to the complexity of sport injuries, athletes' physical readiness to return to gymnastics does not always coincide with their psychological readiness to return to training and competition. Having a multidisciplinary treatment team comprised of medical professionals, psychologists, nutritionists, strength and conditioning coaches, and athletic coaches available to injured athletes can enhance the experience of both physical and psychological rehabilitation and recovery [29]. A holistic approach to injury rehabilitation and recovery that takes into account the physical, psychological, emotional, and sociocultural components of injury ensures that all facets of the injury are treated, contributing to a greater likelihood of successful reentry into gymnastics.

References

1. Kolt GS, Hume PA, Smith P, Williams MM. Effects of a stress-management program on injury and stress of competitive gymnasts. Percept Motor Skills. 2004;99(1):195–207.
2. Ray R, Wiese-Bjornstal DM. Counseling in sports medicine. Champaign: Human Kinetics; 1999.
3. Appaneal RN, Habif S. Psychological antecedents to sport injury. In: Arvinen-Barrow M, Walker N, editors. The psychology of sport injury and rehabilitation. New York: Routledge; 2013. p. 6–22.

4. Fulton J, Wright K, Klley M, Zebrosky B, Zanis M, Dryol C, Butler R. Injury risk is altered by previous injury: a systematic review of the literature and presentation of causative neuromuscular factors. Int J Sports Phys Ther. 2014;9(5):583–95.
5. Selye H. The history of the stress concept. In: Goldberger L, Brenitz S, editors. Handbook of stress: theoretical and clinical aspects. 2nd ed. New York: The Free Press; 1993. p. 7–17.
6. Andersen MB, Williams JM. A model of stress and athletic injury: prediction and prevention. J Sport Exercise Psy. 1988;10(3):294–306.
7. Williams JM, Andersen MB. Psychosocial antecedents of sport injury: review and critique of the stress and injury model. J Appl Sport Psychol. 1998;10(1):5–25.
8. Lazarus RS, Folkman S. Stress, appraisal, and coping. New York: Springer Publishing Company; 1984.
9. MacKinnon DP. Integrating mediators and moderators in research design. Res Soc Work Pract. 2011;21(6):675–81.
10. Brewer BW, Redmond CJ. Psychology of sport injury. Champaign: Human Kinetics; 2017.
11. Appaneal R, Habif S, Washington L, Granquist MD. A systematic review of research examining psychological factors associated with sport injury risk and prevention. Unpublished manuscript. Greensboro: University of North Carolina; 2009.
12. Martens R, Vealey RS, Burton D. Competitive anxiety in sport. Champaign: Human Kinetics; 1990.
13. Krasnow D, Mainwaring L, Kerr G. Injury, stress, and perfectionism in young dancers and gymnasts. J Dance Med Sci. 1999;3(2):51–8.
14. Passer MW, Seese MD. Life stress and athletic injury: examination of positive versus negative events and three moderator variables. J Hum Stress. 1983;9(4):11–6.
15. Perna FM, Antoni MH, Baum A, Gordon P, Schneiderman N. Cognitive behavioral stress management effects on injury and illness among competitive athletes: a randomized clinical trial. Ann Behav Med. 2003;25(1):66–73.
16. Hughes R, Coakley J. Positive deviance among athletes: the implications of overconformity to the sport ethic. Sociol Sport J. 1991;8(4):307–25.
17. Mitrosilis T. 10 iconic sports moments that make us proud to be American. 2016. https://www.foxsports.com/buzzer/gallery/united-states-of-america-usa-best-sports-moments-world-cup-olympics-052715. Accessed 20 Jan 2019.
18. Brewer BW. Psychological consequences of sport injury In: Tenenbaum G, Eklund RC. Encyclopedia of sport and exercise psychology. Los Angeles: SAGE Publications, Inc; 2014. http://du.idm.oclc.org/login?url=https://search.ebscohost.com/login.aspx?direct=true&db=nlebk&AN=713042&site=ehost-live&scope=site. Accessed 22 Jan 2019.
19. Walker N, Heaney C. Psychological responses to injury: a review and critique of existing models. In: Arvinen-Barrow M, Walker N, editors. The psychology of sport injury and rehabilitation. New York: Routledge; 2013. p. 23–39.
20. Brewer BW, Cornelius AE. Psychological factors in sports injury rehabilitation. In: Frontera WR, editor. Rehabilitation of sports injuries: scientific basis. Malden: Blackwell Science; 2003. p. 160–83.
21. Shapiro JL, Brewer BW, Cornelius AE, Van Raalte JL. Patterns of emotional response to ACL reconstruction surgery. J Clin Sport Psychol. 2017;11:169–80. https://doi.org/10.1123/jcsp.2016-0033.
22. Udry E, Gould D, Bridges D, Beck L. Down but not out: athlete responses to season-ending injuries. J Sport Exerc Psychol. 1997;19:229–48.
23. Wadey R, Evans L, Evans K, Mitchell I. Examining the antecedents and mechanisms underlying the perceived benefits following sport injury. J Appl Sport Psychol. 2011;23:142–58.
24. Park CL, Cohen LH, Murch RL. Assessment and prediction of stress-related growth. J Pers. 1996;64:71–105.
25. Kubler-Ross E. On death and dying. New York: Macmillan; 1969.
26. Evans L, Hardy L. Sport injury and grief responses: a review. J Sport Exerc Psychol. 1995;17:227–45.

27. Wiese-Bjornstal DM, Smith AM, Shaffer SM, Morrey MA. An integrated model of response to sport injury: psychological and sociological dynamics. J Appl Sport Psychol. 1998;10:46–69.
28. Brewer BW, Andersen MB, Van Raalte JL. Psychological aspects of sport injury rehabilitation: toward a biopsychosocial approach. In: Mostofsky DL, Zaichkowsky LD, editors. Medical and psychological aspects of sport and exercise, vol. 2002. Morgantown: Fitness Information Technology; 2002. p. 160–83.
29. Clement D, Arvinen-Barrow M. Sport medicine team influences in psychological rehabilitation: a multidisciplinary approach. In: Arvinen-Barrow M, Walker N, editors. The psychology of sport injury and rehabilitation. New York: Routledge; 2013. p. 156–70.
30. Arvinen-Barrow M, Massey WV, Hemmings B. Role of sport medicine professionals in addressing psychosocial aspects of sport-injury rehabilitation: professional athletes views. J Athl Train. 2014;49:764. https://doi.org/10.4085/1062-6050-49.3.44.
31. Association for Applied Sport Psychology: Certification. https://appliedsportpsych.org/certification/. Accessed 21 Jan 2019.
32. Brewer BW, Petitpas AJ, Van Raalte JL. Referral of injured athletes for counseling and psychotherapy. In: Ray R, Wiese-Bjornstal DM, editors. Counseling in sports medicine. Champaign: Human Kinetics; 1999. p. 127–41.
33. Dator J. A comprehensive timeline of the Larry Nassar case. 2019. https://www.sbnation.com/2018/1/19/16900674/larry-nassar-abuse-timeline-usa-gymnastics-michigan-state. Accessed 21 Jan 2019.
34. James RK, Gilliland BE. Crisis intervention strategies. 8th ed. Boston: Cengage Learning; 2016.
35. Dalenberg CJ, Straus E, Carlson EB. Defining trauma. In: Gold SN, editor. APA handbook of trauma psychology, Foundations in knowledge, vol. 1. Washington, D.C.: American Psychological Association; 2017. p. 15–31.
36. American Psychiatric Association. Diagnostic and statistical manual of mental health disorders. 5th ed. Washington, D.C.: American Psychiatric Publishing; 2013.
37. Abrams M, Bartlett M. Trauma and college student-athletes. In: Loughran M, editor. Counseling and psychological services for college student-athletes. 2nd ed. Morgantown: Fitness Information Technology; 2019. p. 105–22.
38. US Department of Health and Human Services: Child welfare information gateway. https://www.childwelfare.gov/topics/systemwide/laws-policies/state/. Accessed 28 Dec 2018.
39. Washington- Lofgren L, Westerman BJ, Sullivan PA, Nashman HW. The role of the athletic trainer in the post-injury psychological recovery of collegiate athletes. Int Sport J. 2004;8:94–104.
40. Hamson-Utley J, Martin S, Walters J. Athletic trainers' and physical therapists' perceptions of the effectiveness of psychological skills within sport injury rehabilitation programs. J Athl Train. 2008;43:258–64.
41. Stiller-Ostrowski JL, Hamson-Utley JJ. Athletic trainers' educational satisfaction and technique use within the psychosocial intervention and referral content area. Athl Train Educ J. 2010;5:4–11.
42. Bartlett ML. The need for sport psychologists in the athletic training room. J Sports Med Doping Stud. 2012;02 https://doi.org/10.4172/2161-0673.1000e120.
43. Arvinen-Barrow M, Pack S. Social support in sport injury rehabilitation. In: Arvinen-Barrow M, Walker N, editors. The psychology of sport injury and rehabilitation. New York: Routledge; 2013. p. 117–31.
44. Taylor J, Taylor S. Psychological approaches to sports injury rehabilitation. Gaithersburg: Aspen Publishers, Inc; 1997.
45. Podlog L, Heil J, Podlog S. Sport injury: psychological consequences and management strategies. In: Mugford A, Cremades JG, editors. Sport, exercise and performance psychology: theories and applications. New York: Routledge; 2019. p. 127–52.
46. Clement D, Shannon V, Connole IJ. Performance enhancement groups for injured athletes, part 1: preparation and development. Int J Athl Ther Train. 2012;17(3):34–6.

47. Clement D, Shannon V, Connole IJ. Performance enhancement groups for injured athletes, part 2: implementation and facilitation. Int J Athl Ther Train. 2012;17(5):38–40.
48. Locke EA, Shaw KN, Saari LM, Latham GP. Goal setting and task performance. Psychol Bull. 1981;90:125–52.
49. Theodorakis Y, Malliou P, Papaioannou A, Beneca A, Filactakidou A. The effect of personal goals, self-efficacy, and self-satisfaction on injury rehabilitation. J Sport Rehabil. 1996;5:214–23.
50. Evans L, Hardy L. Injury rehabilitation: a goal setting intervention study. Res Q Exerci Sport. 2002;73:310–9.
51. Arvinen-Barrow M, Hemmings B. Goal setting in sport injury rehabilitation. In: Arvinen-Barrow M, Walker N, editors. The psychology of sport injury and rehabilitation. New York: Routledge; 2013. p. 56–70.
52. Weinberg RS, Gould D. Foundations of sport and exercise psychology. 7th ed. Champaign: Human Kinetics; 2019.
53. Walker N, Heaney C. Relaxation techniques in sport injury rehabilitation. In: Arvinen-Barrow M, Walker N, editors. The psychology of sport injury and rehabilitation. New York: Routledge; 2013. p. 86–102.
54. Cupal DD, Brewer BW. Effects of relaxation and guided imagery on knee strength, reinjury anxiety, and pain following anterior cruciate ligament reconstruction. Rehabil Psychol. 2001;46:28–43.
55. Crossman J. Coping with sport injuries: psychological strategies for rehabilitation. New York: Oxford University Press Inc; 2001.
56. Jacobson E. Progressive relaxation. Chicago: University of Chicago Press; 1938.
57. Van Raalte JL. Self-talk. In: Hanrahan SJ, Andersen MB, editors. Routledge handbook of applied sport psychology: a comprehensive guide for students and practitioners. Abingdon: Routledge; 2010. p. 510–7.
58. Theodorakis Y, Beneca A, Malliou P, Antoniou P, Goudas M, Laparidis K. The effect of a self-talk technique on injury rehabilitation [Abstract]. J Appl Sport Psychol. 1997;9(Suppl):S164.
59. Beneka A, Malliou P, Gioftsidou A, Kofotolis N, Rokka S, Mavromoustakos S, Godolias G. Effects of instructional and motivational self-talk on balance performance in knee injured. Eur J Phys. 2013;15:56–63. https://doi.org/10.3109/21679169.2013.776109.
60. Walker N. The meaning of sports injury and re-injury anxiety assessment and intervention. Unpublished doctoral thesis. Aberystwyth: University of Wales; 2006.
61. Naoi A, Ostrow A. The effects of cognitive and relaxation interventions on injured athletes' mood and pain during rehabilitation. Athl Insight. 2008;10:1–25.
62. Arvinen-Barrow M, Clement D, Hemmings B. Imagery in sport injury rehabilitation. In: Arvinen-Barrow M, Walker N, editors. The psychology of sport injury and rehabilitation. New York: Routledge; 2013. p. 71–85.
63. Ievleva L, Orlick T. Mental links to enhanced healing: an exploratory study. Sport Psychol. 1991;5:25–40.
64. Gould D, Udry E, Bridges D, Beck L. Coping with season-ending injuries. Sport Psychol. 1997;11:379–99.
65. Hamson-Utley JJ, Vazquez L. The comeback: rehabilitating the psychological injury. Athl Ther Today. 2008;13(5):35–8.
66. Walsh M. Injury rehabilitation and imagery. In: Morris T, Spittle M, Watt AP, editors. Imagery in sport. Champaign: Human Kinetics; 2005. p. 267–84.
67. Kabat-Zinn J. Wherever you go, there you are: mindfulness meditation in everyday life. New York: Hyperion; 1994.
68. Birrer D, Röthlin P, Morgan G. Mindfulness to enhance athletic performance: theoretical considerations and possible impact mechanisms. Mindfulness. 2012;3(3):235–46. https://doi.org/10.1007/s12671-012-0109-2.
69. Josefsson T, Ivarsson A, Lindwall M, Gustafsson H, Stenling A, Böröy J, et al. Mindfulness mechanisms in sport: mediating effects of rumination and emotion regulation on sport-specific coping. Mindfulness. 2017;8(5):1354–63. https://doi.org/10.1007/s12671-017-0711-4.

70. Mohammed WA, Pappous A, Sharma D. Effect of mindfulness based stress reduction (MBSR) in increasing pain tolerance and improving the mental health of injured athletes. Front Psychol. 2018;9:1–10. https://doi.org/10.3389/fpsyg.2018.00722.
71. Shapiro SL, Carlson LE, Astin JA, Freedman B. Mechanisms of mindfulness. J Clin Psychol. 2006;62(3):373–86. https://doi.org/10.1002/jclp.20237.
72. Jones MI, Parker JK. A conditional process model of the effect of mindfulness on 800-m personal best times through pain catastrophising. J Sports Sci. 2015;34(12):1132–40. https://doi.org/10.1080/02640414.2015.1093648.
73. Crossman J. Psychological rehabilitation from sports injuries. Sports Med. 1997;23(5):333–9. https://doi.org/10.2165/00007256-199723050-00005.
74. Podlog L, Eklund RC. The psychosocial aspects of a return to sport following serious injury: a review of the literature from a self-determination perspective. Psychol Sport Exerc. 2007;8(4):535–66. https://doi.org/10.1016/j.psychsport.2006.07.008.
75. Chase MA, Magyar TM, Drake BM. Fear of injury in gymnastics: self-efficacy and psychological strategies to keep on tumbling. J Sports Sci. 2007;23(5):465–75. https://doi.org/10.1080/02640410400021427.
76. Podlog L, Banham SM, Wadey R, Hannon JC. Psychological readiness to return to competitive sport following injury: a qualitative study. Sport Psychol. 2015;29(1):1–14. https://doi.org/10.1123/tsp.2014-0063.
77. Podlog L, Eklund RC. A longitudinal investigation of competitive athletes' return to sport following serious injury. J App Sport Psychol. 2006;18(1):44–68. https://doi.org/10.1080/10413200500471319.

Chapter 6
Medical Illness in Gymnasts

Aubrey Armento and Emily Sweeney

6.1 Infections

Infectious diseases can occur in gymnasts, similar to other athletes. Up to 50% of all high school and college training room visits are due to infectious diseases [1]. Infections can impair the physiological and psychological performance of gymnasts, though there are very few studies that quantify performance deficits in athletes with infections [2]. Poor personal or equipment hygiene, excessive training, and close contact with other athletes can increase the risk of infections in gymnasts. Skin infections may occur by direct contact with another infected athlete or with a mat, or other piece of equipment. Respiratory infections may also occur commonly in gymnasts, especially in poorly ventilated areas. Gastroenteritis-related infections tend to occur in athletes who share water bottles or who have poor hand hygiene. Because infections that occur in gymnasts are not well studied and are very similar to athletes in dance, wrestling, and swimming, some of the concepts in this section are based on studies not specific to gymnasts.

Infections are more likely to occur in the 24-hour period that occurs after acute, intense exercise. This is because intense exercise leads to decreased numbers of natural killer (NK) cell numbers, IgA concentrations, lymphocyte and neutrophil counts, and lower B cell function, all of which suppress immune function [1]. In addition, prolonged intense training periods, especially indoors, can also lead to more subacute and chronic immune depression [3]. Nevertheless, moderate physi-

A. Armento (✉)
University of Colorado, School of Medicine, Aurora, CO, USA

Children's Hospital Colorado, Sports Medicine Center, Aurora, CO, USA
e-mail: Aubrey.Armento@childrenscolorado.org

E. Sweeney
Department of Orthopedics, University of Colorado School of Medicine,
Children's Hospital Colorado, Sports Medicine Center, Aurora, CO, USA
e-mail: Emily.Sweeney@childrenscolorado.org

cal activity stimulates the immune system by increasing neutrophil and NK counts as well as IgA secretions [1, 3]. Encouraging gymnasts to have good personal hygiene, making sure mats and equipment are frequently cleaned, and educating athletes and staff about infections can decrease the risk of developing infections [3].

Skin infections are common in athletes. The most common skin infections reported in athletes are due to community-associated methicillin-resistant *Staphylococcus aureus* (MRSA) [3]. MRSA typically occurs due to direct physical contact between gymnasts and is more likely to occur if there is some form of skin trauma or if equipment like towels are shared [3]. Ninety percent of community-associated MRSA cases lead to skin or soft tissue infections such as cellulitis (Fig. 6.1) or abscesses [4, 5]. These lesions may have purulent drainage or a more superficial erythema without drainage [5]. The NCAA recommends athletes with MRSA be on systemic antibiotics for at least 72 hours before returning to practice or competition [3]. Tinea corporis (ringworm) and tinea pedis (athlete's foot) can also occur in gymnasts and is due to *Trichophyton* [3]. These lesions have a circular appearance with a central clearing and a scaly border (Fig. 6.2). Gymnasts with tinea should be on topical antifungals for at least 72 hours prior to returning to practice or competition [3].

Upper respiratory infections (URIs) are very common in athletes and are typically caused by viruses. Eighty percent of gymnasts at one college developed a URI over the course of a 2-month period, suggesting that URIs are very common [6]. Prevention with handwashing, good nutrition and hydration, and adequate sleep and recovery can decrease the risk of URIs. In addition, the influenza vaccine should be given to athletes annually as long as there are no contraindications [7].

Epstein-Barr virus (EBV) may cause URI-like symptoms but can also cause infectious mononucleosis (IM). EBV is spread by direct contact from saliva, and in IM causes pharyngitis, posterior cervical lymphadenopathy, fever, malaise, and fatigue [1, 8]. Labs typically show lymphocytosis with >10% atypical lymphocytes. Heterophile antibody test and EBV-specific antibodies may also be used to diagnose IM [8]. Splenomegaly typically occurs in IM, however, clinical and ultrasound (US)

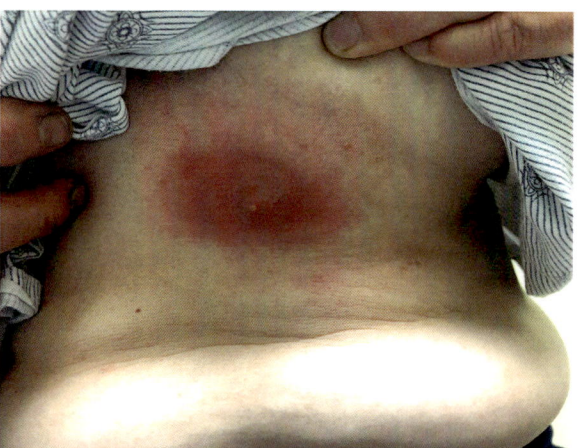

Fig. 6.1 Cellulitis from methicillin-resistant *Staphylococcus aureus* (MRSA)

6 Medical Illness in Gymnasts

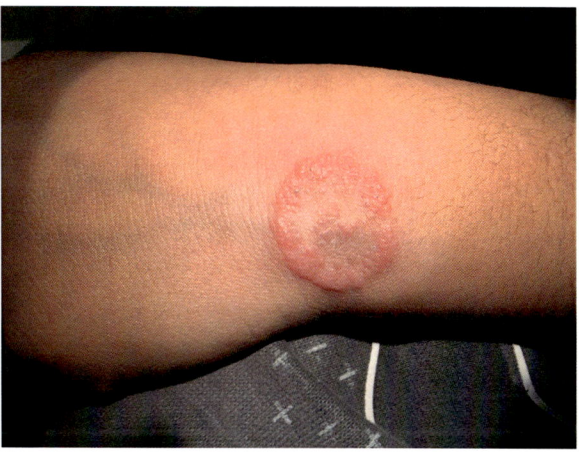

Fig. 6.2 Ringworm on the leg of a teenage athlete

measurements of splenomegaly are unreliable [8]. Therefore, a single US measurement showing "normal" spleen size in a patient with IM does not mean that athlete is ready to return to training. Splenomegaly increases the risk of splenic rupture, which is especially possible in contact athletes as well as gymnasts. If a gymnast falls on her abdomen or performs skills where her abdomen may come into contact with a piece of equipment, splenic rupture is more likely. Gymnasts with IM should limit physical activity for a minimum of 3–4 weeks and until symptoms resolve. In addition, they should not return to training until the spleen is not palpable or when serial spleen measurements by US show regression of spleen size [1, 8].

Measles is a very contagious viral infection that leads to fever, cough, rhinorrhea, and conjunctivitis; however, with appropriate immunization, it can be prevented. There has been one reported outbreak of measles at an international gymnastics competition in 1991 that resulted in three athletes developing measles [3].

Blood-borne illnesses are very rare in athletics and in gymnastics. There are reports of hepatitis B virus (HBV) being transmitted in contact sports, but it is very unlikely for human immunodeficiency virus (HIV) or hepatitis C virus (HCV) to be transmitted, especially in gymnastics.

6.2 Noninfectious Skin Conditions

In addition to skin infections, gymnasts may develop noninfectious causes of skin problems. One small study of collegiate gymnasts found that 32% of gymnasts developed some kind of skin issue over the course of a 2-month period. The most common causes were fungal infections and noninfectious dermatitis caused by chalk [6]. In addition, gymnasts commonly develop calluses on their hands [9] (Fig. 6.3). These calluses can be protective against the gymnast developing a "rip" on her hand (Fig. 6.4) due to frictional forces from the bars. Rips can be very painful, especially when swinging on the bars or rings. Gymnasts with a rip should stop

Fig. 6.3 Gymnast with multiple calluses and old, healing rips on her hands

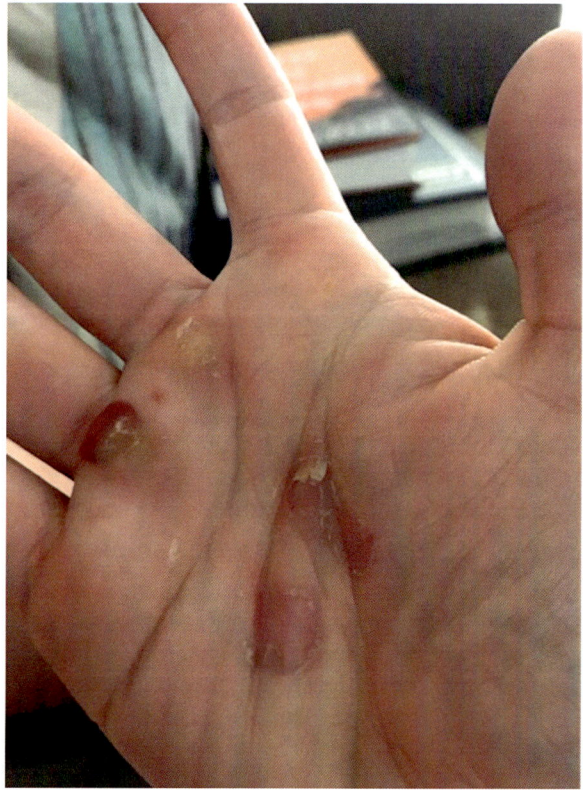

Fig. 6.4 Gymnast with new rips due to friction while performing on bars

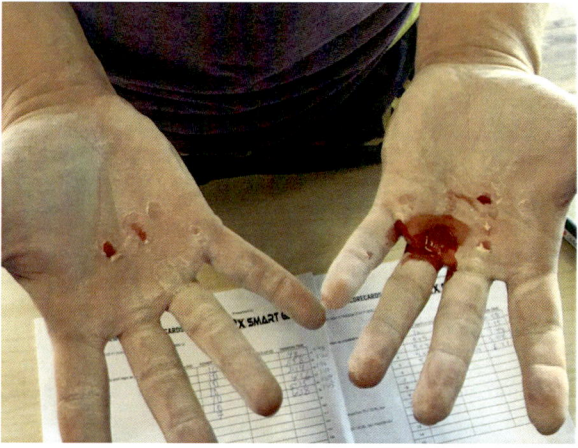

participation, and universal precautions should be taken if blood is present. Gymnasts should clip any loose skin to prevent further tearing and clean then cover the wound. Using a pumice stone to file down calluses, keeping the hands moisturized while not participating in gymnastics, and using hand grips while training on bars and rings can decrease the risk of rips.

6.3 Respiratory Conditions

Gymnasts may have respiratory conditions that can affect their performance. Asthma and exercise-induced bronchoconstriction (EIB) are common condition in athletes; however, gymnasts have lower risk of these conditions compared to endurance athletes, swimmers, and those whose sports occur outdoors [10]. Asthma is a chronic, inflammatory condition consisting of bronchial hyper-responsiveness and bronchoconstriction, while EIB is transient airway narrowing that occurs typically after 5–8 minutes of exercise [10–12]. EIB is more common in athletes with a previous asthma diagnosis; however, EIB may occur in athletes with no other asthma symptoms [11, 12]. EIB is also more common in athletes with allergic rhinitis [12]. Athletes with asthma or EIB may present with cough, shortness of breath, wheezing, or chest tightness. Although pulmonary function tests may be normal at baseline, athletes with EIB will have evidence of airway obstruction with direct or indirect bronchoprovocation testing [10, 11]. First-line treatment of EIB without underlying asthma includes short-acting bega-agonists 15 minutes prior to exercise. Leukotriene receptor agonists such as montelukast (Singulair) have been shown to be effective if adequate control of EIB cannot be achieved with short-acting beta-agonists alone. Management for asthma typically includes using daily inhaled corticosteroids with short-acting inhaled β_2-agonists when needed before exercise [11, 12].

Vocal cord dysfunction (VCD) may be mistaken for EIB in athletes. VCD is due to closure of the vocal cords during inspiration and typically presents with shortness of breath on inspiration, wheezing, and coughing [12]. Diagnosis is made by direct visualization with endoscopy [12]. Athletes with VCD typically have high levels of stress, so modification of stressors, counseling, and breathing techniques can help them manage this condition [12].

6.4 Diabetes Mellitus

Diabetes mellitus (DM) is the most common metabolic disorder in athletes, and in gymnasts, it is typically due to type 1 DM. Type 1 DM is due to loss of insulin secretion. Athletes with DM are at risk for acute issues such as hypoglycemia and hyperglycemia with ketoacidosis, but they are also at risk for chronic conditions such as peripheral vascular disease, neuropathy, vision issues, and kidney complications [13, 14]. Gymnasts with type I DM should check their glucose levels prior to exercising and then at 30-minute intervals during gymnastics. After training or competition, glucose levels should be monitored every 2 hours for up to 4 hours in order to monitor for delayed hypoglycemia [13]. Prior to exercise, glucose levels should be 100–180 mg dL^{-1} [13]. Glucose levels lower than this should be treated with carbohydrate supplementation. If an athlete has pre-exercise glucose levels between 180 and 250 mg dL^{-1}, he or she should consume a noncarbohydrate beverage and continue to monitor levels [13]. If pre-exercise glucose levels are in excess of 250 mg dL^{-1} and ketones are present, the gymnast should not participate in sports [13].

Gymnasts with type 1 DM are also at risk of hypoglycemia. Symptoms of hypoglycemia include hunger, anxiety, sweating, tremor, vision changes, confusion, tachycardia, and palpitations [13]. Gymnasts and coaches should be able to recognize symptoms of hypoglycemia and should promptly check the glucose and treat with 15–20 g of simple carbohydrates [13].

Gymnasts' routines are typically short, anaerobic-type exercises which are less problematic for diabetic athletes than those who participate in long endurance events [13]. However, the long practices of many gymnasts may mean they could have complications if glucose levels are not monitored throughout practice. When gymnasts travel, they should have unused syringes, blood glucose meters, lancets, test strips, alcohol swabs, insulin, a glucagon emergency kit, and ketone testing supplies with them [13].

Gymnasts and other athletes with type 1 DM who have concerns about their weight occasionally withhold insulin in order to lose weight [13]. However, this can lead to risk of ketoacidosis; therefore, athletes should be warned about the dangers of not properly dosing insulin.

6.5 Rhabdomyolysis

Exertional Rhabdomyolysis (ER) is due to muscle tissue breaking down after exercise. Gymnasts with ER may present with severe muscle pain and limited motion of the affected body areas which are out of proportion to the exercises performed. Diagnosis is made based on clinical presentation in conjunction with creatine kinase (CK) levels more than five times the normal range, along with the presence of myoglobinuria. Research has shown, however, that the finding of myoglobinuria is only 80% sensitive for ER [15, 16]. Athletes may be at increased risk for ER if they have sickle cell trait, history of exertional heat illness, or are dehydrated [15]. Although there are no documented cases of ER in gymnasts in the literature, a recent systematic review found that most cases of ER occurred in adolescent or early adult athletes with a high fitness level [16]. Thus, gymnasts may be especially susceptible to ER. Athletes with suspected ER should have a full clinical exam including neurological, musculoskeletal, and skin examinations [15]. Treatment typically involves intravenous fluids [16]. Complications of ER include kidney injury, acute compartment syndrome, and rarely, fatal arrhythmias. Therefore, prevention and early diagnosis of ER are key [15, 16].

6.6 The Female Athlete Triad

The female athlete triad involves three components: low energy availability with or without disordered eating, menstrual dysfunction, and low bone mineral density (BMD). It is described as a spectrum with clinical eating disorders, amenorrhea, and osteoporosis as the serious end points of each component if early intervention is not taken. It is recommended that athletes should be screened for the triad risks factors annually at their preparticipation physicals. Screening includes obtaining a history of menstrual irregularity, stress fractures, critical comments about eating or weight from the athlete, coach, or teammate, dieting, pressure to lose weight, overtraining, early start to sport-specific training, and symptoms of depression [17].

6.6.1 Energy Availability and Disordered Eating

Energy availability is defined as the energy intake (Kcal) minus the energy expenditure (Kcal) divided by kilograms of fat-free mass (FFM) or lean body mass. It can be difficult to use this index to measure energy availability outside of a laboratory, so other options such as dietary recall logs or food frequency questionnaires can be used for most gymnasts and other athletes. Stable body weight or a normal body mass index (BMI) are not necessarily indicative of adequate energy availability, so it cannot be used to exclude an energy availability deficit. Low weight (as measured by an athlete's weight in relation to the 50th BMI percentile) does not necessarily indicate low energy availability but warrants further questioning by the medical provider in order to detect poor eating behaviors including eating disorders [17].

It is important that clinicians screen for eating disorders as they lead to the highest degree of mortality among all mental health disorders. Early detection of eating disorders in young athletes is critical to reduce the risk of developing a chronic, lifelong disorder with associated comorbidities. Eating disorders in children and adolescents can lead to nutritional deficiencies, growth and pubertal delay or arrest, social isolation, and depression. Risk factors for eating disorders include family history of eating disorders, parental dieting or disordered eating behaviors, personality traits of perfectionism, and being in a sport that emphasizes low weight and slim appearance, such as gymnastics [18].

Abnormal eating behaviors in gymnasts may fall on a spectrum ranging from subclinical disordered eating to severe clinical diagnoses including anorexia nervosa and bulimia nervosa. Studies show a high prevalence of disordered eating in elite athletes participating in aesthetic or "appearance-focused" sports such as gymnastics, figure skating, and dance [19]. There is pressure in gymnastics as an aesthetic sport to fit an "ideal" body type, which can be especially difficult for prepubertal girls who may gain a significant amount of body fat as they go through puberty [20]. Gymnastics can create a high-risk environment for the development of eating disorders due to the young age at which many gymnasts reach the elite level, the strong influence of coaches who may pressure athletes to obtain a slim physique, and the aesthetic judging of the sport that idealizes a slim physique. Studies demonstrate an increased prevalence of disordered eating behaviors and attitudes among high-performance gymnasts, in both females and males. Higher levels of depressive symptoms, along with increased psychosocial stress, are also associated with greater severity of eating disorder symptoms [18, 19].

High-performance athletes demonstrate perfectionistic, obsessional, and highly self-disciplined personality traits comparable to those in the normal population with anorexia nervosa. However, contrary to the normal population with anorexia nervosa, disordered eating in athletes tends to stem from the goal of improving performance [18]. The assumption that a lean body leads to improved performance is a risk factor for disordered eating. The desire to be leaner to improve sports performance can be predictive of disordered eating in aesthetic sports [19]. A common reason for athletes to diet is to lose weight in order to enhance performance.

Athletes also report pressure to lose weight from a coach or teacher at a higher rate than non-athletes [20].

Interestingly, athletes, in general, may not demonstrate disordered eating at a higher frequency than non-athletes. In fact, some studies show that there is lower prevalence of disordered eating in adolescent athletes as compared to their non-athlete peers. Athletes tend to have higher self-esteem than non-athletes, which could lower the risk of disordered eating [20]. However, in comparing sport types, athletes in aesthetic sports, such as gymnastics, report less positive body self-esteem and greater weight concerns than athletes in nonaesthetic sports [21].

Eating Disorders The two primary eating disorders are anorexia nervosa and bulimia nervosa. The most current diagnostic criteria of anorexia nervosa include (1) restriction of energy intake relative to requirements, leading to a significantly low body weight (as defined by BMI <18.5), (2) intense fear of weight gain, (3) disturbance in the self-perception of one's body weight or shape or the lack of recognition of the seriousness of the current very low body weight [22]. In order to lose or maintain low weight, patients may undergo dieting, fasting, self-induced vomiting, self-induced purging, excessive exercise, or use appetite suppressants, laxatives, or diuretics. Medical complications of anorexia nervosa include cardiovascular problems such as hypotension, bradycardia, arrhythmias, and cardiomyopathy. Cardiac complications of anorexia nervosa are the most common cause of death. Hypothalamic-pituitary-ovarian dysfunction can result from extreme weight loss, excessive exercise, and emotional distress. This leads to decreased release of gonadotropin-releasing hormone (GnRH) from the hypothalamus, which in turn leads to decreased follicle-stimulating hormone (FSH) and luteinizing hormone (LH) release from the pituitary. Decreased LH, FSH, and estradiol levels result in anovulation and amenorrhea. Decreased estradiol levels, along with low progesterone and insulin-like growth factor levels lead to decreased bone formation, osteopenia, and osteoporosis. Other medical complications of anorexia nervosa include hypothermia, constipation, anemia, thrombocytopenia, leukopenia, dry skin and hair, and lanugo [23].

The diagnosis of bulimia nervosa includes (1) recurrent episodes of binge eating that are characterized by eating a much larger amount of food than normal within a 2-hour period, accompanied by a sense of lack of control over eating during the episode; (2) recurrent compensatory purging behaviors to prevent weight gain after binging such as self-induced vomiting, laxatives, excessive exercise, or fasting; (3) binging and purging episodes that occur on average at least once per week for

3 months [22]. Patients with bulimia may have a normal body mass index, in contrast to those with anorexia nervosa, for which very low body weight is a part of the diagnostic criteria. Many medical complications from bulimia nervosa result from self-induced vomiting and include electrolyte abnormalities, enlarged salivary glands, gastroesophageal reflux, and dental caries. Menstrual irregularities are less common in patients with bulimia nervosa [23].

If there is clinical concern for an eating disorder, initial laboratory studies should include complete blood count (CBC) with differential, complete metabolic panel, liver function tests, thyroid function tests, FSH, LH, and estradiol. Other studies such as an electrocardiogram (ECG) and bone density scan (DEXA) should also be considered.

Indications for hospitalization for eating disorders include heart rate <40 beats per minute (bpm) in adults or less than 50 bpm in children, temperature <36.1 C, potassium <3 mmol per liter, symptomatic hypoglycemia, severe dehydration, weight <75% of expected weight, or lack of improvement or worsening while in outpatient treatment. Whether patients undergo inpatient or outpatient treatment, the goal should be safe weight restoration, along with psychological treatment guided by a multidisciplinary team of a physician, nutritionist or dietitian, and psychologist [23].

For those athletes who do not meet clinical criteria for an eating disorder but demonstrate low energy availability, the treatment goal should be to normalize body weight (goal BMI >18.5) and restore normal menses. A baseline energy needs assessment should be performed to determine a target goal for energy availability, with nutritional counseling and meal planning provided to meet the target. Energy intake should be a minimum of 2000 kcal/day with the addition of increased caloric intake to meet the athletes' specific energy demands. Frequent monitoring of body weight should occur, and target intake should be adjusted to variations in the athlete's training and competition schedules [17].

In summary, disordered eating falls on a spectrum ranging from abnormal eating behaviors to eating disorders like anorexia nervosa and bulimia nervosa. Athletes who participate in gymnastics may be more at risk for eating disorders due to increased pressure to be thin. Athletes who maintain a normal weight can still suffer from negative energy balance if they do not take in enough calories to meet caloric demands. The negative energy availability that results from disordered eating can lead to complications such as menstrual disturbances and poor bone health. In addition, anorexia nervosa and bulimia nervosa can lead to even more debilitating and life-threatening medical complications.

6.6.2 Menstrual Dysfunction

Amenorrhea is defined as the absence of menstruation. Primary amenorrhea or delayed menarche is the absence of menstruation by age 15 in girls with secondary sex characteristics. Secondary amenorrhea is defined as the absence of at least three consecutive menstrual cycles after menarche [23]. Published rates of menstrual dysfunction in adolescents ranges from 7% to 54% [24]. Athletic females achieve menarche approximately 1 year later than non-athletic females, regardless of whether they commenced high-level training prior to or after menarche. In some sports, including gymnastics, there may be athletic advantages to late maturation including narrower hips, less weight, and less body fat [23].

Exercise-induced amenorrhea, also called functional hypothalamic amenorrhea, results from a metabolic energy deficit. It is not a normal response to training. Due to insufficient caloric intake to meet energy requirements, GnRH pulse generation is disrupted in the hypothalamus, which leads to decreased LH pulses from the anterior pituitary. Low LH levels result in low estrogen levels and anovulation. The approximate level of energy availability below which menstrual dysfunction is likely to occur is 30 kcal/kg lean body mass per day [23].

Just as eating disorders occur on a spectrum, so can menstrual dysfunction. For example, subclinical menstrual disturbances can occur without overt amenorrhea. Eumenorrheic athletes can have luteal phase deficiency, leading to inadequate progesterone support for endometrial development and impairment of successful implantation of a fertilized egg. Anovulation can also occur without clinically manifesting as amenorrhea. Another type of menstrual dysfunction involves leptin, which is an adipokine that plays a prominent role in reproductive function. Decreased leptin levels can occur with undernutrition. Low leptin levels have been shown in amenorrheic athletes, indicating a relationship between leptin, energy deficit, and menstrual disturbances [25].

Menstrual abnormalities may be more difficult to assess in gymnasts due to the younger population, who may not have established menarche at the time they reach high levels of training, as opposed to older athletes with measurable dysfunction who have already established menstrual cycles [18]. The level of competition and time spent training has an effect on the likelihood of menstrual dysfunction. Elite level gymnasts who train many hours demonstrate delayed menarche more frequently than high school, college, and club-level athletes. It has also been shown that young gymnasts who engage in less than 15 hours per week of training are less likely to have menstrual disturbances or delayed sexual maturation than their counterparts who train more hours. However, even if gymnasts have delayed pubertal onset, they still are likely to retain a normal progression rate of development once puberty begins [25].

Amenorrhea can have a number of negative effects on a gymnast's health. Decreased bone mineral density can occur if amenorrhea has been present for more than 6 months [23]. It is known that decreased BMD does not just result from hypoestrogenic states, but also from altered levels of various hormones including insulin-like growth factor-1 (IGF-1), cortisol, and leptin. Although increased weight-bearing activity can promote bone formation, increased physical activity in the setting of amenorrhea can lead to decreased BMD. In addition, BMD decreases proportionally with the number of missed menstrual cycles. Thus, athletes who are amenorrhoeic are at increased risk for stress injuries and fractures [25]. Furthermore, studies show there is a positive association with menstrual dysfunction and higher rates of musculoskeletal injury. It is recommended that females be screened for menstrual dysfunction during preparticipation physicals, but physicians should also consider menstrual screening for females presenting for both acute and chronic musculoskeletal injuries [24].

If an athlete presents with primary or secondary amenorrhea, workup should include testing for pregnancy and other endocrinopathies such as thyroid dysfunction, hyperprolactinemia, primary ovarian insufficiencies, or polycystic ovarian syndrome. Amenorrhea secondary to low EA is a diagnosis of exclusion after ruling out possible organic etiologies [17]. Assessment of menstrual dysfunction in athletes involves taking a thorough medical history including menstrual history, training schedule, diet, injury history, drug use, and psychological stress. Laboratory studies include a pregnancy test, LH, FSH, prolactin, and thyroid-stimulating hormone (TSH). Primary amenorrhea caused by outflow obstruction can be ruled out by performing a progestin challenge test or estrogen/progesterone test.

In patients with secondary amenorrhea, the mainstay of treatment involves nonpharmacological measures including reduction in training intensity and increased caloric intake with the goal of achieving spontaneous menstruation. The time course of treatment to achieve resumption of menses is unclear. It has been shown that weight gain and increased energy availability can lead to recovery of menstrual function within months or can take longer than 1 year. Pharmacological measures such as oral contraceptives (OCPs) can be considered if there is a lack of spontaneous menstruation or if new fractures occur despite 1 year or more of nonpharmacological therapy. In general, the use of OCPs to treat athletes with the triad is controversial, as they do not actually restore spontaneous menses but rather may falsely reassure the patient, family, and clinician that menses are normal. If OCPs are used for treatment, it should be done so after at least a year of nonpharmacological therapy. In addition, athletes should still continue nonpharmacological therapy [17]. Finally, clinicians, athletes, and parents should recognize that OCPs may restore menses without actually normalizing ovulation.

In conclusion, menstrual dysfunction in the form of primary or secondary amenorrhea can occur in the setting of negative energy availability. Gymnasts may be at increased risk for menstrual disturbances, particularly at high competitive levels, resulting from overtraining and/or disordered eating that is influenced by the aesthetic pressures of the sport. Hormonal changes as a consequence of menstrual abnormalities put athletes at increased risk for poor bone health and stress fractures.

6.6.3 Low Bone Mineral Density

Low bone mass in athletes is related to menstrual dysfunction and low energy availability. Amenorrhea leads to low estrogen levels, which in turn causes accelerated bone resorption. Other hormones related to bone metabolism, including growth hormone, thyroid hormone, leptin, and IGF-1, can be affected by energy deficit [23].

Low BMD should be tested for with DEXA scanning in high-risk athletes. Risk stratification as determined by the 2014 Female Athlete Triad Coalition is noted below:

- ≥1 "High-risk" Triad Risk Factors:
  - History of diagnosed eating disorder
  - BMI ≤17.5 kg/m^2, ≤85% estimated weight, or recent weight loss of ≥10% in 1 month
  - Menarche ≥16 years of age
  - Current or history of <6 menses over 12 months
  - Two prior stress reactions/fractures, one high-risk stress reaction/fracture (femoral neck, pelvis, sacrum), or a low-energy nontraumatic fracture
  - Prior Z-score of < −2.0 (after at least 1 year from baseline DEXA)

- ≥2 "Moderate risk" Triad Risk Factors:
  - Current or history of disordered eating for 6 months or greater
  - BMI between 17.5 and 18.5, <90% estimated weight, or recent weight loss of 5–10% in 1 month
  - Menarche between ages 15 and 16 years
  - One prior stress reaction/fracture
  - Prior Z-score between −1.0 and −2.0 (after at least 1-year interval from baseline DEXA)

For women ≥20 years of age, DEXA scanning of all weight-bearing sites should be performed. For girls and adolescents <20 years of age, spine as well as whole body less head should be obtained if possible [17]. Z-scores should be obtained for all patients to evaluate for low BMD.

The International Society of Clinical Densitometry defines osteoporosis in patients 5–19 years old as a Z-score ≤ −2.0 (as adjusted for age, gender, and body size) plus a clinically significant fracture history including a lower extremity long bone fracture, vertebral compression fracture, or two or more upper extremity long bone fractures. Diagnosis of low BMD as defined by the American College of Sports Medicine incudes a Z-score that is less than −1.0 in female athletes in weight-bearing sports [17].

Treatment of osteopenia and osteoporosis focuses on the underlying factors including menstrual dysfunction and low energy availability. Athletes should be referred to a dietitian and supplementation with 1500 mg of calcium, and 400–1000 IU of vitamin D daily should be prescribed. The role of further pharmacological therapy is not well-established and should be considered only after a failed response to at least a year of nonpharmacological therapy. The use of OCPs has not been consistently proven to reverse low BMD, which may be a result of the exogenous estrogen suppressing IGF-1 as it passes through the liver. Other forms of estrogen replacement such as transdermal estradiol replacement that do not suppress IGF-1 are under investigation. There are limited data to support the use of bisphosphonates in athletes with the triad and, if used, should be done so in consultation with an endocrinologist [17]. Other risk factors such as smoking, alcohol intake, and weight-bearing exercises should also be addressed [23].

Despite the risks that gymnasts have for low BMD, it has been found that gymnasts actually have higher BMD compared to non-gymnasts and non-athlete controls secondary to the impact loading forces of the sport [23]. These impact forces can increase BMD and offer some level of protection [23]. Several studies show that gymnasts demonstrate greater bone mineral content than non-gymnasts and that the benefit of increased bone mineral accrual affects both competitive and recreational gymnasts [26]. The effects of increased bone mineral content in premenarchal gymnasts have been shown to last into retirement from gymnastics [26, 27]. In another study of high-level rhythmic gymnasts, there was a high prevalence of delayed menarche and menstrual irregularities as compared to non-gymnasts, but the gymnasts showed improved bone health at weight-bearing sites compared to non-gymnasts [28]. Followed over time, gymnasts continuously gained bone mass as compared to non-gymnasts whose bone mass remained stable, despite higher prevalence of menstrual irregularities in gymnasts. Gymnasts with severely delayed menarche demonstrated lower BMD compared to gymnasts with less delayed menarche but still had higher BMD than non-gymnasts. These results suggest that the benefits of high mechanical loading may counter the negative effect of low estrogen levels that result from menstrual dysfunction [28].

In a study comparing high-level runners and gymnasts, gymnasts had significantly higher BMD than runners despite similar menstrual histories [29]. Gymnasts also had significantly higher muscle strength compared to runners, likely secondary to the osteogenic effects that stem from higher impact loading and muscle contraction in gymnastics compared to running [29]. However, in a large-scale study evaluating the epidemiology of stress fractures in young athletes, girls' gymnastics showed the second highest rate of stress fractures at 7%, after girls' cross-country at 10% [30]. Thus, there have been mixed results regarding bone health in gymnasts.

In summary, gymnasts are at increased risk for poor bone health in the setting of disordered eating and menstrual abnormalities, but the high impact loading of the sport offers protection against bone loss and can lead to increased BMD compared to non-gymnasts. Athletes who demonstrate risk factors for the female athlete triad should be screened for low BMD, with DEXA scanning to confirm the diagnosis of low BMD or osteoporosis.

6.7 Relative Energy Deficiency in Sport (RED-S)

RED-S encompasses a low-energy status in physically active males and females resulting from inadequate energy intake and/or excessive energy expenditure. This energy deficiency can lead to multiple negative consequences including impaired bone health, endocrine dysfunction, decreased athlete performance, increased injury risk, and mood disturbance (Fig. 6.5) [31–33]. The International Olympic Committee (IOC) produced the first consensus statement on RED-S in 2014 to replace their

2005 consensus statement on the female athlete triad in order to provide "a more comprehensive, broader term for the overall syndrome" [32]. The components of the female athlete triad including menstrual dysfunction, decreased bone health, and decreased energy availability fall within the realm of RED-S, but RED-S is an expanded concept with a wider range of outcomes that can also apply to the male athlete, including cardiovascular, hematological, gastrointestinal, immunological, and psychological detriments [31, 32]. Although most of the literature focuses on female athletes, there is emerging evidence that male athletes also suffer from energy deficiency and its negative consequences including poor bone health and increased risk of stress fractures [31, 32].

Low energy availability is the foundation of RED-S. As previously mentioned, it is difficult to determine accurate energy availability for athletes outside of a laboratory assessment. Self-reported questionnaires are typically used, and although they have inaccuracies, they may be the most practical tool for providers to evaluate those at risk for RED-S [31]. The approach to evaluation and treatment of RED-S and the associated decreased energy availability, menstrual dysfunction, and bone health is very similar to what was previously described for the female athlete triad. More research needs to be done to understand the unique effects of RED-S on male athletes and how to approach their treatment [31]. In general, the mainstay of treatment for RED-S involves nonpharmacologic interventions to reverse the energy deficit with dietary and training modifications [31, 32]. Pharmacologic treatments to address menstrual dysfunction and low BMD are discussed in the female athlete triad section. Critics of the 2014 consensus statement on RED-S warn against replacing the term "female athlete triad" with "RED-S" as they argue that the triad

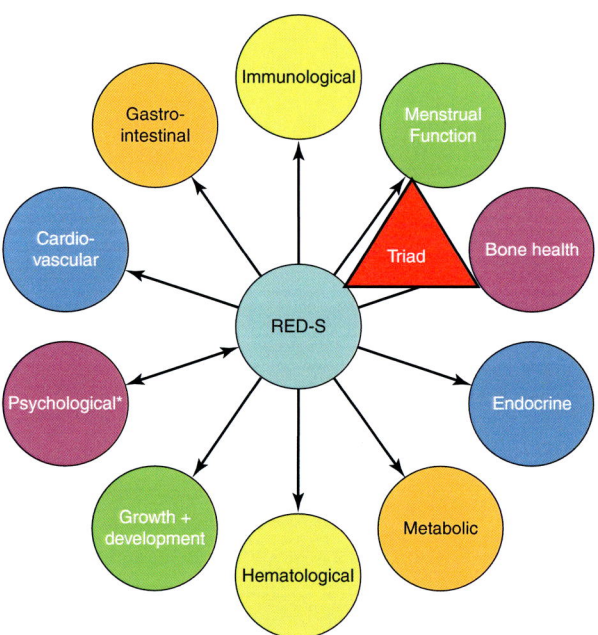

Fig. 6.5 Relative energy deficiency in sport (RED-S) model. (Credits for figure to *International Journal of Sport Nutrition and Exercise Metabolism*)

should be approached as a distinct clinical entity rather than separate health consequences that fall under the umbrella of RED-S [34].

6.8 Vitamin D Deficiency

Although there are few studies investigating the link of vitamin D and gymnasts, there are many known associations between vitamin D and health. Vitamin D plays a critical role in bone health by enhancing intestinal calcium absorption. With low vitamin D levels, parathyroid hormone (PTH) levels increase to stimulate bone turnover in order to release calcium. Increased bone turnover as a result of vitamin D insufficiency leads to higher risk of bony injuries such as stress fractures. Studies show lower levels of vitamin D and high levels of PTH are both risk factors for stress fractures [35, 36].

Vitamin D also plays an important role in protein synthesis and muscle function. Skeletal muscle cells contain vitamin D receptors, indicating that vitamin D is involved in cellular growth and regulation of skeletal muscle. Studies suggest that low vitamin D levels can lead to muscle weakness and that supplementation helps improve muscle strength [36]. This raises the question of the effect of vitamin D on athletic performance, but there is limited research to support vitamin D supplementation as a direct performance enhancer [36].

Vitamin D is also involved in immune function and may help prevent acute and chronic diseases. Low vitamin D levels are associated with cancer, heart disease, and autoimmune diseases, along with more acute illnesses like respiratory tract infections. Research indicates that people with suboptimal vitamin D levels are more likely to suffer from respiratory tract infections [37, 38]. Therefore, not only can vitamin D supplementation improve musculoskeletal health but may also improve immune health as well.

The primary source of vitamin D is sun exposure. Dietary sources of vitamin D include fatty fish, egg yolks, and fortified products such as milk, yogurt, cereal, and juice. Serum 25-(OH)-D concentrations are the best measurement to determine vitamin D status. Vitamin D deficiency is often defined as serum 25 (OH) D level <20 ng/mL, insufficiency as 20–32 ng/mL, and optimal levels >40 ng/mL. Research shows that PTH levels stabilize with 25-(OH)-D levels >75 ng/mL, suggesting higher levels may be necessary to prevent bony fragility that comes from elevated PTH levels [35]. Current guidelines for recommended vitamin D intake suggest that children and adults <70 years old should take in 400–600 IU/day. The Endocrine Society suggests even higher levels up to 1000 IU/day for children 18 years and younger and 1500–2000 IU/day for adults 19–70 years old. Although recommended dosages vary, a common treatment for significant vitamin D deficiency is 50,000 IU/week for 8 weeks [36, 39].

Recent estimates report up to 77% of the general population is vitamin D insufficient, and several studies show a high prevalence of insufficiency and deficiency in athletes [38, 39]. Lack of sun exposure is the main risk factor, which particularly affects gymnasts who train mostly indoors [36]. In a study comparing athletes from indoor and outdoor sports, athletes of indoor sports were almost twice as likely to have vitamin D insufficiency [37]. Low vitamin D levels can lead to loss of athletic participation time due to increased likelihood of stress fractures, muscular injuries, and infections [38]. Vitamin D insufficiency may also preclude peripubertal girls from achieving optimal bone mass [35].

Thus, vitamin D plays a vital role in bone health, which is very important to prevent bony stress injuries, along with muscular strength and immune function. Optimal levels of vitamin D should be a goal for all athletes. Physicians should consider screening athletes of indoor sports, like gymnasts, who are at higher risk for low vitamin D levels due to decreased sun exposure.

6.9 Conclusion

There are a number of medical conditions that affect gymnasts, however, very little research has been published on how these issues affect these athletes. Infections are often due to close contact with other infected individuals. Therefore, clinicians should emphasize proper hygiene for gymnasts and their coaches. In addition, clinicians should be aware of noninfectious medical illnesses that can occur in gymnasts, including diabetes mellitus, asthma, vocal cord dysfunction, and rhabdomyolysis. Finally, it is known that gymnasts are at risk for vitamin D deficiency as well as all the components of RED-S and the female athlete triad including disordered eating, menstrual dysfunction, and low BMD. Clinicians should be aware of these issues and screen for them in gymnasts, especially those with frequent injuries.

References

1. Harris MD. Infectious disease in athletes. Curr Sports Med Rep. 2011;10(2):84–9.
2. Colbey C, Cox AJ, Pyne DB, Zhang P, Cripps AW, West NP. Upper respiratory symptoms, gut health and mucosal immunity in athletes. Sports Med. 2018;48(Suppl 1):65–77.
3. Grosset-Janin A, Nicolas X, Saraux A. Sport and infectious risk: a systematic review of the literature over 20 years. Med Mal Infect. 2012;42(11):533–44.
4. Otto M. Community-associated MRSA: what makes them special? Int J Med Microbiol. 2013;303(6–7):324–30.
5. Loewen K, Schreiber Y, Kirlew M, Bocking N, Kelly L. Community-associated methicillin-resistant Staphylococcus aureus infection: literature review and clinical update. Can Fam Physician. 2017;63(7):512–20.
6. Strauss RH, Lanese RR, Leizman DJ. Illness and absence among wrestlers, swimmers, and gymnasts at a large university. Am J Sports Med. 1988;16(6):653–5.
7. Luke A, d'Hemecourt P. Prevention of infectious diseases in athletes. Clin Sports Med. 2007;26(3):321–44.

8. Shephard RJ. Exercise and the athlete with infectious mononucleosis. Clin J Sport Med. 2017;27(2):168–78.
9. De Luca JF, Adams BB, Yosipovitch G. Skin manifestations of athletes competing in the summer olympics: what a sports medicine physician should know. Sports Med. 2012;42(5):399–413.
10. Bonini M, Silvers W. Exercise-induced bronchoconstriction: background, prevalence, and sport considerations. Immunol Allergy Clin North Am. 2018;38(2):205–14.
11. Boulet LP, O'Byrne PM. Asthma and exercise-induced bronchoconstriction in athletes. N Engl J Med. 2015;372(7):641–8.
12. Wuestenfeld JC, Wolfarth B. Special considerations for adolescent athletic and asthmatic patients. Open Access J Sports Med. 2013;4:1–7.
13. Harris GD, White RD. Diabetes in the competitive athlete. Curr Sports Med Rep. 2012;11(6):309–15.
14. Yardley JE, Colberg SR. Update on management of type 1 diabetes and type 2 diabetes in athletes. Curr Sports Med Rep. 2017;16(1):38–44.
15. Szczepanik ME, Heled Y, Capacchione J, Campbell W, Deuster P, O'Connor FG. Exertional rhabdomyolysis: identification and evaluation of the athlete at risk for recurrence. Curr Sports Med Rep. 2014;13(2):113–9.
16. Manspeaker S, Henderson K, Riddle D. Treatment of exertional rhabdomyolysis in athletes: a systematic review. JBI Database System Rev Implement Rep. 2016;14(6):117–47.
17. De Souza MJ, Nattiv A, Joy E, Misra M, Williams NI, Mallinson RJ, et al. 2014 Female Athlete Triad Coalition consensus statement on treatment and return to play of the female athlete triad: 1st International Conference held in San Francisco, California, May 2012 and 2nd International Conference held in Indianapolis, Indiana, May 2013. Br J Sports Med. 2014;48(4):289.
18. Tan JO, Calitri R, Bloodworth A, McNamee MJ. Understanding eating disorders in elite gymnastics: ethical and conceptual challenges. Clin Sports Med. 2016;35(2):275–92.
19. Krentz EM, Warschburger P. A longitudinal investigation of sports-related risk factors for disordered eating in aesthetic sports. Scand J Med Sci Sports. 2013;23(3):303–10.
20. Martinsen M, Bratland-Sanda S, Eriksson AK, Sundgot-Borgen J. Dieting to win or to be thin? A study of dieting and disordered eating among adolescent elite athletes and non-athlete controls. Br J Sports Med. 2010;44(1):70–6.
21. Varnes JR, Stellefson ML, Janelle CM, Dorman SM, Dodd V, Miller MD. A systematic review of studies comparing body image concerns among female college athletes and non-athletes, 1997–2012. Body Image. 2013;10(4):421–32.
22. American Psychiatric Association., American Psychiatric Association. DSM-5 Task Force. Diagnostic and statistical manual of mental disorders: DSM-5. Washington, D.C.: American Psychiatric Association; 2013. Available from: Connect to resource https://aurarialibrary.idm.oclc.org/login?url=https://dsm.psychiatryonline.org/doi/book/10.1176/appi.books.9780890425596.
23. Madden CC. Netter's sports medicine. Philadelphia: Saunders/Elsevier; 2010. p. 732.
24. Fischer AN, Yang J, Singichetti B, et al. Menstrual dysfunction in females presenting to a pediatric sports medicine practice. Trans J Am College Sports Med. 2017;2(13):79.
25. Roupas ND, Georgopoulos NA. Menstrual function in sports. Hormones (Athens). 2011;10(2):104–16.
26. Erlandson MC, Kontulainen SA, Chilibeck PD, Arnold CM, Baxter-Jones AD. Bone mineral accrual in 4- to 10-year-old precompetitive, recreational gymnasts: a 4-year longitudinal study. J Bone Miner Res. 2011;26(6):1313–20.
27. Erlandson MC, Kontulainen SA, Chilibeck PD, Arnold CM, Faulkner RA, Baxter-Jones AD. Higher premenarcheal bone mass in elite gymnasts is maintained into young adulthood after long-term retirement from sport: a 14-year follow-up. J Bone Miner Res. 2012;27(1):104–10.
28. Maimoun L, Coste O, Georgopoulos NA, Roupas ND, Mahadea KK, Tsouka A, et al. Despite a high prevalence of menstrual disorders, bone health is improved at a weight-bearing bone site in world-class female rhythmic gymnasts. J Clin Endocrinol Metab. 2013;98(12):4961–9.

29. Robinson TL, Snow-Harter C, Taaffe DR, Gillis D, Shaw J, Marcus R. Gymnasts exhibit higher bone mass than runners despite similar prevalence of amenorrhea and oligomenorrhea. J Bone Miner Res. 1995;10(1):26–35.
30. Changstrom BG, Brou L, Khodaee M, Braund C, Comstock RD. Epidemiology of stress fracture injuries among US high school athletes, 2005–2006 through 2012–2013. Am J Sports Med. 2015;43(1):26–33.
31. Mountjoy M, Sundgot-Borgen J, Burke L, Ackerman KE, Blauwet C, Constantini N, et al. International Olympic Committee (IOC) Consensus Statement on Relative Energy Deficiency in Sport (RED-S): 2018 update. Int J Sport Nutr Exerc Metab. 2018;28(4):316–31.
32. Mountjoy M, Sundgot-Borgen J, Burke L, Carter S, Constantini N, Lebrun C, et al. The IOC consensus statement: beyond the Female Athlete Triad–Relative Energy Deficiency in Sport (RED-S). Br J Sports Med. 2014;48(7):491–7.
33. Statuta SM, Asif IM, Drezner JA. Relative energy deficiency in sport (RED-S). Br J Sports Med. 2017;51(21):1570–1.
34. De Souza MJ, Williams NI, Nattiv A, Joy E, Misra M, Loucks AB, et al. Misunderstanding the female athlete triad: refuting the IOC consensus statement on Relative Energy Deficiency in Sport (RED-S). Br J Sports Med. 2014;48(20):1461–5.
35. Lovell G. Vitamin D status of females in an elite gymnastics program. Clin J Sport Med. 2008;18(2):159–61.
36. Ogan D, Pritchett K. Vitamin D and the athlete: risks, recommendations, and benefits. Nutrients. 2013;5:1856–68.
37. Constantini NW, Arieli R, Chodick G, Dubnov-Raz G. High prevalence of vitamin D insufficiency in athletes and dancers. Clin J Sport Med. 2010;20(5):368–71.
38. Sikora-Klak J, Narvy SJ, Yang J, Makhni E, Kharrazi FD, Mehran N. The effect of abnormal vitamin D levels in athletes. Perm J. 2018;22:17–216.
39. Pfotenhauer KM, Shubrook JH. Vitamin D deficiency, its role in health and disease, and current supplementation recommendations. J Am Osteopath Assoc. 2017;117(5):301–5.

Chapter 7
Head and Neck Injuries in Gymnasts

Christine Eng and Steven Makovitch

7.1 Concussion

7.1.1 Epidemiology and Pathophysiology

Concussion, also known as mild traumatic brain injury (mTBI) or mild head injury, is defined as a traumatically induced transient disturbance of brain function caused by complex pathophysiologic processes according to the American Medical Society for Sports Medicine position statement [1]. These processes may include oxidative stress, impaired axonal transport, and altered neurotransmission [2]. Centers for Disease Control and Prevention (CDC) guidelines criteria for concussion include confusion or disorientation, loss of consciousness for 30 minutes or less, post-traumatic amnesia for less than 24 hours or other transient neurologic abnormalities, and Glasgow Coma Scale (GCS) score 13–15 at least 30 minutes after injury [3].

Concussion in sport is currently estimated at about 3.8 million per year in the United States and continues to rise at about an annual rate of 7% per year [4, 5]. Specifically related to gymnastics, a study of children ages 6–17 treated at US hospital emergency departments indicated that concussion/closed head injuries comprised 1.7% of all gymnastics-related injuries. In addition, the frequency of these injuries decreased with increasing age [6]. According to a recent review, concussion comprised 3% of Olympic injuries and up to 8% of all injuries across pooled studies of gymnastics injuries [7, 8]. When looking at NCAA surveillance data from 1988 through 2004, concussions were 2.3% of all injuries in women's gymnastics with a 0.16 injury rate per 1000 athlete exposures [4]. However, self-reported history of

---

C. Eng (✉) · S. Makovitch
Harvard Medical School, Department of Physical Medicine and Rehabilitation, Spaulding Rehabilitation Hospital, Charlestown, MA, USA
e-mail: Ceng1@partners.org; smakovitch@partners.org

concussion symptoms may be up to 15.6–30.2%, possibly suggesting a majority of these are unrecognized and do not present for clinical care [9].

7.1.2 History and Diagnosis

Concussion in sport is often difficult to diagnose, assess, and treat. This is attributed to its complex and often evolving symptomatology, variable prognosis, evolving clinical guidelines, and complex return-to-play factors. Resolution of the clinical and cognitive features typically occurs in a sequential course, but in some cases can be more prolonged [10]. At present, there is no specific biologic marker or imaging study that is reliable for immediate diagnosis, so concussion remains a clinical diagnosis. In addition, loss of consciousness, previously considered to be a hallmark of concussion, only occurs about 10% of the time [1, 10–15].

When diagnosing concussion in sport, acute symptoms may be different from subacute clinical presentation. There are several established guidelines and updated consensus statements which may help clinicians both in the competitive sport environment and in clinic. These include the 2018 CDC guidelines for mTBI in children, the 2017 Concussion in Sport Group consensus statement from Berlin, and previously in 2012 from Zurich [3, 10, 16]. The current in-sport management focuses on prompt identification, rapid screening, and immediate removal from play of those individuals suspected of sustaining concussion [1, 3, 5, 10, 16].

Any gymnast with signs of concussion such as loss of consciousness, tonic posturing, severe headache, or balance disturbance should be immediately removed from participation [10]. The gymnast should be immediately assessed for risk of intracranial injury (ICI) or spine injury. Clinical decision tools may also help to assess the risk of more serious traumatic brain injury (TBI) or ICI. Some risk factors indicating ICI include vomiting, severe mechanism of injury, worsening headache, amnesia, scalp hematoma, skull fracture, and Glasgow Coma Scale (GCS) score less than 15 [2, 3, 17]. Screening with head computed tomography (CT) or magnetic resonance imaging (MRI) is not routinely recommended but may be indicated for higher suspicion of ICI or structural abnormalities [1, 3].

In other cases where concussion is suspected, immediate evaluation of cognitive function is essential and may involve brief neuropsychological testing. Some widely available and validated testing tools include the Sport Concussion Assessment Tool Version 5 (SCAT5), which also incorporates the Maddock's questions, and the Standardized assessment of concussion (SAC) which may be used for those ages 13 and older [10, 18–20]. There is also a child SCAT5 for children ages 5–12 [21]. After removing the gymnast from competition or practice, a more thorough evaluation should be done in an environment with less distractions. Serial assessments are often necessary, and the gymnast should not be left alone after the injury. Gymnasts with suspected concussion should not return to same day practice or competition.

With regard to the pediatric population, recent CDC guidelines for pediatric mTBI recommend using a combination of an age appropriate symptom rating scale with computerized cognitive testing and not solely the SAC alone for children ages 6–18 [2, 3]. Computerized testing after injury may be compared to preseason Immediate Post-Concussion Assessment and Cognitive Testing (ImPACT) scores to help with return to play decisions; however, these tests should not be used as a sole measure for return to play decisions [22]. Preparation for care of athletes with concussion begins with the preparticipation physical exam including a detailed concussion history, history of migraines, and presence of mood, learning, and attention disorders [1, 23, 24].

Gymnasts with concussions should have close follow-up with a medical provider familiar with the most up-to-date concussion management strategies. Thorough assessment of the gymnast with a concussion should include a range of clinical domains such as clinical symptoms, physical signs, cognitive impairment, neurobehavioral features, and sleep-wake cycle disturbance. Somatic symptoms like headache and dizziness are the most common symptoms of concussion. Other symptoms and signs may include cognitive symptoms (e.g., feeling in a fog), emotional lability or behavioral changes, cognitive impairment (e.g., slower reaction time), balance impairment, somnolence, and drowsiness [10]. Examination should include detailed neurological assessment of mental status, cognitive function, vestibulo-oculomotor function, gait, and balance. Serial monitoring of symptom scores, as well as neuropsychological, cognitive, and balance testing, may be helpful to objectively assess resolution to baseline.

New prognostic biomarkers (e.g., S100B, neuronal ubiquitin C-terminal hydrolase-L1, and glial fibrillary acidic protein), diagnostic testing, and advanced imaging modalities are currently being explored for diagnosis and recovery from concussion. Currently, there is no single objective marker to confirm resolution of concussion. There is limited role for these tests in the clinical setting and further research studies are needed to expand their role going forward [1, 3, 10].

7.1.3 Treatment

As noted previously, a gymnast with a diagnosed concussion should not return to same day practice or competition. These gymnasts should have appropriate disposition either to home in a monitored setting or to an emergency setting if needed. Following the injury, the gymnast should be re-evaluated with multimodal clinical assessment and treatment. Those gymnasts with persistent symptoms should be managed with a multidisciplinary approach with providers experienced in sports-related concussion [10].

Most consensus statements and guidelines agree that in the acute period (e.g., 2–3 days) following concussion, primary treatment features a period of relative physical and cognitive rest to help reduce post-concussive symptoms and decrease cognitive demand [1, 3, 10]. In addition, there may be increased risk of recurrent concussion which may have a magnified effect [25]. Cognitive rest includes reduced technology use and screen time and potentially decreased scholastic activities or modified school attendance to be determined on an individualized treatment plan [26]. Following this brief period, the role of strict rest may have a negative role on self-reported symptoms and may delay return to play [27–33]. The exact duration and definitions of relative rest and timing of gradual return to activity have not been fully established [3, 10]. An individualized symptom-limited, supervised, gradual rehabilitation protocol for athletes with continued symptoms in the post-acute period may be beneficial [3, 10, 28, 29].

After concussion, gymnasts may gradually increase the duration and intensity of cognitive and academic activities barring significantly exacerbating symptoms; return to school protocol should be customized with assessment of educational needs and support [3]. Return-to-sport protocol should include a graduated stepwise rehabilitation strategy. Once concussion symptoms resolve, the gymnast may begin progression through a return-to-play protocol first with symptom-limited activity and then light aerobic exercise, sports-specific exercise, noncontact training drills, full practice, and finally full return to play [1, 10]. The athlete may progress through these increasingly demanding activities in a stepwise fashion, provided they do not have exacerbation of symptoms (Table 7.1). The time frame for return will vary based on the athlete's symptoms and skill level. A detailed return-to-play protocol is described in Chap. 12.

Medications that alter mental status should be avoided in the acute setting. There is limited overall evidence to support the role of pharmacotherapy, but medications may be targeted for specific symptoms in more prolonged recovery. There may be some role for non-opioid analgesics like acetaminophen or ibuprofen for headache management, but these may precipitate rebound headaches if used frequently and for longer durations [3, 34]. When assessing for return-to-play, medications that mask symptoms of concussion should be avoided [1, 10].

Concurrent cervical spine, vestibular injury, or other primary and secondary pathologies that contribute to post-concussive symptoms should be managed accordingly [10]. In those with prolonged post-concussive symptoms, formal physical therapy and vestibular rehabilitation as well as collaborative cognitive behavioral therapy should be considered [3, 10, 34]. Sleep disturbance occurs frequently after concussion; lack of adequate sleep may have negative effects on those with concus-

Table 7.1 Gymnastics return-to-play after concussion

Step 1	Limited activity and return to pain-free activities of daily living
Step 2	Light aerobic exercise with increasing exertion without exacerbation of symptoms
Step 3	Return to conditioning – gymnastics specific; avoid inverted skills
Step 4	Progress skills starting with more static skills like handstands with assistance for balance, then integration of light tumbling skills graduating in difficulty. Single low bar skills, progress to rotational and transitions skills, then release skills and finally dismounts. Training with low beam with pads with balance skills and progress to jumps and then aerial skills and dismounts. Vaulting drills perhaps into foam pits or onto landing mats. Then progress to full vaulting skills
Step 5	Return to full practice and then competition. May consider limiting to certain events first, then all around

sion and sleep hygiene should be addressed [3, 35–37]. Management plans should include comprehensive education and cooperative treatment strategies for the gymnast, their parents, coaches, athletic trainers, and school administrators, along with physicians and healthcare professionals experienced in treating concussion.

Prevention of concussion in gymnastics may be multifactorial and may include neck strengthening protocols and alterations to training conditions. At rest, the muscles of the neck provide nearly 80% of the cervical spine's mechanical stability; these muscles may be even more important during trauma [38]. Cervical musculature, therefore, plays an important role in injury prevention [39–41]. However, there is no specific validated neck strengthening program that demonstrates a clear intervention effect and this may only be effective in cases where the gymnast is aware of impending impact [1].

Most often, concussion in the gym may be a result of direct contact with apparatus or mats. There is a general paucity of high-quality data regarding effectiveness of safety measures. Spotting for new or more difficult skills may reduce injury rates and head trauma events. Equipment such as landing mats, crash pads, foam pits, protected beams, and salto or twisting belts may reduce magnitude of force or impact [42].

7.1.4 Prognosis

Prognosis for concussion is generally favorable. Historically, most athletes, especially adults, will have improved symptoms by 3 days, and nearly 80–90% will have resolution of symptoms by 7 days [1, 11, 13, 43, 44]. More recent studies demonstrate a longer recovery time and return to play possibly due to change in medical management, guidelines, and ascertainment bias [10]. Regarding the pediatric population, 70–80% of children with mTBI will not show significant difficulties lasting more than 1–3 months. Among school-aged children with mTBI, 13.7% were symptomatic at 3 months after injury and 2.3% at 1 year after injury [3, 45]. Recovery may be delayed in those with prior concussion, preexisting neurologic or psychiatric disorders, learning difficulties, pre-injury symptoms, lower cognitive ability, intracranial lesions, and those with family and social stressors. Just as there is no single test to diagnose concussion, there is no single marker for resolution. Instead, clinical recovery of concussion is marked by abatement of symptoms, improvement of physical exam to baseline, along with tolerance of physical activity and cognitive exertion.

7.2 Cervical Spine

7.2.1 Epidemiology, Anatomy, and Pathophysiology

Sports-related injuries are among the leading causes of cervical spine injuries in the United States [46, 47]. Cervical spine injuries in gymnastics are not as common as lower or upper extremity injuries, but the possibility of catastrophic injury makes this a crucial aspect of medical care. In addition, female gymnasts have the third highest injury rate of cervical spine injuries at 4.05 per 100,000 athlete exposures, according to a study among high school athletes. Minor cervical spine injuries like soft tissue contusions and muscle sprains are the most common and generally self-limited. While acute spinal cord injuries in athletes are less common, they account for about 2.4% of all athletic hospitalizations [48, 49].

The relatively large range of motion (ROM) of the cervical spine comes at the cost of relative stability. Structural stability of the bones relies on ligamentous structures which all may be prone to injury from a sudden trauma to the neck (Fig. 7.1). Fractures may involve transverse or spinous processes or vertebral compression fractures (Fig. 7.2) [50]. The most common mechanism of acute injury is an axial load applied in a flexed position, but any movement involving hyperflexion or hyperextension may increase functional canal stenosis and mechanical load to the tissues [51].

Trauma to the neck with instability may lead to serious neurologic injury including injury to the spinal cord, exiting nerve roots, brachial plexus, or peripheral nerves. If a gymnast has a narrow canal at baseline either congenitally or acquired due to pathology, this may predispose to neurologic injury [51, 52]. Although less frequent in gymnastics than football, cervical neurologic injuries include stingers and transient quadriparesis. A stinger is generally a transient neuropraxic injury to the cervical roots or brachial plexus leading to unilateral upper extremity neurologic deficit. Transient quadriparesis, also known as spinal cord concussion or cervical

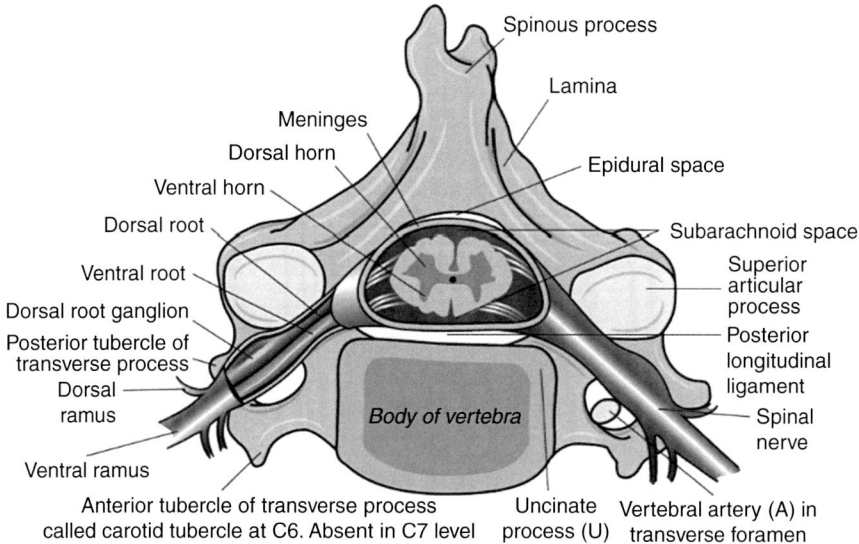

Fig. 7.1 Cross-sectional anatomy of the cervical spine which illustrates the relationship of spinal cord and spinal nerve to the surrounding skeletal elements. (*Adapted from* Lee [63], [Fig. 2.4, page 90])

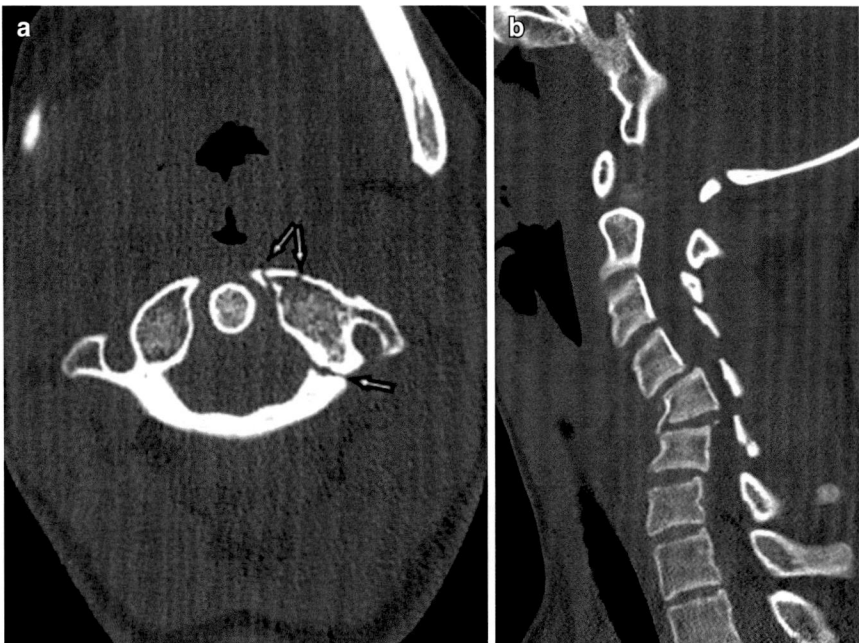

Fig. 7.2 Traumatic cervical spine fractures. (**a**) Axial CT showing comminuted C1 burst fracture through the anterior and posterior arches (Jefferson). (**b**) Sagittal CT showing burst fracture of the C5 and C6 vertebral bodies resulting in focal kyphosis

cord neuropraxia, is an injury to the spinal cord that results in transient paresthesia with varying degrees of weakness. Any gymnast complaining of neurologic symptoms in more than one extremity must be considered for injury to the spinal cord [51, 53–55].

More commonly, gymnasts will present with subacute to chronic nonspecific neck pain. Surrounding musculature provides dynamic stability to the spine and is more commonly injured [50]. Other common injuries include symptomatic disc herniations involving extravasation of the gel-like nucleus pulposus through the injured annulus fibrosis which may occur throughout the spine. This may lead to disc degeneration given the relative avascularity of the disc, the compressive forces, and dehydration over time. Herniation of the disc may also result in compression or irritation of the spinal nerve root producing radicular symptoms [56].

7.2.2 History and Diagnosis

In the acute setting, any gymnast who sustains trauma to the cervical spine, reports tenderness, or has decreased range of motion should have a complete neurologic examination. Medical personnel must maintain a high level of suspicion of spinal cord injury especially in the unconscious athlete. If any structural or neurologic injury is even suspected, the gymnast should be immediately immobilized with a cervical collar and transferred with their neck in a neutral position and spine board to a trauma center. No traction or manipulation of the neck should be performed. The gymnast should only be moved for cardiopulmonary resuscitation (CPR) or for transport with trained medical personnel using practiced lift techniques and proper immobilization equipment. Initially, assessment and maintenance of airway, breathing, and circulation are paramount [47, 48, 57].

After stabilization and transport, a full examination for neurologic injury including assessment of skin discoloration, deformity, step-offs, spinous process tenderness, and testing of strength, sensation, deep tendon reflexes, rectal tone, and bulbocavernosus reflex should be completed [47, 48, 57]. Once fracture and instability are ruled out, range of motion and Spurling's test (Fig. 7.3), which is specific (93%), but not sensitive (30%) for nerve root impingement, may be performed [57, 58].

Evaluation of the gymnast with more nonspecific or subacute to chronic neck pain includes full neurologic and musculoskeletal examination. Examination of the gymnast starts with inspection for deformity, atrophy, step-offs, scoliosis, and assessment of posture. Thorough palpation for spinous process, myofascial, or muscle tenderness and assessment of range of motion should be performed. Next, strength, sensation, and deep tendon reflexes should be tested.

Diagnostic imaging should begin with cervical spine radiographs, potentially including flexion and extension views if the gymnast is neurologically stable. Then, if any fracture or dislocation is suspected, further advanced imaging with CT may be useful. If neurologic injury to the spinal cord or nerve roots is suspected, MRI may be helpful in showing spinal cord edema, nerve root or cord impingement, as

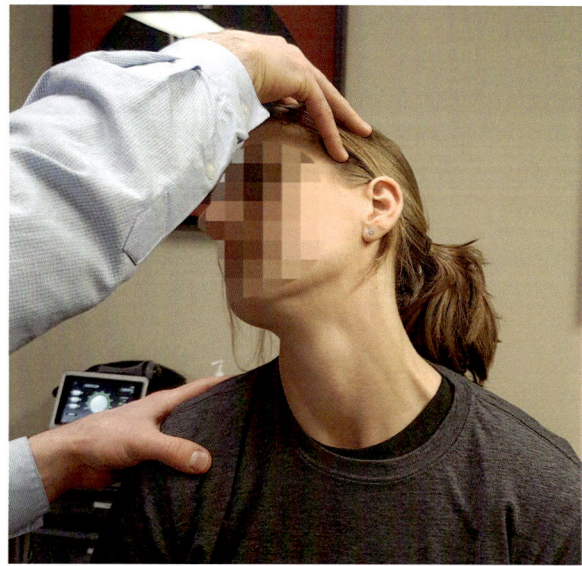

Fig. 7.3 Spurling's neck compression test can be useful in evaluation of radiculitis by increasing nerve root compression. It is designed to reproduce first with cervical extension and ipsilateral rotation to increase stress to the intervertebral disc and narrow the neuroforamina. This test may be done with or without axial compression which may amplify these effects

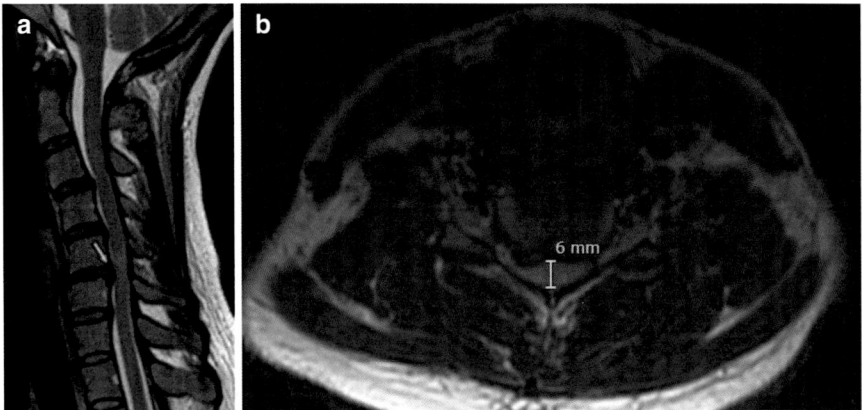

Fig. 7.4 MRI cervical spine. (**a**) Sagittal T2. (**b**) Axial T2 showing disc bulge at C5–6 resulting in compression of the spinal cord and T2 hyperintense intrinsic cord signal changes consistent with myelomalacia

well as identifying disc, facet, ligamentous, and soft tissue pathology (Fig. 7.4) [51]. MRI and CT myelogram may also be useful for assessment of functional stenosis [51, 54]. There may also be a role for somatosensory evoked potentials to evaluate for myelopathy or dorsal column involvement and electromyography for radiculopathy or plexopathy [51].

7.2.3 Treatment and Return to Play

Supervision with increased difficulty of skills along with improved safety equipment may mitigate risk of neck injury. Often, the lack of supervision and the mismatch of level of skill to the ability of the gymnast are cited as risks for injury [59, 60]. In addition, prevention of spine injury is twofold and includes reducing repetitive stresses and reducing risk of acute neck injury. There should be a focus on technique and training of skills which may reduce mechanical load and repetitive stresses to the spine. Some of the most effective prevention strategies include banning unsafe skills, for example, the elimination of Thomas Salto or rollout skills for all gymnasts since 2017.

Treatment of serious acute neck injuries is based on injury type and stability. A summary of injuries and treatment may be found in Table 7.2. Treatment of more minor injuries begins with rest, ice, nonsteroidal anti-inflammatories (NSAIDS), and gentle range of motion. Otherwise, conservative treatment is aimed at symptom management and neuromuscular and mechanical optimization with a rehabilitation protocol. Gymnasts with neck pain may have deficits with muscular recruitment, postural stability, oculomotor control, or have relative mobility deficits in the cervical and thoracic spine or the shoulder girdle. These should be addressed for optimized mechanics and decreased cervical spine load. Other targeted interventions

Table 7.2 Management of cervical spine injuries

Injury	Mechanism-pathophysiology	Presentation	Diagnostic testing	Treatment	Return to play
Cervical radiculopathy from disc herniation	Spinal nerve root compression from acute disc herniation	Unilateral radiating pain, tingling, numbness, weakness in spinal root distribution	MRI, possible EMG for radiculopathy	Symptomatic conservative treatment including physical therapy, medications, epidural steroid injection, possible surgical evaluation (Anterior cervical discectomy and fusion [(ACDF)] most common)	Absolute contra-indication: symptomatic disc herniation, neurologic deficit, decreased ROM. Return to play: asymptomatic may return to play even with ACDF
Cervical stenosis	Congenital or acquired narrowing of central spinal canal (<13 mm) possibly leading to spinal cord impingement	May include signs or symptoms of myelopathy: loss of finger dexterity, balance, upper motor neuron signs, burning pain, sensory loss, +/− weakness	X-ray, MRI, possible CT myelogram	Symptomatic conservative treatment including physical therapy, medications, epidural steroid injection, possible surgical evaluation	Torg ratio <0.8 has poor positive predictive value, but if asymptomatic no contra-indication; absolute contra-indication: cervical myelopathy, decreased ROM, neurologic deficit
Stinger	Traction, compression, or direct trauma, resulting in transient neurapraxic injuries to the brachial plexus or cervical nerve roots most commonly upper trunk, C5-6.	Unilateral upper extremity neurologic deficit, burning pain, +/− weakness	X-ray (flexion/extension), MRI, may consider brachial plexus MRI, EMG for prognosis and diagnosis	Symptomatic rest, pain control, rehabilitation program, eliminate predisposing factors. Unclear evidence for cervical collars, B vitamins, epidural steroid injection	Same day return to play: First episode or second in separate seasons with rapid resolution and normal exam. Evaluation for return/relative contra-indication: 1st or 2nd with persistent signs or symptoms >24 h or ≥3 episodes, absolute contra-indication: Persistent pain, decreased ROM, neurologic deficit

Condition	Etiology	Symptoms	Diagnostics	Treatment	Return to play
Transient quadraparesis	Transient neurologic Episode encompassing sensory symptoms with or without motor changes resolving within 48 hours	Burning pain, numbness, tingling, sensation loss, +/− weakness or complete paralysis	X-ray (flexion/ extension), MRI (for any spinal cord edema, structural abnormalities/compression or functional reserve), possible CT to rule out bony injury, possible somatosensory evoked potential for myelopathy	Initial full cervical precautions, spine board, transfer, management of airway, breathing, circulation. Use of corticosteroids and systemic hypothermia remain controversial Symptomatic treatment with rest, pain control, rehabilitation program, eliminate predisposing factors	May return if 1st episode, resolution of all signs and symptoms, full ROM, no instability for functional stenosis Relative contra-indication: 2nd episode, functional stenosis, single-level Klippel-Feil, healed cervical fracture, single-level cervical decompression and fusion without stenosis, small disc herniation or spondylosis without functional stenosis, absolute contra-indication: >2 episodes, cervical myelopathy, decreased ROM, any neurologic deficit, predisposing os odontoideum, Klippel-Feil fusion >2 levels, atlanto-occipital fusion, or brain stem signs (Arnold-Chiari or basilar invagination)
C1 (Jefferson), C2 (Hangman's) fractures	Axial loading, hyperflexion or hyperextension with vertebral fracture	Localized neck pain +/− neurologic deficit	X-ray, MRI	Cervical immobilization, neurosurgical consultation	Healed fracture with normal ROM may return to play; absolute contra-indication continued instability, C1–2 fusion
Atlanto-axial instability	Congenital (Down syndrome), degenerative (RA, JRA), traumatic, infectious	Unsteady gait, paresthesia, loss of bowel/bladder control	X-ray	Surgical evaluation	Absolute contra-indication: C1–2 fusion or continued hypermobility/instability

Adapted from [48, 51, 54, 55, 61, 62]

MRI magnetic resonance imaging, *CT* computed tomography, *EMG* electromyography, *RA* rheumatoid arthritis, *JRA* juvenile rheumatoid arthritis, *ROM* range of motion, *ACDF* anterior cervical discectcmy and fusion such as manual therapies, massage, dry needling, or trigger point injections for myofascial pain may be helpful.

Currently, there is no high-level evidence regarding return-to-play after cervical spine injury; instead, this decision is made on an individual basis using best clinical judgment. In general, athletes with persistent neurologic injury should not return to activity. Those with stable spinal fusion and complete recovery may return to sport [48, 54]. Most sources indicate that athletes with spinal cord injury or persistent neurologic deficits should not return to contact sports. However, each determination should be made on a case-by-case basis via a shared decision-making model. There is likely a role for adaptive gymnastics activity.

References

1. Harmon KG, Drezner J, Gammons M, Guskiewicz K, Halstead M, Herring S, et al. American Medical Society for Sports Medicine position statement: concussion in sport. Clin J Sport Med. 2013;23(1):1–18.
2. Lumba-Brown A, Yeates K, Sarmiento K, Al E. Diagnosis and management of mild traumatic brain injury in children: a systematic review. JAMA Pediatr. 2018;172:e182847.
3. Lumba-Brown A, Yeates K, Sarmiento K, Al E. Centers for disease control and prevention guideline on the diagnosis and management of mild traumatic brain injury among children. JAMA Pediatrics. 2018;172(11):e182853.
4. Hootman JM, Dick R, Agel J. Epidemiology of collegiate injuries for 15 sports: summary and recommendations for injury prevention initiatives. J Athl Train. 2007;42(2):311–9.
5. Giza CC, Kutcher JS, Ashwal S, Barth J, Getchius TSD, Gioia GA, et al. Summary of evidence-based guideline update: evaluation and management of concussion in sports. Neurology. 2013;80(24):2250–7.
6. Singh S, Smith GA, Fields SK, McKenzie LB. Gymnastics-related injuries to children treated in emergency departments in the United States, 1990–2005. Pediatrics. 2008;121(4):e954–60.
7. Edouard P, Steffen K, Junge A, Leglise M, Soligard T, Engebretsen L. Gymnastics injury incidence during the 2008, 2012 and 2016 Olympic Games: analysis of prospectively collected surveillance data from 963 registered gymnasts during Olympic Games. Br J Sports Med. 2018;52(7):475–81.
8. Thomas RE, Thomas BC. A systematic review of injuries in gymnastics. Phys Sportsmed. 2019;47:96–121.
9. O'Kane JW, Levy MR, Pietila KE, Caine DJ, Schiff MA. Survey of injuries in Seattle area levels 4 to 10 female club gymnasts. Clin J Sport Med. 2011;21(6):486–92.
10. McCrory P, Meeuwisse W, Dvorak J, Aubry M, Bailes J, Broglio S, et al. Consensus statement on concussion in sport—the 5th international conference on concussion in sport held in Berlin, October 2016. Br J Sports Med. 2017;51(11):838 LP-47.
11. McCrea M, Barr WB, Guskiewicz K, Randolph C, Marshall SW, Cantu R, et al. Standard regression-based methods for measuring recovery after sport-related concussion. J Int Neuropsychol Soc JINS. 2005;11(1):58–69.
12. Collins MW, Iverson GL, Lovell MR, McKeag DB, Norwig J, Maroon J. On-field predictors of neuropsychological and symptom deficit following sports-related concussion. Clin J Sport Med. 2003;13(4):222–9.
13. Meehan WP 3rd, d'Hemecourt P, Comstock RD. High school concussions in the 2008–2009 academic year: mechanism, symptoms, and management. Am J Sports Med. 2010;38(12):2405–9.

14. McCrory P, Meeuwisse W, Johnston K, Dvorak J, Aubry M, Molloy M, et al. Consensus statement on concussion in sport – the 3rd international conference on concussion in sport held in Zurich, November 2008. PMR. 2009;1(5):406–20.
15. Mansell JL, Tierney RT, Higgins M, McDevitt J, Toone N, Glutting J. Concussive signs and symptoms following head impacts in collegiate athletes. Brain Inj. 2010;24(9):1070–4.
16. McCrory P, Meeuwisse W, Aubry M, Cantu B, Dvorak J, Echemendia R, et al. Consensus statement on concussion in sport–the 4th international conference on concussion in sport held in Zurich, November 2012. J Sci Med Sport. 2013;16(3):178–89.
17. Osmond MH, Klassen TP, Wells GA, Davidson J, Correll R, Boutis K, et al. Validation and refinement of a clinical decision rule for the use of computed tomography in children with minor head injury in the emergency department. CMAJ. 2018;190(27):E816–e22.
18. McCrea M, Kelly JP, Randolph C, Kluge J, Bartolic E, Finn G, et al. Standardized assessment of concussion (SAC): on-site mental status evaluation of the athlete. J Head Trauma Rehabil. 1998;13(2):27–35.
19. Maddocks DL, Dicker GD, Saling MM. The assessment of orientation following concussion in athletes. Clin J Sport Med. 1995;5(1):32–5.
20. Echemendia RJ, Meeuwisse W, McCrory P, Davis GA, Putukian M, Leddy J, et al. The sport concussion assessment tool 5th edition (SCAT5): background and rationale. Br J Sports Med. 2017;51(11):848–50.
21. Davis GA, Purcell L, Schneider KJ, Yeates KO, Gioia GA, Anderson V, et al. The child sport concussion assessment tool 5th edition (Child SCAT5): background and rationale. Br J Sports Med. 2017;51(11):859–61.
22. Schatz P, Pardini JE, Lovell MR, Collins MW, Podell K. Sensitivity and specificity of the ImPACT Test Battery for concussion in athletes. Arch Clin Neuropsychol. 2006;21(1):91–9.
23. American Academy of Family Physicians, American Academy of Pediatrics, American College of Sports Medicine and American Medical Society for Sports Medicine. Preparticipation physical evaluation. 4th ed; 2010. p. 168.
24. Seto CK. The preparticipation physical examination: an update. Clin Sports Med. 2011;30(3):491–501.
25. Schneider KJ, Leddy JJ, Guskiewicz KM, Seifert T, McCrea M, Silverberg ND, et al. Rest and treatment/rehabilitation following sport-related concussion: a systematic review. Br J Sports Med. 2017;51(12):930–4.
26. Johnson RS, Provenzano MK, Shumaker LM, McLeod TCV, Bacon CEW. The effect of cognitive rest as part of postconcussion management for adolescent athletes: a critically appraised topic. J Sport Rehabil. 2017;26(5):437–46.
27. Thomas DG, Apps JN, Hoffmann RG, McCrea M, Hammeke T. Benefits of strict rest after acute concussion: a randomized controlled trial. Pediatrics. 2015;135(2):213–23.
28. Gagnon I, Grilli L, Friedman D, Iverson GL. A pilot study of active rehabilitation for adolescents who are slow to recover from sport-related concussion. Scand J Med Sci Sports. 2016;26(3):299–306.
29. Gagnon I, Galli C, Friedman D, Grilli L, Iverson GL. Active rehabilitation for children who are slow to recover following sport-related concussion. Brain Inj. 2009;23(12):956–64.
30. Leddy JJ, Kozlowski K, Donnelly JP, Pendergast DR, Epstein LH, Willer B. A preliminary study of subsymptom threshold exercise training for refractory post-concussion syndrome. Clin J Sport Med. 2010;20(1):21–7.
31. Silverberg ND, Iverson GL. Is rest after concussion "the best medicine?": recommendations for activity resumption following concussion in athletes, civilians, and military service members. J Head Trauma Rehabil. 2013;28(4):250–9.
32. Moser RS, Glatts C, Schatz P. Efficacy of immediate and delayed cognitive and physical rest for treatment of sports-related concussion. J Pediatr. 2012;161(5):922–6.
33. Moser RS, Schatz P, Glenn M, Kollias KE, Iverson GL. Examining prescribed rest as treatment for adolescents who are slow to recover from concussion. Brain Inj. 2015;29(1):58–63.

34. Teleanu RI, Vladacenco O, Teleanu DM, Epure DA. Treatment of pediatric migraine: a review. Maedica. 2016;11(2):136–43.
35. Venter RE. Role of sleep in performance and recovery of athletes: a review article. S Afr J Res Sport Ph Edu Recreation. 2012;34(1):167–84.
36. Kemp S, Biswas R, Neumann V, Coughlan A. The value of melatonin for sleep disorders occurring post-head injury: a pilot RCT. Brain Inj. 2004;18(9):911–9.
37. Mollayeva T, Pratt B, Mollayeva S, Shapiro CM, Cassidy JD, Colantonio A. The relationship between insomnia and disability in workers with mild traumatic brain injury/concussion: insomnia and disability in chronic mild traumatic brain injury. Sleep Med. 2016;20:157–66.
38. Panjabi MM, Cholewicki J, Nibu K, Grauer J, Babat LB, Dvorak J. Critical load of the human cervical spine: an in vitro experimental study. Clin Biomech (Bristol, Avon). 1998;13(1):11–7.
39. Eckner JT, Oh YK, Joshi MS, Richardson JK, Ashton-Miller JA. Effect of neck muscle strength and anticipatory cervical muscle activation on the kinematic response of the head to impulsive loads. Am J Sports Med. 2014;42(3):566–76.
40. Collins CL, Fletcher EN, Fields SK, Kluchurosky L, Rohrkemper MK, Comstock RD, et al. Neck strength: a protective factor reducing risk for concussion in high school sports. J Prim Prev. 2014;35(5):309–19.
41. Le Flao E, Brughelli M, Hume PA, King D. Assessing head/neck dynamic response to head perturbation: a systematic review. Sports Med. 2018;48(11):2641–58.
42. Daly RM, Bass SL, Finch CF. Balancing the risk of injury to gymnasts: how effective are the counter measures? Br J Sports Med. 2001;35(1):8–18; quiz 9
43. Makdissi M, Darby D, Maruff P, Ugoni A, Brukner P, McCrory PR. Natural history of concussion in sport: markers of severity and implications for management. Am J Sports Med. 2010;38(3):464–71.
44. Marar M, McIlvain NM, Fields SK, Comstock RD. Epidemiology of concussions among United States high school athletes in 20 sports. Am J Sports Med. 2012;40(4):747–55.
45. Barlow KM, Crawford S, Stevenson A, Sandhu SS, Belanger F, Dewey D. Epidemiology of postconcussion syndrome in pediatric mild traumatic brain injury. Pediatrics. 2010;126(2):e374–81.
46. Clarke KS. Epidemiology of athletic neck injury. Clin Sports Med. 1998;17(1):83–97.
47. Puvanesarajah V, Qureshi R, Cancienne JM, Hassanzadeh H. Traumatic sports-related cervical spine injuries. Clin Spine Surg. 2017;30(2):50–6.
48. Schroeder GD, Vaccaro AR. Cervical spine injuries in the athlete. J Am Acad Orthop Surg. 2016;24(9):e122–33.
49. Nalliah RP, Anderson IM, Lee MK, Rampa S, Allareddy V, Allareddy V. Epidemiology of hospital-based emergency department visits due to sports injuries. Pediatr Emerg Care. 2014;30(8):511–5.
50. Chang D, Bosco JA. Cervical spine injuries in the athlete. Bull NYU Hosp Jt Dis. 2006;64(3–4):119–29.
51. Concannon LG, Harrast MA, Herring SA. Radiating upper limb pain in the contact sport athlete: an update on transient quadriparesis and stingers. Curr Sports Med Rep. 2012;11(1):28–34.
52. Cantu RC. Stingers, transient quadriplegia, and cervical spinal stenosis: return to play criteria. Med Sci Sports Exerc. 1997;29(7 Suppl):S233–5.
53. Torg JS, Corcoran TA, Thibault LE, Pavlov H, Sennett BJ, Naranja RJ Jr, et al. Cervical cord neurapraxia: classification, pathomechanics, morbidity, and management guidelines. J Neurosurg. 1997;87(6):843–50.
54. Jeyamohan S, Harrop JS, Vaccaro A, Sharan AD. Athletes returning to play after cervical spine or neurobrachial injury. Curr Rev Musculoskelet Med. 2008;1(3–4):175–9.
55. Nagoshi N, Tetreault L, Nakashima H, Nouri A, Fehlings MG. Return to play in athletes with spinal cord concussion: a systematic literature review. Spine J. 2017;17(2):291–302.
56. Yamaguchi JT, Hsu WK. Intervertebral disc herniation in elite athletes. Int Orthop. 2019;43(4):833–40.

57. Snyder RL. Neck injuries. In: Madden CC, Putukian M, McCarty E, Young C, editors. Netter's sports medicine. 2nd ed. Philadelphia: Elsevier, Inc.; 2018.
58. C Tong H, J Haig A, Yamakawa K. The Spurling test and cervical radiculopathy. Spine. 2002;27(2):156–9.
59. Silver JR, Silver DD, Godfrey JJ. Injuries of the spine sustained during gymnastic activities. Br Med J (Clin Res Ed). 1986;293(6551):861–3.
60. Kruse D, Lemmen B. Spine injuries in the sport of gymnastics. Curr Sports Med Rep. 2009;8(1):20–8.
61. Sedgley MD, Cothran VE. Cervical spine injuries. Curr Sports Med Rep. 2017;16(6):379–80.
62. Joaquim AF, Hsu WK, Patel AA. Cervical spine surgery in professional athletes: a systematic review. Neurosurg Focus. 2016;40(4):E10.
63. Lee SW. Musculoskeletal injuries and conditions: assessment and management. New York: Demos Medical; 2017.

Chapter 8
Spine Injuries in Gymnasts

Steven Makovitch and Christine Eng

8.1 Thoracic and Lumbar Spine

8.1.1 Epidemiology

Low back pain is common in the general population, with a lifetime prevalence as high as 84% [1]. The complaint of low back pain by the gymnast is no exception and is also highly prevalent. Studies have documented the prevalence of back pain in the gymnast ranging anywhere from 25% to 85% [2–8]. This wide variation exists due to the heterogeneity of study populations. A Swedish study of high-level athletes which included 26 females and 26 males from the national gymnastics team reported the prevalence of back pain at 65.4% and 84.6% in females and males, respectively. Back pain was defined as prior or present pain in the thoracic or lumbar spine of greater than 1 week or of recurrent episodes regardless of duration. Male gymnasts had the highest percentage of pain rated as severe as compared with other sports [7]. A high incidence of low back pain has also been noted in rhythmic gymnastics. A small, prospective study of 7 adolescent, elite rhythmic gymnasts found 6 out of 7 participants (86%) reported back pain at some point during the 7-week study period [9].

Reports of spine injuries in the gymnast are also common. An epidemiological study of female collegiate gymnasts from the 1988–1989 through 2003–2004 seasons revealed that low back strains were the third most common practice and competition injury reported at 6% and 3% of all injuries, respectively. However, this injury surveillance data only captured acute injuries [10]. Another 18-month prospective study of Australian elite and sub-elite female gymnasts found that lower back injuries were the second most common injury reported at 14.9% of all injuries

---

S. Makovitch (✉) · C. Eng
Harvard Medical School, Department of Physical Medicine and Rehabilitation, Spaulding Rehabilitation Hospital, Charlestown, MA, USA
e-mail: smakovitch@partners.org; Ceng1@partners.org

[11]. A more recent analysis of women's gymnastics data from the NCAA Injury Surveillance Program during the 2009–2010 through 2013–2014 academic years reported trunk injuries as the third most frequent injury at 13.4%. Trunk injuries included the chest, abdomen, upper back, and lower back [12]. Data from a single institution over a 21-year period in precollegiate female gymnasts found an overall incidence of back injuries of 11.1% [13]. A study of level 4–10 female gymnasts, which classified injuries into acute and overuse, found that 8.8% of acute injuries involved the mid and low back and 18% of overuse injuries involved the low back [14]. Further large-scale studies are needed to specify back injury patterns related to gender, age, competitive level, type of injury, and location.

Given the high prevalence of back-related pain and injuries in the active gymnast, there is concern for repercussions later in life. Conflicting data exists on this question, although it appears most studies suggest no difference in back pain compared with the general population. A study of 64 former elite female gymnasts who competed during the 1970s showed no increased prevalence of back pain compared to age-matched controls. However, the authors do point out that over time, the demands of gymnastics training have become more complex with increased stress to the spine [15]. Another study looked at both former elite male and female athletes, including gymnasts, with a mean follow-up of 13 years. Despite significantly more radiographic abnormalities in the thoracic and lumbar spine, there was no increased report of back pain compared to controls. In fact, the frequency of back pain in male gymnasts decreased from 85% to 67% [16].

8.1.2 Biomechanics

The mechanical load of the spine in gymnastics has been noted to reach or be close to the limits of tissue tolerances [17]. Modern gymnastics tends to emphasize high-speed extension and flexion motions. This is particularly apparent with release skills, such as a Tkatchev release on high bar and uneven bars, and dismounts. Landings with partially completed somersaults and twists increase these rapid forces [18]. Injury or tissue damage occurs when the limits of tissue tolerances are exceeded in one traumatic failure or in repeated micro-failures [17].

Biomechanical studies have shown incredible amounts of force generation in the gymnasts' spine. During a giant swing on uneven bars or high bar prior to a Tkatchev release, shear force at L5-S1 is about 4 times one's body weight. Average compressive landing forces at the L5-S1 level in the gymnast's spine have been calculated at 11.6 and 14.8 times body weight for a forward and backward salto, respectively. Maximum compressive forces were found during a backward salto landing at 40 times body weight. Average landing shear forces at the L5-S1 level have also been calculated at 1.4 and 2.2 times body weight for a forward and backward salto, respectively [19].

Given the high compressive and shear forces to the spine, proper landing mechanics in gymnastics are vital. Maximum shear forces occur at 40–45 ms immediately after touchdown and were found to be 5.5 times body weight during a backward somersault landing. Appropriate core strength also cannot be understated as the load to the erector spinae musculature has been calculated at 14 times body weight [19].

Examination of a gymnast's everyday posture has been found to correlate with their landing mechanics. A biomechanical study completed in female elite gymnasts found the static posture of the lower lumbar spinal segments (L3–L5) was highly predictive of spinal postures during various landings. Gymnasts were found to land with a lower lumbar spinal posture close to or beyond their active end range of spinal flexion and experienced ground reaction forces 5–13 times their body weight [20].

The notable increased spinal loading in gymnastics does confer some benefits and has been found to be a powerful osteogenic stimulus. A study comparing elite prepubertal female gymnasts to swimmers found that the gymnasts had a significantly higher bone mineral density of the spine tested at L2–L4 [21]. Gymnastics exposure has also been found associated with shorter, wider vertebral bodies (tested at L3), yielding greater axial compressive strength and lower fracture risk [22].

8.1.3 History and Examination

A detailed history and physical examination is the first step in the evaluation of the gymnast with back pain. As with any pain history, factors to explore include timing, location, quality, severity, frequency, exacerbating or alleviating factors, and associated signs or symptoms. The clinician should determine if the pain is due to a traumatic injury versus a more chronic condition. Whether or not there is a mechanical bias for onset or relief of pain, such as flexion, extension, or rotation of the gymnast's spine, may not only lend support to a diagnosis but also help with directing a rehabilitation plan. Referral patterns of pain and presence of associated neurological symptoms such as numbness, tingling, or weakness should be obtained. An important task of the history is to always help rule out rare, but serious causes of back pain, commonly referred to as "red flag" symptoms. Questioning the presence of red flag symptoms such as weakness, bowel or bladder changes, weight loss, and fever should always be part of the history.

Specific details of pain referral patterns can be helpful in narrowing down the differential diagnosis. In the thoracic spine region, there is the possibility of referred pain from the cervical spine or visceral organs. The classic example is gallbladder disorders referring to the inferior angle of the scapula region. However, many visceral structures can refer pain to the thoracic region, such as the heart (C8-T4), esophagus (T4–6), stomach and duodenum (T6–10), and spleen (T7–10) [23]. It is also important to elucidate a history of systemic symptoms including fevers, skin rashes, and a history of inflammatory bowel disorders or rheumatological disorders.

Examination of the spine should be thorough and include inspection, palpation, range of motion, a detailed neurological examination, and special provocative maneuvers. Visualization of the spine and posture wearing a gown open to the back is important to look for scoliosis, exaggerated lumbar lordosis or thoracic kyphosis, pelvic tilt, and superficial skin conditions. The spine of a gymnast is typically extremely flexible, and if focal restriction is noted, further investigation is warranted. Palpation should include the spinous processes, paraspinal musculature, ribs, gluteal musculature, sacrum, and sacroiliac joints. The spine and surrounding muscles such as the paraspinals, quadratus lumborum, and gluteal musculature should be palpated for pain and myofascial trigger points. A detailed neurological examination should be conducted including reflexes, strength, and sensation, especially in the setting of any lower limb or radicular symptoms. The presence of dural tension should also be evaluated with straight leg raise or seated slump testing (Fig. 8.1).

The examiner must also consider the interaction of hip and sacroiliac joint-related conditions and their potential role in causing low back pain. Likewise, examination of the shoulder must be considered in the gymnast with thoracic pain. Even in the clinic setting, simple gymnastics-specific screening maneuvers such as a static bridge may be performed. This allows for evaluation of functional motion across the gymnast's shoulders, thoracolumbar spine, and hip regions looking for hypomobility or hinge points (Fig. 8.2).

8.1.4 Diagnostics and Imaging

It is well documented that imaging findings of spinal pathology in the general population are common even in asymptomatic individuals, especially with increasing age [24]. Therefore, correlating imaging findings with a detailed history and examination is of great value. However, one must keep in mind that back pain in the pediatric and adolescent population is unique and has been found to correlate more closely with pathological imaging findings [7, 25]. Diagnosing a gymnast with a simple muscular strain without conducting an appropriate investigation runs the risk of delaying proper diagnosis and management [25].

Multiple studies have shown a correlation between imaging findings and back pain in the gymnast. A prospective study of 19 Olympic-level female gymnasts using MRI found current low back pain to significantly correlate with findings of spondylolysis and spondylolisthesis. Bilateral pedicle bone marrow edema and muscle strain were also only found in the symptomatic gymnasts [26]. Another study of high-level female gymnasts not only found a correlation of back pain with MRI abnormalities but also found that MRI abnormalities increased with older age and with training greater than 15 hours per week [2]. Other studies found that male gymnasts have increased disc degeneration when compared to nonathletes, which also correlated with back pain [7, 8].

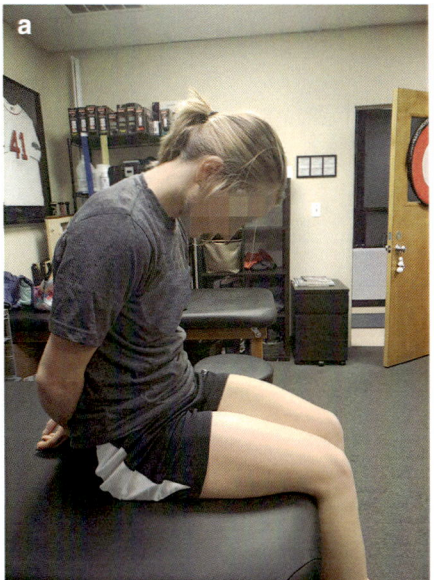
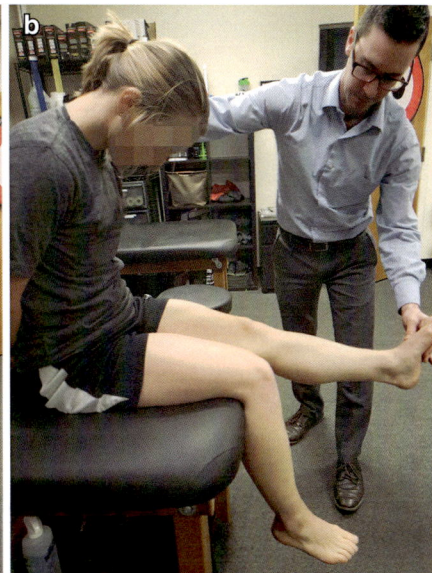
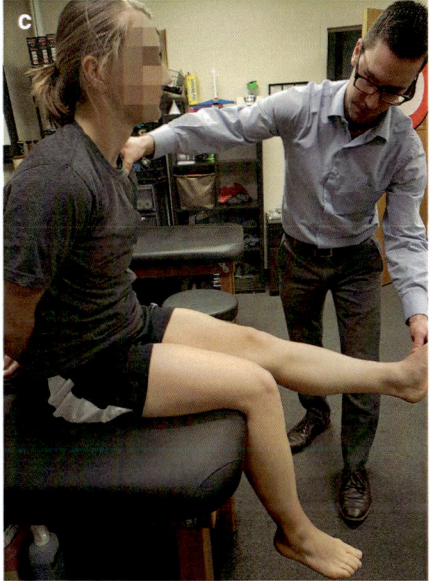

Fig. 8.1 Seated slump test is a neural tension test thought to examine irritability of structures including meninges, spinal nerve roots, and sciatic nerve. It also can be used to evaluate for acute disc herniation. (**a**) Position 1: patient in slumped position at edge of table with head forward. (**b**) Position 2: examiner may add gentle overpressure with gentle knee extension and ankle dorsiflexion with reproduction of typical symptoms. (**c**) Position 3: cervical extension in the slumped position with improvement of symptoms

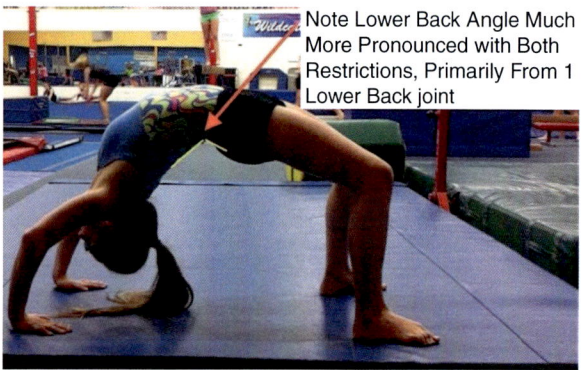

Fig. 8.2 Bridge evaluation with single hinge point, poor shoulder angle, and hip restriction

There are multiple imaging modalities of interest in evaluating the gymnast's spine which will be discussed according to workup for each specific spinal pathology. For a general overview of diagnostic options, refer to the cervical spine section in Chap. 7. In addition to imaging, the presence of any red flag symptoms or in the appropriate clinical setting, further laboratory workup should also be considered. Basic labs to consider include complete blood count with differential, blood cultures, erythrocyte sedimentation rate (ESR), and C-reactive protein (CRP). Additional neurological testing to consider in the setting of weakness or radicular symptoms include electrodiagnostic testing with electromyography and nerve conduction studies. There may also be a role for somatosensory evoked potentials to evaluate for myelopathy or dorsal column involvement [27].

8.1.5 Specific Conditions

8.1.5.1 Spondylolysis and Spondylolisthesis

Spondylolysis is a defect through the pars interarticularis of the vertebral arch which may occur unilaterally or bilaterally (Fig. 8.3). This may progress to spondylolisthesis, either anterior (anterolisthesis) or posterior (retrolisthesis), which is translation of one vertebrae on another. Spondylolisthesis can be classified into five different types including dysplastic (congenital), isthmic, degenerative, traumatic, and pathological [28]. The isthmic type of spondylolisthesis is the most common form seen in gymnasts and includes any defect to the pars interarticularis [29].

Spondylolysis is generally thought to result from traumatic microfracture with subsequent progressive fracture from repetitive stress or a fatigue fracture from repetitive overload, especially hyperextension [30]. Cadaveric studies have shown that repetitive mechanical fatigue can cause the neural arch to fracture when the cellular bone repair mechanisms are outpaced by damage. Also, adolescents and children have a more elastic intervertebral disc which allows increased stress through the bony pars [31]. Spondylolysis can also be thought of as existing on a

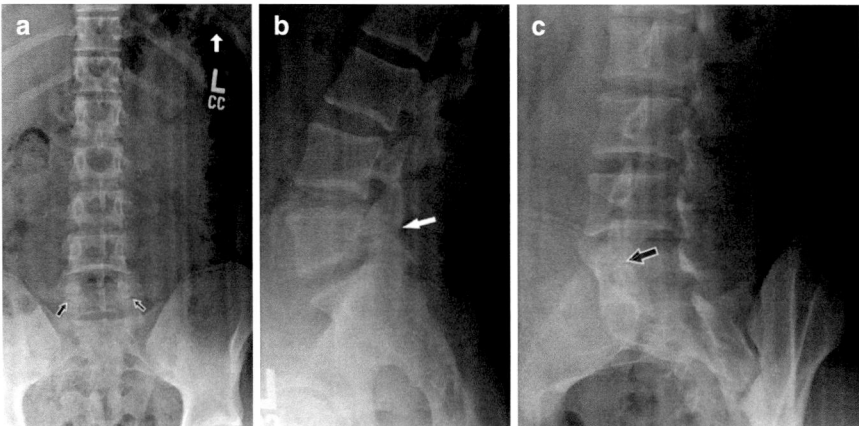

Fig. 8.3 Spondylolysis radiographs demonstrating bilateral spondylolysis pars defects at L5. (**a**) AP. (**b**) Lateral. (**c**) oblique view not typically necessary

continuum of pathology with three different subtypes. First, stress reactions are described as intraosseous edema with surrounding sclerosis of the pars, lamina, or pedicle without clear cortical or trabecular disruption. Second, a stress fracture is disruption of trabecular or cortical bone of the pars without a bony gap or lysis. Third, true spondylolysis or nonunion of the pars is when there is complete disruption of the pars interarticularis with a gap and surrounding sclerosis at the edges of the defect [32].

Spondylolysis has been reported to account for up to 40–50% of the cases of low back pain in the pediatric and adolescent sports orthopedic population [25, 33]. The diagnosis must therefore be considered in every adolescent gymnast who presents with functionally limiting low back pain [34]. In gymnasts, these lesions are most likely resultant from repetitive flexion and extension of the spine at the extreme ranges of motion, in addition to twisting maneuvers. The vast majority of lesions, up to 95%, occur at the L5 level [35]. The incidence of spondylolysis in the general population has been reported to be up to 8% [35, 36].

Spondylolisthesis is graded by the percentage of anterior displacement of one vertebrae on another, with grade I defined as 0–25%, grade II defined as 25–50%, grade III defined as 50–75%, grade IV defined as 75–100%, and grade V referring to complete anterior displacement, also known as spondyloptosis [37]. In most cases of spondylolisthesis, the majority of slippage has already occurred at the time of initial presentation [38]. The presence of spondylolisthesis in athletes with spondylolysis has been reported at about 30% [39].

Clinical presentation of spondylolysis and spondylolisthesis typically includes dull, achy, axial low back pain which can radiate into the buttocks and posterior thighs. Additionally, spondylolisthesis may present with radicular symptoms including numbness, tingling, or even weakness to the lower limbs due to nerve root compression. Pain is typically improved with rest and worsens with activity especially extension-based maneuvers.

Inspection typically reveals hyperlordosis of the lumbar region, but in some cases of spondylolisthesis, a kyphotic posture may be compensatory to reduce mechanical nerve root irritation [30]. With palpation, one should look for any indication of a step-off of the spinous processes indicating spondylolisthesis. Examination should include lumbar extension to see if typical pain is reproduced. A study in adolescent athletes found that pain with lumbar extension had a sensitivity and specificity of 81% and 40%, respectively, for detecting spondylolysis and therefore could serve as a good screening measure [40]. Historically, the one-legged hyperextension test is performed; however, this has not been shown reliable for detection of active spondylolysis [41]. Tight hamstrings may also be present, although the mechanism is not completely understood [42]. A detailed neurological examination of the lower limbs should also be conducted especially in the setting of any lower limb radicular symptoms including strength, reflexes, and evidence of dural tension signs (Fig. 8.1).

Imaging for Spondylolysis and Spondylolisthesis

Several imaging modalities have been described in identifying pars lesions including plain radiographs, bone scintigraphy (bone scan), CT, single-photon emission CT (SPECT) or SPECT-CT, and MRI [43]. There is controversy within the literature about the optimal use of each of these imaging modalities [34]. Standing anteroposterior and lateral radiographs are likely the most reasonable initial imaging evaluation. Although oblique radiographs have long been the standard for assessing pars defects, this adds increased radiation exposure, and no significant change in sensitivity or specificity has been noted between four-view and two-view radiographs [44]. Plain radiographs are neither sensitive nor specific. In gymnasts, rates of spondylolysis on plain radiographs have been found to range from 11% to 33% [3, 39, 45]. If X-rays are normal but clinical suspicion of a pars lesion is high, further imaging modalities are required.

Multiple algorithms exist for imaging choice after plain radiographs, and there is no clear consensus. Some recommend SPECT imaging, followed by CT with thin cuts through the level of pathology [6]. Others recommend MRI for early detection and CT in more persistent courses [43]. Each of these approaches has both advantages and shortcomings.

Although bone scans have been shown to have a relatively high sensitivity (84%), they also provide seven to nine times the effective radiation dose as a two-view radiograph. In addition, bone scans have the highest organ-specific absorbed dose compared to other modalities [46]. Given these findings, initial workup with a bone scan is not recommended especially in the younger gymnast.

CT scans, on the other hand, have been shown to provide double the radiation dose as a two-view radiograph [46]. CT is widely regarded as the gold standard for demonstrating the bony anatomy of the neural arch and best demonstrates incomplete and complete fractures [47]. Compared with a bone scan, they are unable to provide functional information about the rate of bone turnover and progression to a full pars fracture. In addition, approximately one in five stress injuries to the pars interarticularis will be missed on CT scans in pediatric patients with new-onset back pain [48].

Single-photon emission computed tomography (SPECT) is considered an extremely sensitive technique for early diagnosis of acute lysis [49]. SPECT is a nuclear medicine tomographic imaging technique detecting gamma ray emission which allows for three-dimensional reconstruction of images [50]. Increased radionuclide uptake in an intact pars, lamina, or pedicle is consistent with a stress reaction, and a relative decrease in tracer has been correlated with improvement of clinical symptoms. Therefore, SPECT may be predictive of the ability for lysis to heal [51]. Unfortunately, it is nonspecific, poor at detecting chronic lesion, and cannot distinguish between stress reaction and overt fractures [49]. In addition, it exposes the patient to increased ionizing radiation and provides little in the way of evaluation of other anatomic structures that may play a role in pain generation [52].

MRI has been shown to be superior in detecting early pars stress reactions that cannot be seen on plain films or CT and avoids radiation exposure entirely [49]. It also allows good visualization of other potential causes of low back pain such as a disc herniation [6]. Unfortunately, not all MRI protocols are optimal and vary depending on the institution. Fat suppressed fast spin T2-weighted images in the sagittal plane are considered critical in making the diagnosis on MRI [53]. Another sequence on MRI that has been shown helpful is the 3D volumetric interpolated breath-hold examination (VIBE). The VIBE sequence increases spatial resolution, improves image contrast, and appears to correlate well with CT in demonstrating the extent of fracture lines [52]. One study comparing CT to MRI with VIBE sequences showed that the MRI results were 100% accurate in detecting complete pars fractures [54]. Preferably, this is performed using a 3 T MRI magnet [52]. A grading system of pars fracture morphology using MRI has been described by Hollenberg and ranges from grade 0 to 4 (Table 8.1).

Although CT best demonstrates fracture size and extent, MRI is more likely to detect acute spondylolysis by way of marrow edema on fat-saturated T2-weighted images (Fig. 8.4) [47]. With advances in MRI technology, detection of spondylolysis has improved. In general, MRI should be considered first, given the lack of ionizing radiation and ability to detect other spinal pathology in the gymnast. If MRI is negative and clinical suspicion is high, it may be necessary to progress to CT or

Table 8.1 Hollenberg MRI classification for spondylolysis

Grade	Findings
0	Normal
1	Bone edema with intact cortices compatible with stress reaction
2	Incomplete stress fracture
3	Complete active fracture with accompanying bone marrow edema
4	Complete fracture without accompanying bone marrow edema, consistent with a chronic defect

Adapted from Ref. [55]

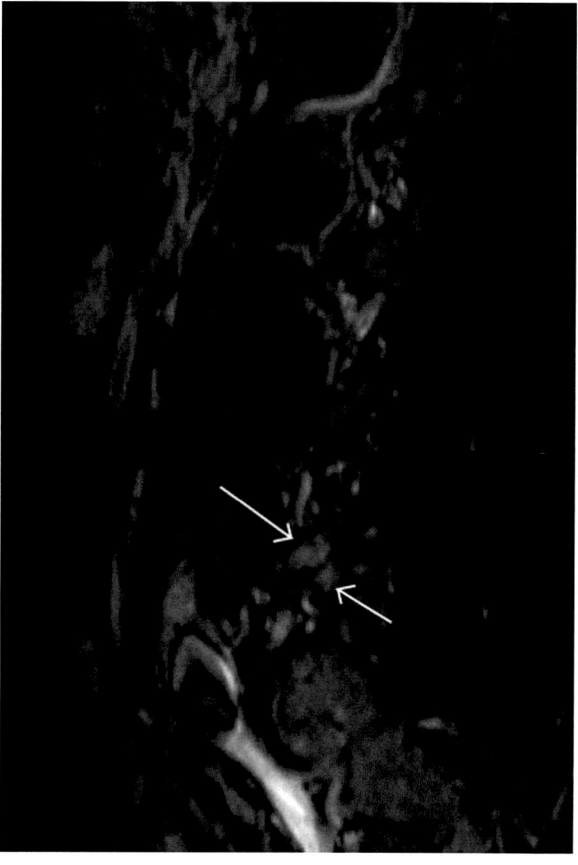

Fig. 8.4 MRI sagittal STIR sequence demonstrating left L5 pars defect (spondylolysis) with surrounding bone marrow edema suggestive of acute process

SPECT. In high-level gymnasts who need to return quickly, a CT at 3 months may be considered to assess healing progression.

Prognosis of Spondylolysis and Spondylolisthesis

Much about the natural history of spondylolysis and spondylolisthesis can be elucidated from a 45-year follow-up study of 500 first-grade children followed into adulthood. At the age of 6 years, 22 subjects (4.4%) were found to have either unilateral or bilateral pars defects. Healing of the pars defect was only found in three subjects, all with unilateral defects. All subjects with unilateral defects did not have spondylolisthesis [56].

Rate of progression was found to be low, and rates slowed over each decade after diagnosis. Initially, evidence of spondylolisthesis with an average translation of 11% was noted in 10–16 subjects with bilateral pars defects. Over the first decade, average progression was only 7%. Then for the second and third decade, it was 4% followed by 2% in the fourth decade [56]. Progression typically occurs during the growth spurt in adolescence and is more common in females. Also, progression is more common in a child or adolescent if initial translation is greater than 50%. After skeletal maturity, progression is usually minimal [38].

Prognosis in those with low-grade spondylolisthesis (grade I or II) is generally good and follows a similar clinical course to that of the general population [56]. A study of 86 athletes (24 of which were gymnasts) with a diagnosis of spondylolysis or spondylolisthesis ages 6–20 was followed for 5 years. In 36 of the athletes, no progression of spondylolisthesis was noted, and in 7 athletes, a decrease in translation was found. Of the 33 athletes who had progression, it was on average only 10.5%. Despite intensive daily training, the athletes had no symptoms during this period of observation [57]. Thus, most experts agree that there is no justification in general for advising children and adolescents with asymptomatic spondylolysis and low-grade spondylolisthesis to not participate in competitive sports [34, 38, 56, 57]. The same is true in gymnasts.

Regarding patients with grade III or IV spondylolisthesis, a long-term follow-up study over an average of 18 years was conducted. In those treated nonoperatively, disabling neurological deficits, disabling pain, or incontinence of the bowel or bladder did not develop. The patients were noted to lead surprisingly active lives, limiting themselves from few recreational endeavors [58].

Treatment of Spondylolysis and Spondylolisthesis

In general, the great majority of individuals with spondylolysis have excellent results with conservative management and are able to return to sport in 3–6 months [59]. There is, however, overall lack of consensus on the optimal management of spondylolysis. Treatment can be divided into those with the opportunity for bony healing and those with low chance of healing as determined by imaging findings. There is reasonable chance for healing if imaging demonstrates stress reaction, sclerosis only, hairline fracture, or minimal separation with or without cystic margins but no cortication. On the other hand, there is a low chance of healing with widely separated pars lesions and those with well corticated fracture margins [6, 60, 61].

Looking from another perspective, there is some evidence that radiographic healing is not required for good outcome. Retrospective studies have demonstrated that 70–90% of athletes with symptomatic spondylolysis and spondylolisthesis achieved good to excellent long-term outcomes and return to play even without radiographic bony fusion [59, 60, 62, 63].

In gymnasts with low healing potential, treatment is largely symptomatic. Rest is only prescribed until they are asymptomatic and have full spinal range of motion. After this point, they may be progressed more rapidly as tolerated [6].

For those with a chance for bony healing (unilateral defect, stress reaction only), consider starting with an initial period of rest from gymnastics followed by a graded rehab program [6]. Historically, it has been recommended to have strict rest for 3 months after diagnosis. However, a recent retrospective study of 196 adolescent athletes demonstrated earlier initiation of a physical therapy program at around

2 months resulted in quicker return to sport, on average 25 days sooner. There was no increased risk of adverse outcomes with this more aggressive protocol [64].

Physical therapy should be individualized to the gymnast's needs but in general should start with neutral spine stabilization exercises and low-impact aerobic exercise. When pain-free, the gymnast should gradually progress to increasing spinal motion to end range and then dynamic and plyometric strengthening. Final steps of the protocol should focus on integration of specific gymnastics skills with graded difficulty and increasing dynamic spinal motion with focus on correction of biomechanics to prevent injury (see Chaps. 11 and 12 for more information on rehab and return to sport).

Much debate exists regarding bracing, likely due to absent high-quality studies [59]. If there is a chance for bony healing, some authors advocate for bracing. Various brace types have been recommended and range from rigid braces such as a lumbosacral orthosis, to soft corsets. Overall, the results tend to be similar regardless of the type of brace and duration of brace use [34, 65, 66]. Rate of compliance with activity modification and rest is likely more important to clinical improvement than use of a brace [63]. If a brace is used, most clinicians recommend a period of 3 months, and gymnasts may be weaned out of the brace once asymptomatic, regardless of bony union on imaging [59].

Biomechanical data comparing various braces has shown that bracing reduced spinal load with certain movements, while other movements caused increased load, and no brace was found to be superior [67, 68]. Another biomechanical study found that use of a soft or rigid lumbosacral orthosis actually increased intersegmental spinal motion at the lumbosacral junction [69]. Bracing may restrict gross body motion and activity more so than stabilize the actual fracture site [34]. Therefore, its main role may be to serve as a reminder to the gymnast.

Conservative management of a gymnast with low-grade spondylolisthesis is similar to that of spondylolysis, given that translations rarely progress. Indications for surgical intervention include failure of a comprehensive conservative treatment plan for more than 6 months, persistent back pain, and pars nonunion at 9–12 months [70]. Additional indications include increasing pain, worsening neurological impairment, and progressive spondylolisthesis [71]. A pars repair can be considered for spondylolysis or grade I spondylolisthesis in the presence of normal disc height [70]. Direct repair is thought to be advantageous as it preserves spinal motion. There are several different surgical techniques used and all seem to demonstrate excellent results with 80–100% of athletes returning to their previous athletic activities [59]. Surgical fusion is considered with a grade II or higher spondylolisthesis, significant disc degeneration at the level of lysis, and patient age greater than 20 years old (Fig. 8.5) [71]. There is no clear recommendation with regard to return to play after fusion surgery for spondylolisthesis [72]. Most surgeons recommend return at 6 months for noncontact, low-impact sports and 12 months for contact sports [71].

Routine follow-up imaging is not necessary for older adolescents with isolated, unilateral defects who progress appropriately through treatment. However, the presence of spondylolisthesis, bilateral pars defects, or, possibly, a unilateral

Fig. 8.5 Grade IV spondylolisthesis in a competitive gymnast and diver who required surgical intervention

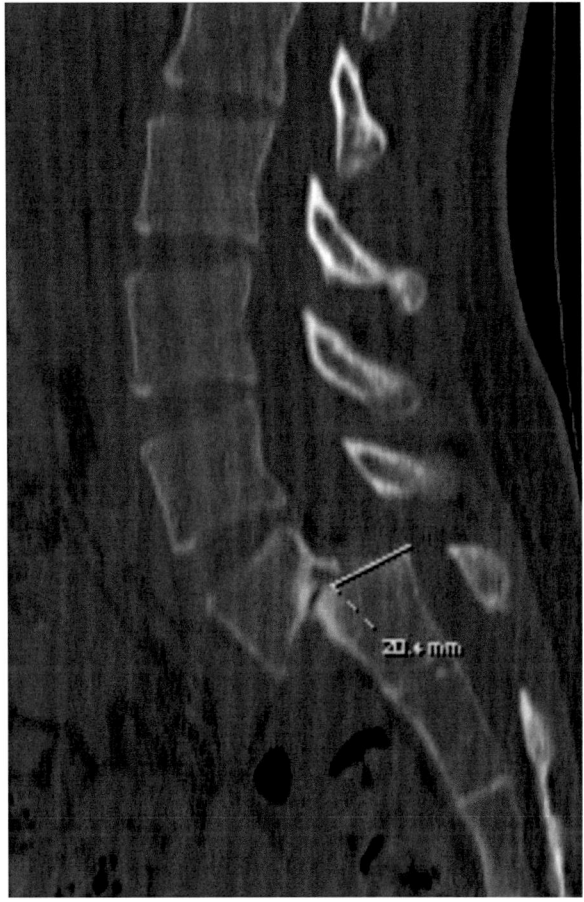

defect in a very young athlete has a higher risk of progression. Progression may be monitored with routine standing lateral radiographs every 6–12 months until skeletal maturity is reached [34, 73].

8.1.5.2 Scheuermann's Disease

Scheuermann's disease was first described in 1920 as a rigid kyphosis of the thoracic or thoracolumbar spine occurring in adolescents [74]. The disorder is characterized by radiographic findings of vertebral body wedging, vertebral endplate irregularity, diminished anterior vertebral growth, and intervertebral disc herniation (Schmorl's nodes) (Fig. 8.6) [75]. The most widely accepted diagnostic criteria was proposed by Sorensen which includes three adjacent wedged vertebrae, angled by at least 5 degrees [76]. For some authors, one wedged vertebra is sufficient for diagnosis if associated with irregular vertebral endplates [77]. Prevalence is about equal in

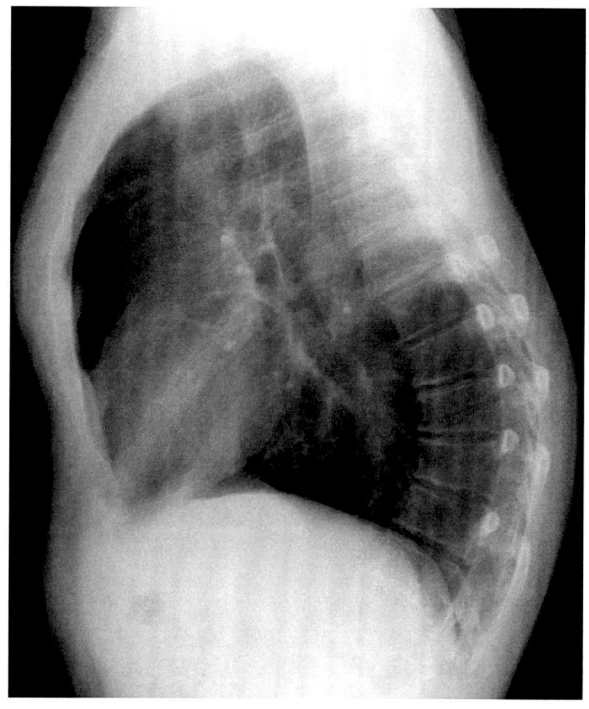

Fig. 8.6 Scheuermann's kyphosis on lateral view radiograph showing increased kyphosis, anterior wedging, and irregular vertebral endplates

males and females [74]. Two distinct patterns have been described. The thoracic pattern, type I, is the most common and generally involves more than one level. More rarely, type II occurs in the lumbar spine with less severe wedging and affects a single level [75, 78].

The exact etiology of Scheuermann's kyphosis is still unknown. A study of twins indicates that there is a major genetic contribution [79]. Histopathological studies have shown disorganized enchondral ossification, a reduction in collagen, and an increase in mucopolysaccharides in the endplates [80, 81]. There is also implication of either acute or repeated trauma to an immature spine especially in a sport such as gymnastics which involves repetitive loading of a flexed spine [82]. The prevalence of radiographic endplate abnormalities has been shown to be higher in athletes, particularly those involved in gymnastics [7, 83].

Clinical presentation most commonly includes a painful, fixed, dorsal kyphosis. Pain is typically mild to moderate, worse toward the end of the day or after physical activity, and relieved by rest [82]. Excessive dorsal kyphosis generally leads to non-structural lumbar hyperlordosis, pelvic anteversion, and rounding of the shoulders [76]. Long-term follow-up studies have shown an increased prevalence of back pain when compared to controls, which was unrelated to the degree or apex level of kyphosis [84, 85].

Workup with plain radiographs reveals the majority of diagnostic structural abnormalities. However, MRI is helpful in demonstrating Schmorl's nodes and disc prolapse beneath the vertebral apophyses and also helps to exclude discitis [75].

The majority of patients do well with conservative management. Treatment is aimed at reducing load to the anterior aspect of the spine and reducing pain. One study showed that an intensive rehabilitation program including physical therapy, osteopathy, postural education, and psychological support offered significant reduction in pain scores [86]. The focus of physical therapy should be on correcting pelvic tilt to reduce lumbar lordosis, increasing the strength of thoracic extensor musculature, and stretching tight musculature which typically includes the pectoralis major and hamstrings [77, 87].

Bracing should only be considered in an adolescent with a thoracic kyphosis over 55 degrees or a thoracolumbar kyphosis over 40 degrees. Bracing does not have an impact on more mature adolescents with a Risser sign of 4 or 5. Use of a thoracolumbosacral orthosis is preferred and should be worn for a minimum of 20 hours per day for 18 months [78]. A recent study showed that brace treatment with an average time of 14 hours per day for 23 months was not only effective in halting progression but also in partially correcting the degree of kyphosis even in severe cases of up to 90 degrees [87].

Surgical indications include neurological deficits due to spinal pathology. Relative indications for surgery include symptomatic thoracic kyphosis greater than 80 degrees and thoracolumbar kyphosis greater than 65 degrees when pain is unrelieved by conservative measures and when there is rapid curve progression [78].

8.1.5.3 Vertebral Ring Apophysis Fracture

Vertebral ring apophysis fracture, also known as limbus vertebra, is a defect in the vertebral body, caused by anterior, lateral, or posterior herniation of the nucleus pulposus through an immature ring apophysis, resulting in a triangular avulsion fragment [88]. Fracture of the vertebral ring apophysis is a rare but important cause of low back pain in the gymnast and generally occurs on the anterior portion of the vertebral body. The vertebral ring apophyses are located outside the epiphyseal plates of the vertebra both cranially and caudally. They start to appear around 5 years of age and fuse with rest of the body at 18–20 years. Due to this late closure, the apophyseal ring remains a weak point during adolescence [88].

Two mechanisms have been suggested to explain traumatic abnormalities of the vertebral ring apophysis: intravertebral disc herniation (marginal Schmorl's node) and failure in tension-shear forces [89]. Most cases of vertebral apophysis injuries have been found to occur in young, physically active individuals likely from trauma or muscular overload [89]. One study found that these injuries occurred only in athletes and were most commonly found in female elite gymnasts [89]. Another study of Olympic-level female gymnasts found anterior ring apophyseal injuries in 9 out of 19 gymnasts on MRI. The study also found a correlation between anterior ring apophyseal injuries and development of mild to moderate disc disease at the affected level [26].

Clinical presentation overall is variable. Some patients are asymptomatic while others complain of back pain or have positive dural tension signs. Those with avulsion of the posterior ring apophysis are more likely to have neurological symptoms due to irritation of the spinal cord [88]. Besides location, one study found that fragments of smaller size had no clinical significance, while large apophyseal fragments with associated disc herniation led to a greater chance of chronic back pain [90].

Initial imaging with plain radiographs may show an avulsion fragment. CT scan is the imaging modality of choice for diagnosis of an apophyseal fracture and will best demonstrate the size, shape, and location of the fracture (Fig. 8.7). CT imaging further helps to differentiate calcified or noncalcified fractures from lumbar disc herniations. However, MRI best shows the presence of a disc herniation or extrusion and whether there is neurological compression [91].

Surgical indications include a failed trial of conservative care (6–12 weeks), decline in neurological status, intolerable low back and/or leg pain, severely affected function (e.g., unable to participate in activities of daily living), and any signs of cauda equina syndrome. Currently, posterior discectomy with excision of a mobile osseous fragment without fusion is the preferred approach [92].

Unless red flag symptoms like neurological compromise are present, conservative management incudes rest, analgesics, and activity modification either with or

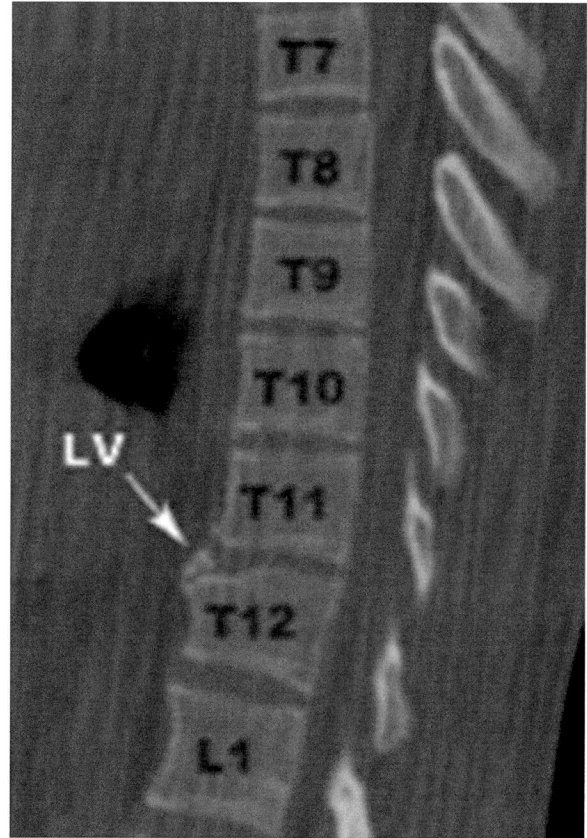

Fig. 8.7 Anterior ring apophysis fracture with anterior superior endplate deformity of T12 demonstrated on CT sagittal view. (*Adapted from Imaging Anatomy of the Human Spine. A Comprehensive Atlas Including Adjacent Structures. Scott E. Forseen MD, Neil M. Borden MD [image 4, page 160, Limbus vertebra]*)

without use of a spinal orthosis brace. The goal is to reduce and centralize pain, restore mobility, address functional limitations, and safely return the athlete to gymnastics. As with other spinal injuries in the skeletally immature athlete, an emphasis is placed on lumbopelvic stability, proper posture, and facilitating proper loading of the spine [93]. Less favorable responses to conservative management have been noted when both an apophyseal ring fracture and disc herniation are present with larger osseous fragments [92].

8.1.5.4 Scoliosis

Scoliosis is a deformity of the spine defined as a lateral curvature of the spine greater than 10 degrees. Scoliosis is traditionally categorized into pathological, degenerative, congenital, neuromuscular, and idiopathic forms. Most common in the gymnast is the idiopathic type which accounts for 75–80% of all scoliosis cases. Idiopathic scoliosis can be further characterized based on the timing of presentation into infantile (<3 years), juvenile (4–9 years), and adolescent (>10 years). The adolescent type accounts for about 90% of all idiopathic scoliosis cases with an estimated worldwide prevalence ranging from 0.47% to 5.2%. Females are affected twice as commonly as males and also have a greater risk of curvature progression [94].

Although a paucity of studies exists in gymnasts, a high incidence of scoliosis has been found specifically in female rhythmic gymnasts at 12%. The authors proposed that a triad of factors may contribute to this finding in gymnasts, including increased joint laxity, delayed growth and maturity, and chronic asymmetrical loading of the spine [95]. Another study looked at why those with idiopathic scoliosis may participate more in gymnastics. The authors found that idiopathic scoliosis was associated with higher joint laxity. Those with higher joint laxity have better adaptation to the sport and continued to practice gymnastics. Furthermore, the authors explain that gymnastics may be beneficial to patients with scoliosis by reinforcing the deep spinal muscles with proprioceptive activities. One must note that participation in sport was only about 2 hours per week, much lower than typical in competitive gymnastics [96].

Idiopathic scoliosis is typically noted due to a cosmetic deformity with asymmetry in the shoulders, hips, or trunk prompting referral for evaluation. There are mixed findings on whether pain is significantly associated with idiopathic scoliosis; however, it does not seem to be a problem for the majority of those affected. In most studies, pain has not shown a strong correlation with degree of curvature, untreated cases fare reasonably well from the perspective of back pain, and patients' self-perception of their image correlates with pain [97]. On the other hand, a 23-year follow-up of adolescents treated conservatively with bracing found significant limitations in everyday activities due to low back pain and neck-related impairment compared to healthy controls. In addition, back pain was found to be associated with curve progression [98].

The Adam's forward bend test (Fig. 8.8) is used as a screening exam to assess for rotational deformity as an indicator of scoliosis. The examiner stands behind the

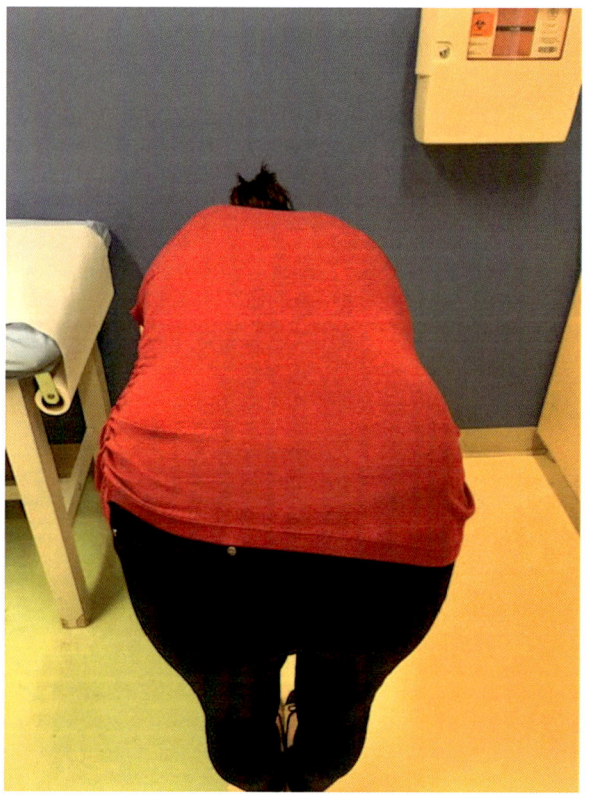

Fig. 8.8 Adam's forward bend test showing a left thoracic prominance

patient as they bend forward. Rotation of the thoracic vertebrae causes rotation and deformity of the attached ribs with elevation on the side of convexity and depression on the side of concavity [99]. A scoliometer can be used to measure the degree of rotational deformity. A reading of 5 degrees of rotation has been found to correspond to 20 degrees of coronal rotation on radiographs [100]. The Scoliosis Research Society (SRS) recommends an axial trunk rotation of 5–7° as a threshold for referral for X-ray [101].

The gold standard for visualizing scoliosis curvature is a standing PA radiograph of the spine. The coronal curvature can be evaluated by measuring the Cobb angle (Fig. 8.9). In the Cobb method, a line is drawn through the superior surface of the uppermost vertebra and inferior surface of the lowest vertebrae of the curve. The angle at the intersection of lines drawn perpendicular to the above two lines is the Cobb angle or the curvature of the scoliosis [102].

Curves progress in about two-thirds of patients before reaching skeletal maturity (Risser sign of ≥4 in females or 5 in males). However, progression is generally small, and only one-third of patients with scoliosis will experience more than a 10 degree increase in curve magnitude. Less than 10% will have an increase of 30 degrees or more [103]. The likelihood of progression varies depending on sex, curve magnitude, curve location, and maturity or remaining growth potential [103].

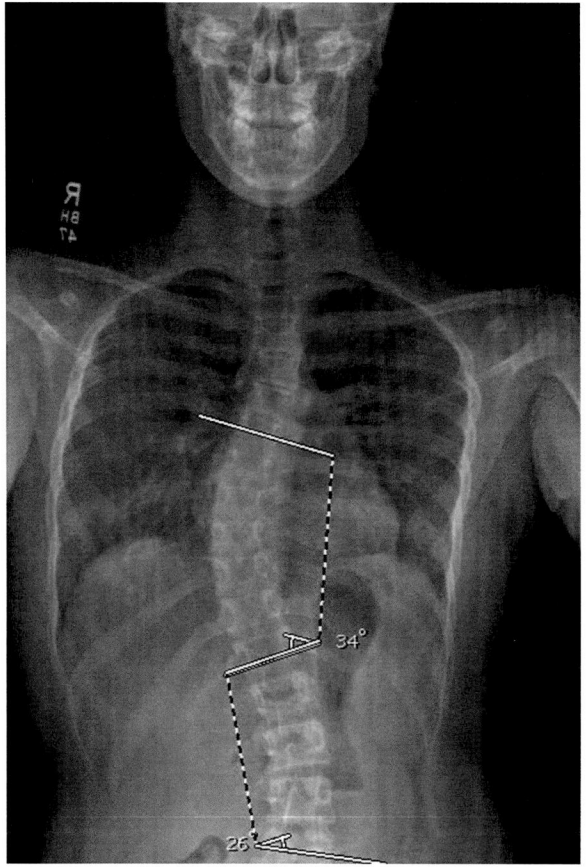

Fig. 8.9 Upright radiograph of scoliosis demonstrating Cobb angle in the thoracic and lumbar spine

Curves less than 30 degrees at skeletal maturity are less likely to continue to progress [104]. During the first 2 years of puberty when the peak growth velocity increases (11–13 years in girls and 13–15 years in boys), there is increased risk of progression. These gymnasts should be monitored more closely at 6-month intervals [105]. Progression may be monitored by way of axial trunk rotation using a scoliometer. This both reduces healthcare cost and reduces radiation exposure from follow-up radiographs [106].

Those with a Cobb angle of less than 20 degrees are usually observed, and exercise treatment is recommended. Bracing should be implemented with a Cobb angle of 30–40 degrees or if there is a Cobb angle of 20–29 degrees with substantial growth remaining (Risser sign 0–2) or curve progression (≥ 5 degrees over 3–6 months). Those with a Cobb angle of 40–50° may be managed with bracing or surgery, and those with a Cobb angle greater than 50° usually require surgical intervention [103].

Exercise therapy has long been advocated for mild cases of scoliosis (Cobb angle of 10–20°). Compared to standard therapy (core exercises, stretching, and spinal mobilization), a program of active, self-correction, and task-oriented exercises in mild scoliosis was shown to actually improve Cobb angle measurements [107]. A recent meta-analysis looked at the effect of the Schroth method, which was first developed in 1920 as an individualized treatment program designed to shift one's spinal curvature toward a normal pattern. Correction is achieved through a combination of stretching, strengthening, and breathing in reverse directions of all existing abnormal curvatures based on a patient's unique spinal curvature. Mental imagery, external stimuli, and mirror control are also employed to facilitate postural correction which is encouraged throughout routine daily living [108]. The overall effect size was found to be high in those with spinal curvatures of 10–30 degrees when exercises were performed over a period of at least 6 months [109].

Asymptomatic athletes are allowed unrestricted sport participation. Participation decision should be individualized in consultation with a spine specialist for those with painful high degree curves, those being treated with bracing, and those who had surgical correction [102]. There are no current guidelines for return to sport after surgical correction for scoliosis. A survey study of spinal deformity surgeons noted that postsurgical correction, most patients were allowed to return to sport with running at 3 months, noncontact and contact sports at 6 months, and collision sports at 12 months [110]. No specific guidelines exist specifically in return to gymnastics after surgical correction.

8.1.5.5 Discogenic Pain and Radiculopathy

The intervertebral disc can be a common cause of acute and chronic back pain in the gymnast. The intervertebral disc consists of a firm, collagenous exterior annulus fibrosis and a gelatinous interior nucleus pulposus. The intervertebral disc offers shock absorption and allows for the dispersion of axial and torsional forces at each spinal level. Discogenic causes of low back pain typically include internal disc disruption, annular fissure, disc herniation, and degenerative disc disease. With internal disc disruption, the internal architecture of the disc is disrupted, but its external surface remains essentially normal. It is characterized by degradation of the nucleus pulposus and radial fissures that extend to the outer third of the annulus. An annular fissure is disruption in the outer annular fibrosis and has been found to highly correlate with pain [111]. A disc bulge (displacement >50% of the disc circumference) or disc herniation (<50%) is described as disc material that extends beyond the intervertebral disc space [112]. Degenerative disc disease is a broad term used to describe the aging process and includes findings such as desiccation, fibrosis, narrowing of the disc space, diffuse bulging, and osteophyte formation [113].

It is postulated that gymnasts are at greater risk of disc injury due to extreme degrees of spinal motion and mechanical loading. Disc pathology on imaging has been found to be higher in gymnasts and also correlates with back pain. An increased incidence and frequent coexistence of disc and vertebral body abnormalities in this population strongly suggest a traumatic and mechanical overloading etiology [7]. Animal models have demonstrated that repetitive flexion and extension movements result in disc herniations [114]. Cadaveric studies have demonstrated that a herniated disc is associated with loads in a fully flexed posture likely in conjunction with poor spinal muscular control [115]. Also, the combination of axial rotation combined with flexion may lead to radial lesions within the annulus fibrosis [116]. With these findings in mind, it is clear how the gymnast may be at an increased risk for intervertebral disc pathology given the repetitive loading in a flexed, extended, and rotated posture. A common example would be during the takeoff or landing in a backward full twisting salto.

Presentation of discogenic pain can vary but typically includes axial low back pain that starts after a flexion or twisting-based maneuver with an associated sensation of a pop in the lower back. Pain is typically a deep ache with spasm to the back muscles and may radiate into one or both gluteal regions. In general, pain is worse with sitting and flexion or twisting maneuvers. Increasing intradiscal pressure such as with coughing or sneezing may acutely increase symptoms [117]. Standing and extension-based maneuvers or lying flat may improve the pain. If a disc herniation is located more laterally within the neural foramen, pain may radiate into the lower extremities in a dermatomal distribution due to irritation of the associated spinal nerve root. In these cases, pain may actually be located to one of the lower extremities instead of the back, referred to as radicular pain. Even without mechanical compression, the herniated nucleus pulposis may generate a large inflammatory reaction and cause radicular symptoms [112].

Examination may reveal acute spinal shift, paraspinal and gluteal muscular hypertonicity, and reduced spinal motion due to pain. A complete neurological examination including assessment for radiculopathy with weakness and/or reflex changes in a spinal nerve distribution should be performed especially in the setting of lower limb symptoms. Provocative dural tension maneuvers are more indicative of disc-related pain.

Radiographs are often performed as a first step; however, they lack sensitivity and specificity for disc-related pathology. Provocative discography remains the gold standard for the diagnosis of discogenic lower back pain. This is an invasive procedure that involves placement of a needle into the disc under fluoroscopy to illicit the patient's typical pain response. However, this is rarely performed in clinical practice due to its invasive nature, risk of infection, and risk of increasing degenerative changes in long term [117]. Therefore, MRI is usually the next best step after radiographic films due to its ability to provide high resolution of disc pathology without using ionizing radiation (Fig. 8.10).

As previously noted, it is well documented that imaging pathology is common among the asymptomatic general population [24] and even the pediatric population, with up to 20% of asymptomatic patients having abnormal disc findings [118]. There is evidence, however, linking abnormal intervertebral disc imaging findings with back pain specifically in the gymnast. In one such study, MRI findings for elite athletes across multiple sports including gymnastics were analyzed for abnormalities. A significant correlation was found between the severity of an athlete's back pain and findings of reduced disc height, Schmorl's nodes, and vertebral body configuration changes [8]. Another study specifically compared 24 elite male gymnasts to nonathlete controls using MRI of the thoracic and lumbar spine. Signs of disc

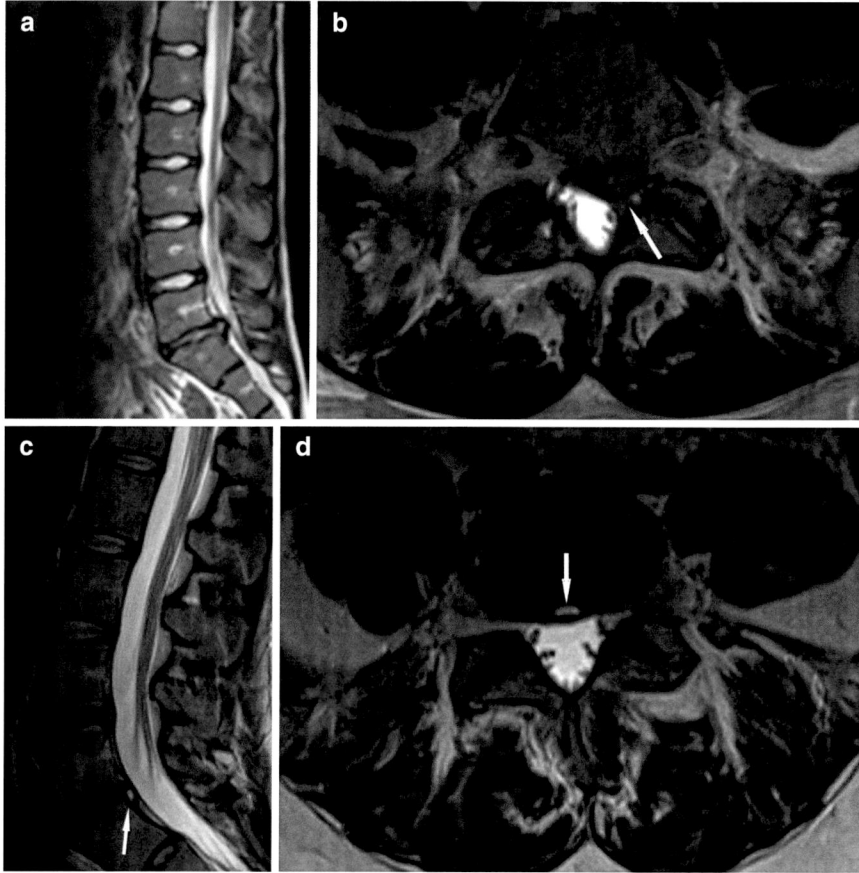

Fig. 8.10 Disc pathology on MRI. (**a**) Sagittal T2-weighted image of L5-S1 disc herniation. (**b**) Axial T2 of left paracentral disc herniation. (**c**) Sagittal. (**d**) Axial T2-weighted images of annular tear and disc degenerative changes in 20-year-old gymnast

degeneration were significantly more common among gymnasts than nonathletes (75% versus 31%). Gymnasts were also found to have a higher number of affected discs and a higher degree of signal reduction than nonathletes [7].

The goal of treatment of a disc herniation or other disc pathology in the gymnast is to return to gymnastics without pain or neurological deficit and with full function [119]. In the majority of cases, pain will resolve with time. However, there are several treatment options to consider. Non-pharmacological treatment should always be employed first and includes superficial heat, massage, acupuncture, and spinal manipulation. If needed, a short course of NSAIDs may offer pain relief in the acute period. Skeletal muscle relaxants may also prove helpful especially with difficulty sleeping due to pain. In cases of severe pain, a short course of oral steroids is commonly prescribed, although evidence for this is lacking [120]. In the setting of significant radicular symptoms, neuropathic modulatory medications such as gabapentin may be considered.

A detailed therapy program for treatment of a disc herniation in the gymnast should be employed. The program may be divided into four phases which include an acute inflammatory phase (I), a repair phase (II), a remodeling phase (III), and finally a very individualized return to gymnastics phase (IV).

Phase I should focus on pain reduction and relative rest by reducing excess mechanical stresses imparted to the disc. The gymnast should be educated on muscular spinal stabilization like an abdominal bracing technique. Education should also be provided on appropriate posture control for their daily activities. A good example is learning "hip hinging" which involves bending at the hips with appropriate lumbar lordosis posture rather than by spinal flexion [121]. Another simple treatment strategy in the initial phase is the use of mechanical diagnosis and therapy (MDT), commonly known as directional preference, or the McKenzie method. This employs repetitive spinal motions in the direction which reduces pain and avoidance of motion which exacerbates pain. Most commonly with a disc herniation, this involves extension-based movements but should be very individualized to each gymnast. In the setting of radicular pain, the concept of centralization should be taught, which involves reducing leg symptoms to a more proximal location by way of a spinal directional preference [122].

Phase II involves exercises that carefully load the spine in a neutral position in order to stimulate collagen repair. It includes exercises that resist frontal and rotational movements. An example is a static plank exercise with progression to a single-leg plank. Phase III involves full integration of dynamic rotational movements which aid in the alignment, organization, and cross-linking of collagen fibers. Examples include lunges with a twisting motion and rotational chops and lifts using resistance bands. Finally, phase IV is gymnastics-specific rehabilitation which should progress the athlete through full, dynamic spinal motion exercises. The gymnast must be able to move freely in all three planes of motion with good mobility, motor control, efficiency, and power [123].

When conservative treatment has failed to provide significant relief, epidural steroid spinal injection options are considered. Indications for epidural steroid injections according to the most recent North American Spine Society guidelines include lumbar radicular pain, evidence of nerve root impingement on imaging, or failure of at least 4 weeks of conservative management. Epidural steroids are also considered for high-level athletes with axial only back pain especially during the midst of a competitive season. Evidence in high-level athletes does show quicker return to sport when compared to surgery [119]. Indications for surgical referral include moderate to severe weakness, progressive weakness, symptoms of cauda equina, and uncontrolled pain despite conservative management strategies.

8.1.5.6 Facet Pain

Each spinal segment contains two posterolateral zygapophysial joints, often referred to as facet joints (Fig. 8.11). The facet joints are formed by the superior and inferior articular processes of adjacent vertebrae and have features of a classic synovial joint

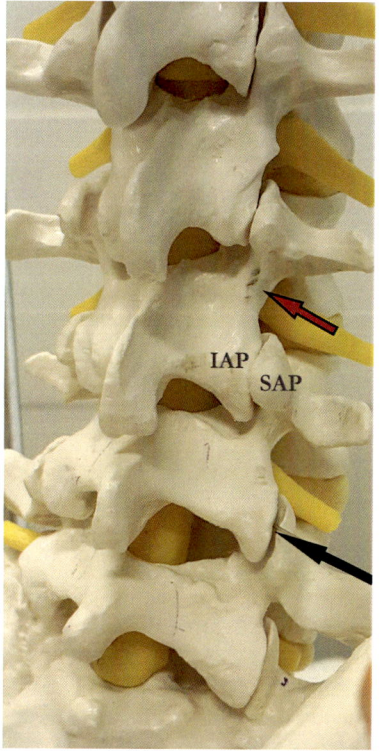

Fig. 8.11 Facet joint anatomy: inferior articular process (IAP), superior articular process (SAP). Facet joint is indicated by the black arrow and the pars interarticularis is indicated by the red arrow

including hyaline cartilage, a synovial membrane, and a joint capsule [124]. Each facet joint receives afferent nerve fibers from the medial branch of the spinal nerve exiting at that level, as well as from the level above.

Facet pain may also be referred to as posterior element overuse syndrome, hyperlordotic low back pain, and mechanical low back pain [125]. Facet pain is defined as pain that arises from any structure that is part of the facet joints, including the fibrous capsule, synovial membrane, hyaline cartilage, and bone. Most commonly, facet pain develops from repetitive stress and/or cumulative trauma which leads to inflammation of the joint. Degenerative changes may be seen in the older athlete [119]. Typically, the stress on the facet joint comes from repetitive extension and rotation of the spine, both of which are extremely common in gymnastics. Overall, there is a paucity of literature on facet pain in the gymnast. Distinguishing pain from the facet joints versus other structures in the low back can be challenging [126].

The presentation of facet pain is very similar to that of spondylolysis. The most common complaint is axial low back pain, unilateral or bilateral, which is typically worse with standing and extension of the spine. Pain originating from the upper lumbar facet joints may extend into the flank, hip, and lateral thigh, whereas pain from the lower facet joints may radiate into the posterior thigh. Referral of pain distal to the knee is rarely associated with facet pathology [127]. Examination may reveal tenderness over the paraspinals in the region of pathology. Pain may increase with facet loading maneuvers (Fig. 8.12).

Fig. 8.12 Facet loading exam maneuver

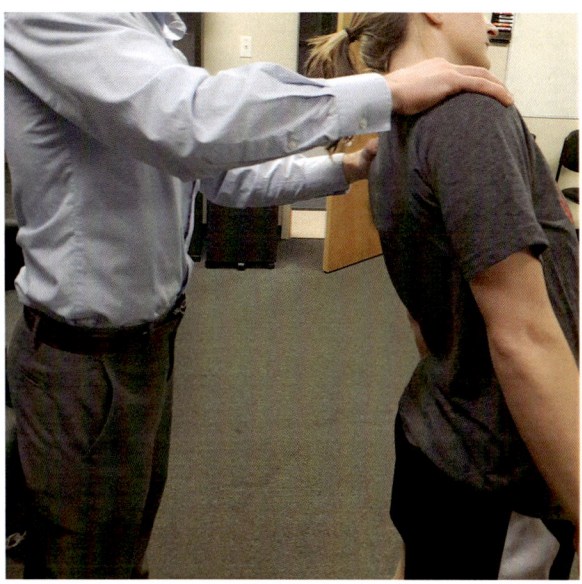

Plain films, CT, and MRI historically have low predictive value for pain associated with the facets. Bone scans have high sensitivity but low diagnostic specificity. The overlay of a CT scan of the area of interest with a bone scan with SPECT imaging can provide the anatomic resolution of a CT scan plus the sensitivity of the bone scan [128]. Unfortunately, this provides a high amount of ionizing radiation. Fat suppression sequences (STIR) on MRI may allow for better visualization of facet edema, which has been found to correlate with back pain (Fig. 8.13) [129]. A gold standard for diagnosis is still lacking. A more invasive option is the use of diagnostic facet joint blocks or medial branch blocks under fluoroscopic guidance [126].

The rehabilitation strategy of facet-mediated pain is similar in concept to that of spondylolysis. Initially, the program should start with a period of relative rest with avoidance of extension-based movements or other maneuvers which reproduce pain. A short course of anti-inflammatories may be considered. A program that focuses on neuromuscular re-education to reduce dysfunctional extension-based movement patterns is also recommended [130].

For the gymnast who has not responded to a detailed course of conservative treatment, providers may consider facet joint injections or medial branch blocks and subsequent radiofrequency denervation. There are limited studies in the athletic population regarding these procedures and no studies in gymnasts. Debate exists over the utility of facet joint steroid injections versus undergoing radiofrequency denervation of the medial branches; however, there is some evidence of equal outcome at 6 months [131]. One must keep in mind that the medial branches innervate the multifidus muscles which are important for spinal stability. The clinician treating gymnasts should use great caution in recommending radiofrequency denervation, and if completed, it is recommended to keep the neurotomy to less than three spinal segments [132].

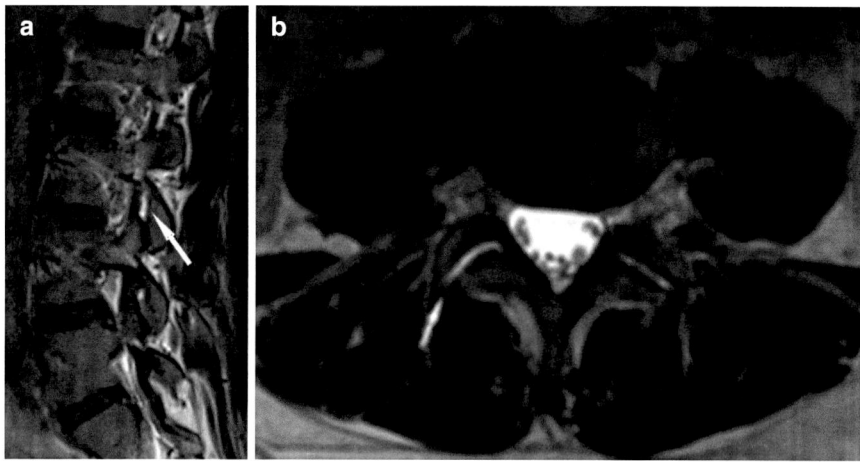

Fig. 8.13 Facet joint imaging: MRI T2 weighted. (**a**) Sagittal and (**b**) axial images of facet joint with mild effusion

8.1.5.7 Myofascial Pain and Other Considerations

Even after a thorough history, examination, and diagnostic workup, the etiology of back pain in the gymnast may be elusive. The clinician should investigate other causes or contributing factors including the myofascial complex. This is especially important to consider when pain and referral patterns are not dermatomal or myotomal, do not correspond with spinal pathology on imaging, or do not respond to typical treatment.

Fascia is defined as the soft tissue component of the connective tissue system that permeates the human body and is seen as one interconnected tensional network that adapts its fiber arrangement, length, and density according to local tensional demands [133]. The thoracolumbar fascia, for example, has been found to contain free nerve endings and sympathetic fibers [134], along with mechanoreceptors, [135] which suggests its role as a pain generator and cause of altered proprioceptive awareness. It is imperative that the clinician examine the myofascial structures of the back as focal fascial restriction may lead to biomechanical inefficiency and global dysfunction [136]. Treatment may include stretching, massage, myofascial release, and trigger point injections.

8.2 Sacrum and Sacroiliac Joints

8.2.1 *Epidemiology, Anatomy, and Pathophysiology*

The sacroiliac (SI) joint, the largest axial joint in the body, refers to the large, irregularly shaped, and mostly diarthrodial joint formed by the union of the sacrum and ilium. Its main function is to dampen the forces of ambulation and

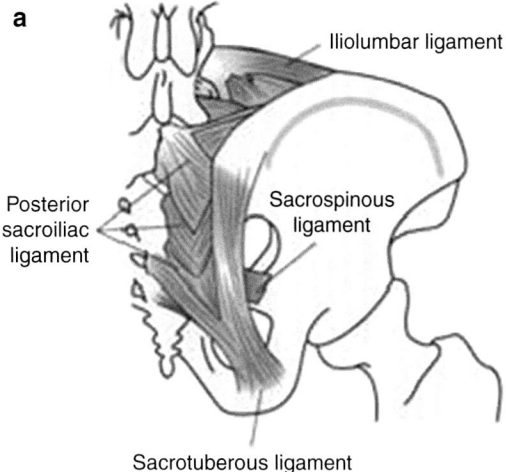

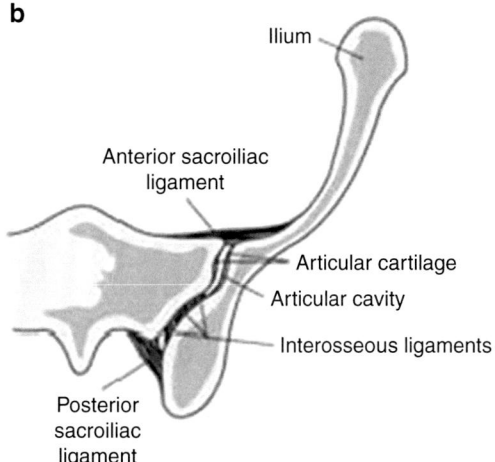

Fig. 8.14 Sacroiliac anatomy showing basic schematic of ligamentous structures of the sacroiliac joint. (*Adapted from* Lee [168]. *[Figure 6.5, page 250]*)

assist in load transmission from the legs across the pelvis, spine, and trunk. The irregular shape of the joint potentially provides an elegant force closure to act as keystones for the pelvic ring [137]. Furthermore, the joint is lined by a fibrous capsule and surrounded by several strong ligaments which impart much of its stability while limiting motion, thought to be around 2 degrees in all three planes (Fig. 8.14) [137].

The SI joint is thought to cause 15–25% of all low back pain, yet it is often an underappreciated source of axial back pain, partly because diagnosis may be challenging [138]. Although the exact prevalence in gymnasts is not yet established, SI joint dysfunction and pain is thought to have a higher incidence in this population due to repetitive asymmetric load and shear stress to the pelvis as well as the fact that SI pain commonly coexists with hypermobility [139, 140].

Pain in the SI region may be conferred from the joint itself or the important surrounding structural ligaments and myofascial structures. SI joint dysfunction or mechanical incompetence of the SI joint complex may arise from disruption of any of these structures or their functional interplay. SI joint dysfunction in gymnastics is most often seen as a result of acute trauma or repetitive microtrauma secondary to either increased laxity or excessive joint compression stiffness. There is a sexual dimorphism between male and female gymnasts after puberty that affects the joint structure, motion, and progression of degeneration which must be considered [137], as gender-related differences in SI joint development can lead to higher rates of misalignment and pain in young females [141]. Structural issues, decreased myofascial stability, or deficiency of neuromuscular control may lead to SI dysfunction and are important to consider in treatment modalities for the gymnast [124, 137, 139, 142].

8.2.2 History and Diagnosis

A gymnast with SI pain may present with a single acute injury most commonly involving sudden rotation and axial load to the pelvis; but most often they will present with a more gradual progression of low back pain [138–140]. Symptoms of SI joint pain are varied, but athletes may often present with aching low back or gluteal region pain, or clicking/popping in the posterior pelvis [138–140]. This is often worse with transitional motions, running, stair climbing, or single-leg activities. Occasionally, the gymnasts may point to the SI joint when indicating the area of pain with a single finger, which is described as the Fortin finger test. However, pain may also radiate into the groin or lower extremities and may be accompanied by tingling and numbness, making it difficult to distinguish from other etiologies of pain [138, 140, 143].

Certain conditions can mimic SI dysfunction. Pain that is worse at night, associated with morning stiffness, and improved by exercise is suspicious for rheumatological etiology and spondyloarthropathy [140, 144]. Although rarer, sacroiliitis from sources including rheumatological conditions, infection, gout, and hematological malignancies must not be overlooked, and any gymnast with systemic symptoms including multiple joint involvement or fever should have further diagnostic workup [140, 144]. If sacroiliitis is suspected, further laboratory tests including blood cultures, erythrocyte sedimentation rate (ESR), C-reactive protein (CRP), and human leukocyte antigen (HLA)-B27 may be obtained. In addition, consideration of a rheumatology consult is also recommended for the adolescent gymnast [140, 144].

Examination of the gymnast with suspected SI dysfunction should include assessment of strength, flexibility, neurological testing, all the elements of the lumbar physical examination, and evaluation of the hip joints in addition to specific SI joint testing. A thorough palpatory exam for tenderness at the posterior superior iliac crest, along the long dorsal ligament, and muscular attachment sites should be performed. Testing for relative tightness of hamstrings and adductors should be performed. Evaluation of dynamic hip girdle stability can be assessed with single-leg activities (Fig. 8.15). There is no single physical exam maneuver that is sensitive or

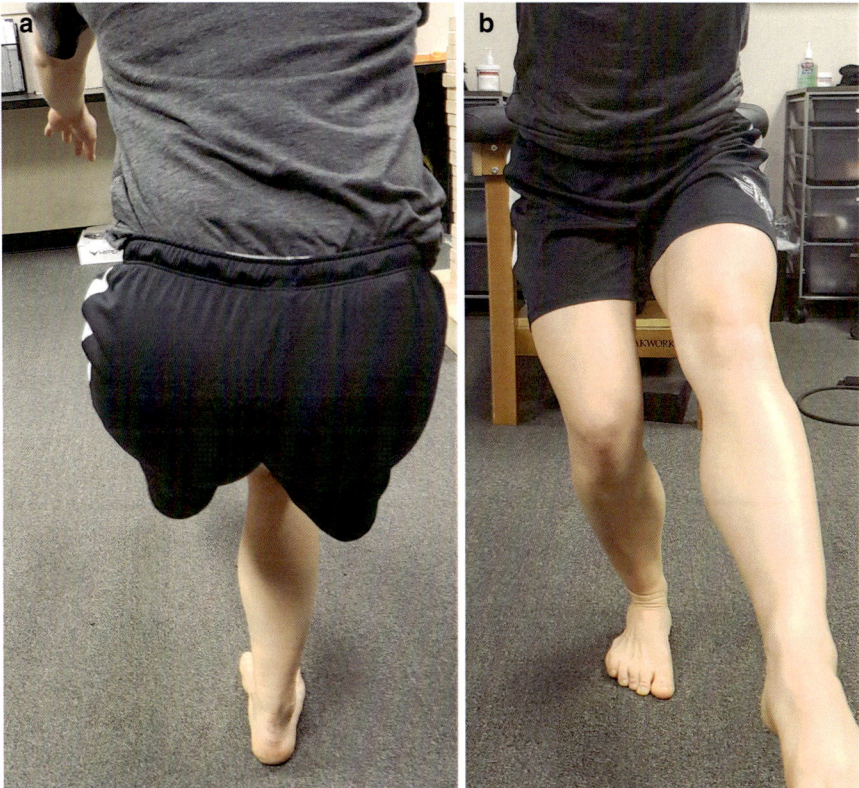

Fig. 8.15 Evaluation of single-leg squat looking for pelvic positioning and tilt, knee valgus, trunk shift, and functional instability. (**a**) Posterior. (**b**) Anterior

specific in diagnosis of SI joint pain; instead, the presence of three positive physical exam maneuvers has a sensitivity of 85–94% and specificity 77–79% [138, 140, 145, 146]. Common exam maneuvers include thigh thrust or posterior pelvic pain provocation test, sacral thrust, Gaenslen's, distraction, compression, Patrick's/FABER, and active straight leg raise (Fig. 8.16).

For most mechanical SI joint pain, imaging studies may be normal and are most useful for ruling out other more serious issues like malignancy, inflammation, fracture, or infection. It is best to start with plain anterior-posterior pelvis radiographs especially if there is history of acute trauma. MRI is useful for delineating inflammatory processes, stress fractures, or structural lesions. There has also been recent evidence of using a specialized hybrid SPECT scan with fused X-ray CT for the diagnosis of mechanical dysfunction of the SI joint [147].

For years, the diagnostic image-guided SI joint injection has been held as a paradigm for SI joint pain. However, there is evidence that a larger proportion of patients will have a false negative with intra-articular injections if they have more mechanical ligamentous SI dysfunction. Peri-articular injection has been demonstrated as possibly more effective for those with positive physical exam maneuvers [148, 149].

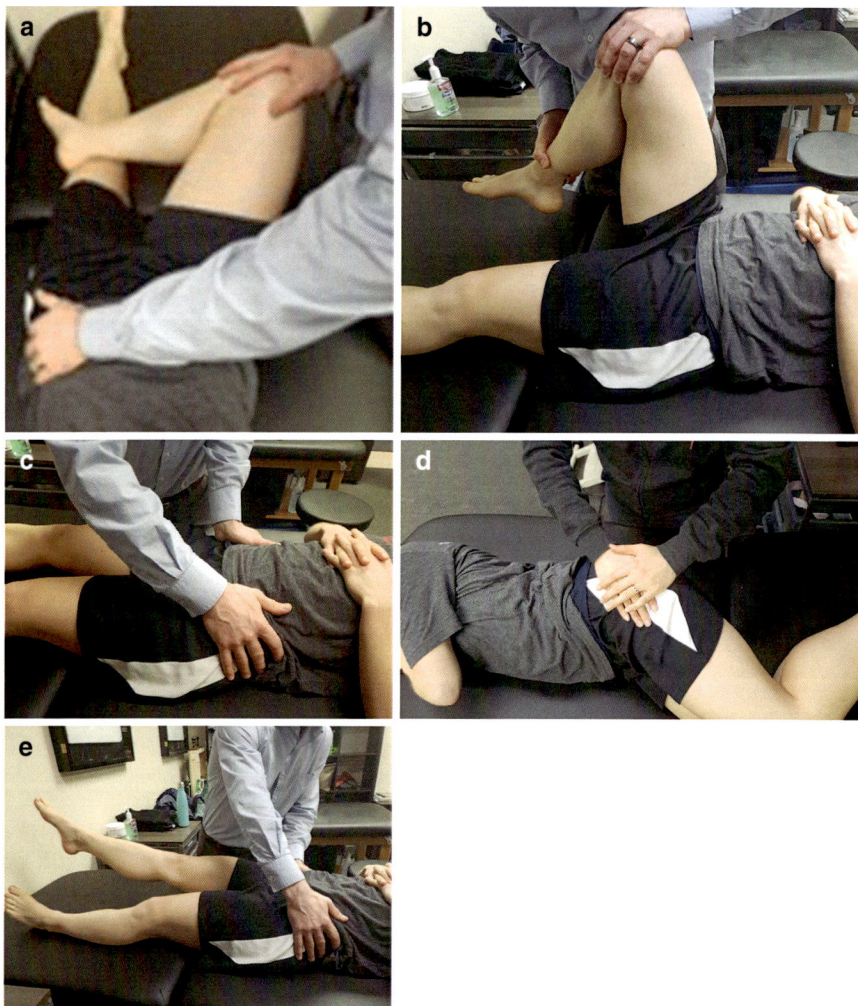

Fig. 8.16 Common sacroiliac joint physical exam maneuvers. (**a**) Patrick's FABER. (**b**) Thigh thrust or posterior pelvic pain provocation test. (**c**) Pelvic distraction provocation. (**d**) Compression provocation. (**e**) Active straight leg raise

8.2.3 Treatment

Treatment of the gymnast with suspected SI joint dysfunction should start conservatively. Use of an SI joint belt or brace may be effective in short-term pain relief but is not generally advocated for long-term function [150]. The use of manual therapy and manipulation by a trained clinician is relatively low risk and may be helpful in pain reduction [138]. A comprehensive rehabilitation program should focus on pelvic-hip girdle mechanics and dynamic movement patterns especially with single-leg activities which may increase shear stress. Anti-inflammatory and topical medications may be useful for analgesic effects in the acute setting.

There are many described interventional options for SI joint pain and dysfunction; high-quality evidence is still lacking for many of these. As discussed previously, both intra-articular and extra-articular injections may be useful for diagnosis, and treatment with a corticosteroid injection may have a role in acute pain relief. The use of orthobiological injections, specifically dextrose prolotherapy and platelet-rich plasma, is potentially beneficial in the hypermobile gymnast. A few lower-quality studies suggest longer-term improvement in pain and function in comparison to steroid injections [151–154]. In regard to SI nerve blocks, the innervation to the SI region is complex and variable, which accounts for the multiple described techniques and potentially variable results. There is a limited role for radiofrequency ablation for the SI joint in the gymnast based on lower-quality and limited evidence for its efficacy in the SI joint and more invasive nature of the treatment [155].

Surgery for the SI joint includes multiple approaches for joint fusion for stability. Again, there are limited high-quality studies and mixed results [156, 157]. This should only be considered as a last resort in carefully selected athletes if all other treatment options have been exhausted.

8.3 General Treatment of the Gymnast's Spine

As previously noted, gymnasts sustain extremely high compressive forces to the spine which can be a target for prevention of injury. Initial energy at touchdown, body position at landing, and trunk angular momentum prior to landing have been shown to determine the compressive and shear forces at the lumbar spine on landing. A proper technique with an upright trunk position, well-tuned leg muscle stiffness for muscular energy absorption, and a soft landing mat may reduce spinal loading at landing. In addition, the use of a soft complementary mat on top of the landing mat can reduce spinal load by about 20% [19].

Foot position is another important aspect of gymnastics landings. Landing with a heels-first technique results in higher vertical ground reaction forces compared with a toes-first technique. Gymnasts should be trained to land softly with a toes-first technique in addition to using leg muscles for energy absorption [158].

Besides landings, skills of particular interest in the gymnast include those employing spinal hyperextension. Training of spinal hyperextension typically begins early in childhood with performing a dynamic backbend skill or static bridge. A literature review on this topic has not found backbends to be a threat to spine health in young gymnasts [159]. However, proper training of a backbend and static bridge hold provides a pivotal screening tool and teaching point in a young gymnast's career and during rehabilitation after a spinal injury. Ideally, moving to and from an extended or arched position (e.g., back walkover or back handspring) begins with shoulder extension, then progresses with extension of the upper thoracic segments, and moves sequentially to the lower thoracic and then lumbar segments (Fig. 8.17) [159].

Fig. 8.17 Evaluation of back handspring. (**a**) Correct positioning and loading. (**b**) Closed shoulder angle, thoracolumbar hinge point, with inadequate distribution of ground reaction forces

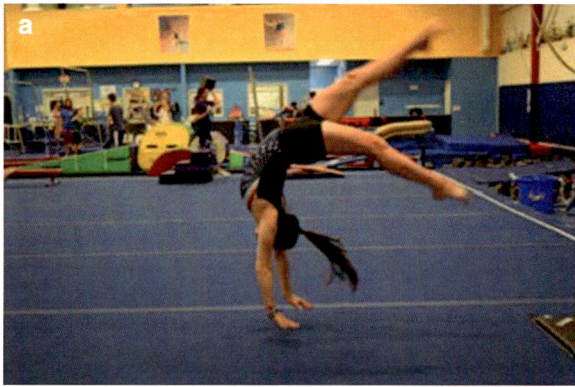

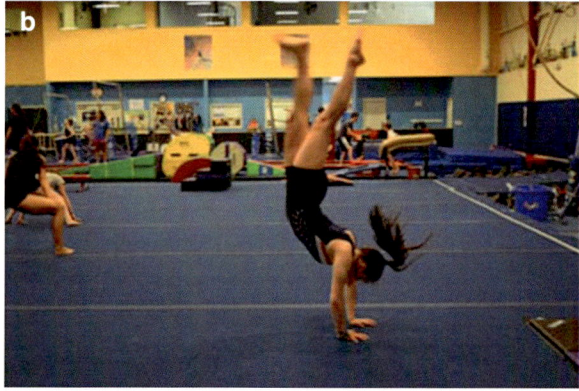

It is common for gymnasts to develop a "hinge" point at only a few segments of the spine instead of more optimally distributing motion throughout the spine. This may theoretically lead to increased injury such as spondylolysis due to overload at a particular spinal segment. This concept of a "hinge" point may develop due to tight hip flexors, reduced shoulder flexibility, or abnormal neuromuscular control of the core. As discussed previously, these factors can be easily screened for in the office setting by having the gymnast perform a bridge (Fig. 8.18).

Core stability exercises remain a cornerstone in the rehabilitation of the gymnast's spine. Despite having incredible strength and flexibility, gymnasts can still have core muscle imbalances or weakness [160]. Clinicians should also understand the concepts of functional spinal stability and their role in postural abnormalities. Bergmark proposed that spinal stability is maintained by two main muscle subsystems which include a local and a global subsystem. The local stabilizing subsystem is composed of muscles that provide the stiffness necessary to stabilize individual spinal motion segments and aid in controlling lumbar spinal postures (i.e., multifidus, transversus abdominus). The global subsystem includes the primary movers of the spine (i.e., iliopsoas, rectus abdominus) [161].

Gymnasts with spinal-related pain commonly demonstrate consistent underactivity of the local system but show variable overactivity of the global system in the

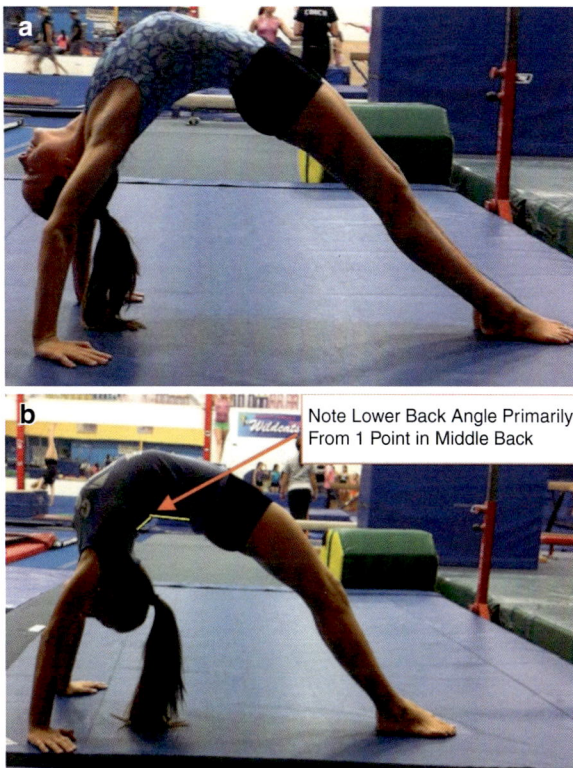

Fig. 8.18 Bridge evaluation (**a**) correct bridge mechanics (**b**) Single hinge point at thoracolumbar region

strategies they adopt for posture and movement. This mismatch manifests as a "crossed pelvic syndrome." Gymnasts typically have a posterior pelvic crossed syndrome with underactivity of the multifidus, abdominal wall, glutei, and inefficient diaphragm activity. In contrast, they have hyperactivity in the thoracolumbar erector spinae, iliopsoas, and hip rotators [162].

The gymnast must be treated from a functional model of spinal stability where all muscles (both local and global) are evaluated and treated in order to allow the spine to move appropriately and accept loads in all directions necessary for the performance of all aspects of a certain skill [162, 163]. Electromyography patterns of well-trained gymnasts show they are able to appropriately activate the erector spinae musculature in order to reduce spinal compression with a more homogeneous pressure distribution on the intervertebral disc and endplates [19]. When returning a gymnast back to sport, protocols should be graduated in difficulty to ensure they are activating the musculature correctly.

It has also been found that individuals with low back pain may have a deficiency in lumbar proprioceptive awareness [164]. These patients do best with a program focused on correcting dysfunctional movement patterns to reduce excessive forces to painful structures [165]. Strategies to control painful lumbar extension include increasing hip or thoracic extension and tilting the pelvis posteriorly. It is proposed that learning to control lumbar extension movements with gymnastics-specific skills and understanding pain may lead to more effective and efficient recovery [130].

It is important to educate gymnasts on maintaining proper spinal posture during everyday movements while outside of training periods. There is evidence that abnormal static and dynamic spinal postures may be linked with low back pain [20]. As previously discussed, the static posture of the lower lumbar spine in gymnasts may be predictive of spinal postures during dynamic skills and landings [20]. Focusing on posture outside the gym may help to translate into better landing mechanics in the gym.

8.4 Discussion and Psychosocial Factors

It is clear that back pain in the gymnast may often be complex and multifactorial. In contrast, standard treatment approaches generally focus solely on pathoanatomy and biomechanical correction. As discussed previously, tissue pathology and the pain that athletes experience may not always correlate. Nociception from injury directed mainly via C-fibers and A-delta fibers from the back are transmitted to the central nervous system. Over time, these nerves may become hyperexcitable resulting in peripheral sensitization leading to heightened sensitivity to stimuli in the region. Due to the sensitivity of persistent input, this may result in central sensitization whereby the spinal cord, brain stem, and brain become the source of dysfunction even without further peripheral input [166].

In addition, it is well established that the experience of pain and suffering is not purely due to nociception but influenced by numerous factors such as beliefs, pain behaviors, culture, and the psychosocial aspects of the athlete [167]. Pain and pain patterning may even impact performance of the athlete. Therefore, gymnasts with persistent or disabling pain should be treated through the lens of a biopsychosocial model. This has been well described by Puentedura and Louw to include "aspects of anatomy, pathoanatomy, biomechanics, brain representation of injury, the nervous system's processing of information, psychological issues associated with pain, evolutionary biology, and fear avoidance" [167].

The gymnast should be asked about the psychosocial aspects of their pain including fear and anxiety, and any maladaptive coping strategies, such as guarding and hypervigilance, must be explored. In this way, the interdisciplinary treatment team may determine factors associated with the individual gymnast's pain state and then address and decouple them from interfering with the gymnast's full recovery.

References

1. Walker BF. The prevalence of low back pain: a systematic review of the literature from 1966 to 1998. J Spinal Disord. 2000;13(3):205–17.
2. Goldstein JD, Berger PE, Windler GE, Jackson DW. Spine injuries in gymnasts and swimmers. An epidemiologic investigation. Am J Sports Med. 1991;19(5):463–8.

3. Jackson DW, Wiltse LL, Cirincoine RJ. Spondylolysis in the female gymnast. Clin Orthop Relat Res. 1976;117:68–73.
4. Micheli LJ. Back injuries in gymnastics. Clin Sports Med. 1985;4(1):85–93.
5. Sands WA, Shultz BB, Newman AP. Women's gymnastics injuries. A 5-year study. Am J Sports Med. 1993;21(2):271–6.
6. Standaert CJ. New strategies in the management of low back injuries in gymnasts. Curr Sports Med Rep. 2002;1(5):293–300.
7. Sward L, Hellstrom M, Jacobsson B, Nyman R, Peterson L. Disc degeneration and associated abnormalities of the spine in elite gymnasts. A magnetic resonance imaging study. Spine. 1991;16(4):437–43.
8. Sward L, Hellstrom M, Jacobsson B, Peterson L. Back pain and radiologic changes in the thoraco-lumbar spine of athletes. Spine. 1990;15(2):124–9.
9. Hutchinson MR. Low back pain in elite rhythmic gymnasts. Med Sci Sports Exerc. 1999;31(11):1686–8.
10. Marshall SW, Covassin T, Dick R, Agel J. Descriptive epidemiology of collegiate women's gymnastics injuries: National Collegiate Athletic Association Injury Surveillance System, 1988-1989 through 2003-2004. J Athl Train. 2007;42(2):234–40.
11. Kolt GS, Kirkby RJ. Epidemiology of injury in elite and subelite female gymnasts: a comparison of retrospective and prospective findings. Br J Sports Med. 1999;33(5):312–8.
12. Kerr ZY, Hayden R, Barr M, Klossner DA, Dompier TP. Epidemiology of National Collegiate Athletic Association Women's Gymnastics Injuries, 2009-2010 Through 2013-2014. J Athl Train. 2015;50(8):870–8.
13. Saluan P, Styron J, Ackley JF, Prinzbach A, Billow D. Injury types and incidence rates in precollegiate female gymnasts: a 21-year experience at a single training facility. Orthop J Sports Med. 2015;3(4):2325967115577596.
14. O'Kane JW, Levy MR, Pietila KE, Caine DJ, Schiff MA. Survey of injuries in Seattle area levels 4 to 10 female club gymnasts. Clin J Sport Med. 2011;21(6):486–92.
15. Tsai L, Wredmark T. Spinal posture, sagittal mobility, and subjective rating of back problems in former female elite gymnasts. Spine. 1993;18(7):872–5.
16. Lundin O, Hellstrom M, Nilsson I, Sward L. Back pain and radiological changes in the thoraco-lumbar spine of athletes. A long-term follow-up. Scand J Med Sci Sports. 2001;11(2):103–9.
17. Brüggemann G-P. Neuromechanical loading of biological tissues. In: Jensen R, Ebben W, Petushek E, Richter C, Roemer K, editors. Marquette; 2010. p. 164–82. https://ojs.ub.uni-konstanz.de/cpa/issue/view/ISBS2010; https://ojs.ub.uni-konstanz.de/cpa/article/view/4394.
18. Prassas S, Kwon YH, Sands WA. Biomechanical research in artistic gymnastics: a review. Sport Biomech. 2006;5(2):261–91.
19. Brüggemann G. Sport-related spinal injuries and their prevention. In: Biomechanics in sport. Oxford: Blackwell Science Ltd; 2000. p. 550.
20. Wade M, Campbell A, Smith A, Norcott J, O'Sullivan P. Investigation of spinal posture signatures and ground reaction forces during landing in elite female gymnasts. J Appl Biomech. 2012;28(6):677–86.
21. Courteix D, Lespessailles E, Peres SL, Obert P, Germain P, Benhamou CL. Effect of physical training on bone mineral density in prepubertal girls: a comparative study between impact-loading and non-impact-loading sports. Osteoporos Int. 1998;8(2):152–8.
22. Dowthwaite JN, Rosenbaum PF, Scerpella TA. Mechanical loading during growth is associated with plane-specific differences in vertebral geometry: a cross-sectional analysis comparing artistic gymnasts vs. non-gymnasts. Bone. 2011;49(5):1046–54.
23. Ombregt L, Bisschop P, Ter Veer HJ, Van de Velde T. A system of orthopaedic medicine. Philadelphia: Churchill Livingstone; 2003.
24. Boden SD, Davis DO, Dina TS, Patronas NJ, Wiesel SW. Abnormal magnetic-resonance scans of the lumbar spine in asymptomatic subjects. A prospective investigation. J Bone Joint Surg Am. 1990;72(3):403–8.
25. Micheli LJ, Wood R. Back pain in young athletes. Significant differences from adults in causes and patterns. Arch Pediatr Adolesc Med. 1995;149(1):15–8.

26. Bennett DL, DeLano MC. Lumbar spine MRI in the elite-level female gymnast with low back pain. Skelet Radiol. 2006;35(7):503–9.
27. Concannon LG, Harrast MA, Herring SA. Radiating upper limb pain in the contact sport athlete: an update on transient quadriparesis and stingers. Curr Sports Med Rep. 2012;11(1):28–34.
28. Wiltse LL, Newman PH, Macnab I. Classification of spondylolysis and spondylolisthesis. Clin Orthop Relat Res. 1976;117:23–9.
29. Caine DJ, Russell K, Lim L. Handbook of sports medicine and science. Gymnastics: Wiley; 2013.
30. Gagnet P, Kern K, Andrews K, Elgafy H, Ebraheim N. Spondylolysis and spondylolisthesis: a review of the literature. J Orthop. 2018;15(2):404–7.
31. Cyron BM, Hutton WC. The fatigue strength of the lumbar neural arch in spondylolysis. J Bone Joint Surg Br. 1978;60-b(2):234–8.
32. Herman MJ, Pizzutillo PD. Spondylolysis and spondylolisthesis in the child and adolescent: a new classification. Clin Orthop Relat Res. 2005;434:46–54.
33. Nitta A, Sakai T, Goda Y, Takata Y, Higashino K, Sakamaki T, et al. Prevalence of symptomatic lumbar spondylolysis in pediatric patients. Orthopedics. 2016;39(3):e434–7.
34. Standaert CJ, Herring SA. Expert opinion and controversies in sports and musculoskeletal medicine: the diagnosis and treatment of spondylolysis in adolescent athletes. Arch Phys Med Rehabil. 2007;88(4):537–40.
35. Grogan JP, Hemminghytt S, Williams AL, Carrera GF, Haughton VM. Spondylolysis studied with computed tomography. Radiology. 1982;145(3):737–42.
36. Brooks BK, Southam SL, Mlady GW, Logan J, Rosett M. Lumbar spine spondylolysis in the adult population: using computed tomography to evaluate the possibility of adult onset lumbar spondylosis as a cause of back pain. Skelet Radiol. 2010;39(7):669–73.
37. Randall RM, Silverstein M, Goodwin R. Review of pediatric spondylolysis and spondylolisthesis. Sports Med Arthrosc Rev. 2016;24(4):184–7.
38. Lonstein JE. Spondylolisthesis in children. Cause, natural history, and management. Spine. 1999;24(24):2640–8.
39. Soler T, Calderon C. The prevalence of spondylolysis in the Spanish elite athlete. Am J Sports Med. 2000;28(1):57–62.
40. Akira H, Tsuneo T, Mitsunori Y, Kazunori I, Tosihiko Y, Kazuhiko N. Characteristics of clinical and imaging findings in adolescent lumbar spondylolysis associated with sports activities. J Spine. 2012;1:124.
41. Masci L, Pike J, Malara F, Phillips B, Bennell K, Brukner P. Use of the one-legged hyperextension test and magnetic resonance imaging in the diagnosis of active spondylolysis. Br J Sports Med. 2006;40(11):940–6.
42. Kayser R, Mahlfeld K, Heyde CE, Grasshoff H, Mellerowicz H. Tight hamstring syndrome and extra- or intraspinal diseases in childhood: a multicenter study. Eur Spine J. 2006;15(4):403–8.
43. Tofte JN, CarlLee TL, Holte AJ, Sitton SE, Weinstein SL. Imaging pediatric spondylolysis: a systematic review. Spine. 2017;42(10):777–82.
44. Beck NA, Miller R, Baldwin K, Zhu X, Spiegel D, Drummond D, et al. Do oblique views add value in the diagnosis of spondylolysis in adolescents? J Bone Joint Surg Am. 2013;95(10):e65.
45. Rossi F. Spondylolysis, spondylolisthesis and sports. J Sports Med Phys Fitness. 1978;18(4):317–40.
46. Miller R, Beck NA, Sampson NR, Zhu X, Flynn JM, Drummond D. Imaging modalities for low back pain in children: a review of spondylosis and undiagnosed mechanical back pain. J Pediatr Orthop. 2013;33(3):282–8.
47. Dunn AJ, Campbell RS, Mayor PE, Rees D. Radiological findings and healing patterns of incomplete stress fractures of the pars interarticularis. Skelet Radiol. 2008;37(5):443–50.
48. Yang J, Servaes S, Edwards K, Zhuang H. Prevalence of stress reaction in the pars interarticularis in pediatric patients with new-onset lower back pain. Clin Nucl Med. 2013;38(2):110–4.
49. Campbell RS, Grainger AJ, Hide IG, Papastefanou S, Greenough CG. Juvenile spondylolysis: a comparative analysis of CT, SPECT and MRI. Skeletal Radiol. 2005;34(2):63–73.

50. Levin CS. Primer on molecular imaging technology. Eur J Nucl Med Mol Imaging. 2005;32(Suppl 2):S325–45.
51. Anderson K, Sarwark JF, Conway JJ, Logue ES, Schafer MF. Quantitative assessment with SPECT imaging of stress injuries of the pars interarticularis and response to bracing. J Pediatr Orthop. 2000;20(1):28–33.
52. Mushtaq R, Porrino J, Guzman Perez-Carrillo GJ. Imaging of spondylolysis: the evolving role of magnetic resonance imaging. PM R. 2018;10(6):675–80.
53. Rush JK, Astur N, Scott S, Kelly DM, Sawyer JR, Warner WC Jr. Use of magnetic resonance imaging in the evaluation of spondylolysis. J Pediatr Orthop. 2015;35(3):271–5.
54. Ang EC, Robertson AF, Malara FA, O'Shea T, Roebert JK, Schneider ME, et al. Diagnostic accuracy of 3-T magnetic resonance imaging with 3D T1 VIBE versus computer tomography in pars stress fracture of the lumbar spine. Skelet Radiol. 2016;45(11):1533–40.
55. Hollenberg GM, Beattie PF, Meyers SP, Weinberg EP, Adams MJ. Stress reactions of the lumbar pars interarticularis: the development of a new MRI classification system. Spine. 2002;27(2):181–6.
56. Beutler WJ, Fredrickson BE, Murtland A, Sweeney CA, Grant WD, Baker D. The natural history of spondylolysis and spondylolisthesis: 45-year follow-up evaluation. Spine. 2003;28(10):1027–35. discussion 35
57. Muschik M, Hahnel H, Robinson PN, Perka C, Muschik C. Competitive sports and the progression of spondylolisthesis. J Pediatr Orthop. 1996;16(3):364–9.
58. Harris IE, Weinstein SL. Long-term follow-up of patients with grade-III and IV spondylolisthesis. Treatment with and without posterior fusion. J Bone Joint Surg Am. 1987;69(7):960–9.
59. Bouras T, Korovessis P. Management of spondylolysis and low-grade spondylolisthesis in fine athletes. A comprehensive review. Eur J Orthop Surg. 2015;25 Suppl 1:S167–75.
60. Morita T, Ikata T, Katoh S, Miyake R. Lumbar spondylolysis in children and adolescents. J Bone Joint Surg. 1995;77(4):620–5.
61. Sairyo K, Sakai T, Yasui N. Conservative treatment of lumbar spondylolysis in childhood and adolescence: the radiological signs which predict healing. J Bone Joint Surg. 2009;91(2):206–9.
62. Blanda J, Bethem D, Moats W, Lew M. Defects of pars interarticularis in athletes: a protocol for nonoperative treatment. J Spinal Disord. 1993;6(5):406–11.
63. El Rassi G, Takemitsu M, Woratanarat P, Shah SA. Lumbar spondylolysis in pediatric and adolescent soccer players. Am J Sports Med. 2005;33(11):1688–93.
64. Selhorst M, Fischer A, Graft K, Ravindran R, Peters E, Rodenberg R, et al. Timing of physical therapy referral in adolescent athletes with acute spondylolysis: a retrospective chart review. Clin J Sport Med. 2017;27(3):296–301.
65. Alvarez-Diaz P, Alentorn-Geli E, Steinbacher G, Rius M, Pellise F, Cugat R. Conservative treatment of lumbar spondylolysis in young soccer players. Knee Surg Sports Traumatol Arthrosc. 2011;19(12):2111–4.
66. Ruiz-Cotorro A, Balius-Matas R, Estruch-Massana AE, Vilaro AJ. Spondylolysis in young tennis players. Br J Sports Med. 2006;40(5):441–6; discussion 6.
67. Nachemson A, Schultz A, Andersson G. Mechanical effectiveness studies of lumbar spine orthoses. Scand J Rehabil Med Suppl. 1983;9:139–49.
68. van Poppel MN, de Looze MP, Koes BW, Smid T, Bouter LM. Mechanisms of action of lumbar supports: a systematic review. Spine. 2000;25(16):2103–13.
69. Axelsson P, Johnsson R, Stromqvist B. Effect of lumbar orthosis on intervertebral mobility. A roentgen stereophotogrammetric analysis. Spine. 1992;17(6):678–81.
70. Radcliff KE, Kalantar SB, Reitman CA. Surgical management of spondylolysis and spondylolisthesis in athletes: indications and return to play. Curr Sports Med Rep. 2009;8(1):35–40.
71. Drazin D, Shirzadi A, Jeswani S, Ching H, Rosner J, Rasouli A, et al. Direct surgical repair of spondylolysis in athletes: indications, techniques, and outcomes. Neurosurg Focus. 2011;31(5):E9.

72. Kolcun JPG, Chieng LO, Madhavan K, Wang MY. Minimally-invasive versus conventional repair of spondylolysis in athletes: a review of outcomes and return to play. Asian Spine J. 2017;11(5):832–42.
73. Cavalier R, Herman MJ, Cheung EV, Pizzutillo PD. Spondylolysis and spondylolisthesis in children and adolescents: I. Diagnosis, natural history, and nonsurgical management. J Am Acad Orthop Surg. 2006;14(7):417–24.
74. Lowe TG, Line BG. Evidence based medicine: analysis of Scheuermann kyphosis. Spine. 2007;32(19 Suppl):S115–9.
75. Khoury NJ, Hourani MH, Arabi MM, Abi-Fakher F, Haddad MC. Imaging of back pain in children and adolescents. Curr Probl Diagn Radiol. 2006;35(6):224–44.
76. Palazzo C, Sailhan F, Revel M. Scheuermann's disease: an update. Joint Bone Spine. 2014;81(3):209–14.
77. Bradford DS. Vertebral osteochondrosis (Scheuermann's kyphosis). Clin Orthop Relat Res. 1981;158:83–90.
78. Yaman O, Dalbayrak S. Kyphosis and review of the literature. Turk Neurosurg. 2014;24(4):455–65.
79. Damborg F, Engell V, Andersen M, Kyvik KO, Thomsen K. Prevalence, concordance, and heritability of Scheuermann kyphosis based on a study of twins. J Bone Joint Surg Am. 2006;88(10):2133–6.
80. Ippolito E, Bellocci M, Montanaro A, Ascani E, Ponseti IV. Juvenile kyphosis: an ultrastructural study. J Pediatr Orthop. 1985;5(3):315–22.
81. Scoles PV, Latimer BM, DigIovanni BF, Vargo E, Bauza S, Jellema LM. Vertebral alterations in Scheuermann's kyphosis. Spine. 1991;16(5):509–15.
82. Hollingworth P. Back pain in children. Br J Rheumatol. 1996;35(10):1022–8.
83. Epstein NE, Epstein JA. Limbus lumbar vertebral fractures in 27 adolescents and adults. Spine. 1991;16(8):962–6.
84. Harreby M, Neergaard K, Hesselsoe G, Kjer J. Are radiologic changes in the thoracic and lumbar spine of adolescents risk factors for low back pain in adults? A 25-year prospective cohort study of 640 school children. Spine. 1995;20(21):2298–302.
85. Ristolainen L, Kettunen JA, Heliovaara M, Kujala UM, Heinonen A, Schlenzka D. Untreated Scheuermann's disease: a 37-year follow-up study. Eur Spine J. 2012;21(5):819–24.
86. Weiss HR, Dieckmann J, Gerner HJ. Effect of intensive rehabilitation on pain in patients with Scheuermann's disease. Stud Health Technol Inform. 2002;88:254–7.
87. Etemadifar MR, Jamalaldini MH, Layeghi R. Successful brace treatment of Scheuermann's kyphosis with different angles. J Craniovertebr Junction Spine. 2017;8(2):136–43.
88. Nusman C, van Rijn R, Lim L, Maas M. An 11-year-old high-level competitive gymnast with back pain. Br J Sports Med. 2013;47(14):929–32.
89. Sward L, Hellstrom M, Jacobsson B, Karlsson L. Vertebral ring apophysis injury in athletes. Is the etiology different in the thoracic and lumbar spine? Am J Sports Med. 1993;21(6):841–5.
90. Chang CH, Lee ZL, Chen WJ, Tan CF, Chen LH. Clinical significance of ring apophysis fracture in adolescent lumbar disc herniation. Spine. 2008;33(16):1750–4.
91. Kadam G, Narsinghpura K, Deshmukh S, Desai S. Traumatic lumbar vertebral ring apophysis fracture with disk herniation in an adolescent. Radiol Case Rep. 2017;12(2):427–30.
92. Wu X, Ma W, Du H, Gurung K. A review of current treatment of lumbar posterior ring apophysis fracture with lumbar disc herniation. Eur Spine J. 2013;22(3):475–88.
93. Deleo T, Merotto S, Smith C, D'Angelo K. A posterior ring apophyseal fracture and disc herniation in a 21-year-old competitive basketball player: a case report. J Can Chiropr Assoc. 2015;59(4):373–82.
94. Blevins K, Battenberg A, Beck A. Management of Scoliosis. Adv Pediatr. 2018;65(1):249–66.
95. Tanchev PI, Dzherov AD, Parushev AD, Dikov DM, Todorov MB. Scoliosis in rhythmic gymnasts. Spine. 2000;25(11):1367–72.

96. Meyer C, Cammarata E, Haumont T, Deviterne D, Gauchard GC, Leheup B, et al. Why do idiopathic scoliosis patients participate more in gymnastics? Scand J Med Sci Sports. 2006;16(4):231–6.
 97. Balague F, Pellise F. Adolescent idiopathic scoliosis and back pain. Scoliosis Spinal Disord. 2016;11(1):27.
 98. Misterska E, Glowacki J, Okret A, Laurentowska M, Glowacki M. Back and neck pain and function in females with adolescent idiopathic scoliosis: a follow-up at least 23 years after conservative treatment with a Milwaukee brace. PLoS One. 2017;12(12): e0189358.
 99. Bunnell WP. An objective criterion for scoliosis screening. J Bone Joint Surg Am. 1984;66(9):1381–7.
100. Coelho DM, Bonagamba GH, Oliveira AS. Scoliometer measurements of patients with idiopathic scoliosis. Braz J Phys Ther. 2013;17(2):179–84.
101. Hresko MT, Talwalkar V, Schwend R. Early detection of idiopathic scoliosis in adolescents. J Bone Joint Surg Am. 2016;98(16):e67.
102. Patel DR, Kinsella E. Evaluation and management of lower back pain in young athletes. Transl Pediatr. 2017;6(3):225–35.
103. Dunn J, Henrikson NB, Morrison CC, Nguyen M, Blasi PR, Lin JS. U.S. Preventive Services Task Force Evidence Syntheses, formerly Systematic Evidence Reviews. Screening for Adolescent Idiopathic Scoliosis: A Systematic Evidence Review for the US Preventive Services Task Force. Rockville (MD): Agency for Healthcare Research and Quality (US); 2018.
104. Weinstein SL. Natural history. Spine. 1999;24(24):2592–600.
105. Charles YP, Daures JP, de Rosa V, Dimeglio A. Progression risk of idiopathic juvenile scoliosis during pubertal growth. Spine. 2006;31(17):1933–42.
106. Larson JE, Meyer MA, Boody B, Sarwark JF. Evaluation of angle trunk rotation measurements to improve quality and safety in the management of adolescent idiopathic scoliosis. J Orthop. 2018;15(2):563–5.
107. Monticone M, Ambrosini E, Cazzaniga D, Rocca B, Ferrante S. Active self-correction and task-oriented exercises reduce spinal deformity and improve quality of life in subjects with mild adolescent idiopathic scoliosis. Results of a randomised controlled trial. Eur Spine J. 2014;23(6):1204–14.
108. Lehnert-Schroth C, Smith DA. Three-dimensional treatment for scoliosis: physiotherapeutic method for deformities of the spine: Martindale Press; 2007.
109. Park JH, Jeon HS, Park HW. Effects of the Schroth exercise on idiopathic scoliosis: a meta-analysis. Eur J Phys Rehabil Med. 2018;54(3):440–9.
110. Lehman RA Jr, Kang DG, Lenke LG, Sucato DJ, Bevevino AJ. Return to sports after surgery to correct adolescent idiopathic scoliosis: a survey of the Spinal Deformity Study Group. Spine J. 2015;15(5):951–8.
111. Schellhas KP, Pollei SR, Gundry CR, Heithoff KB. Lumbar disc high-intensity zone. Correlation of magnetic resonance imaging and discography. Spine. 1996;21(1):79–86.
112. Braddom RL. Physical medicine and rehabilitation: Elsevier Health Sciences; 2010.
113. Fardon DF, Williams AL, Dohring EJ, Murtagh FR, Gabriel Rothman SL, Sze GK. Lumbar disc nomenclature: version 2.0: recommendations of the combined task forces of the North American Spine Society, the American Society of Spine Radiology and the American Society of Neuroradiology. Spine J. 2014;14(11):2525–45.
114. Callaghan JP, McGill SM. Intervertebral disc herniation: studies on a porcine model exposed to highly repetitive flexion/extension motion with compressive force. Clin Biomech (Bristol, Avon). 2001;16(1):28–37.
115. Adams MA, Hutton WC. Prolapsed intervertebral disc. A hyperflexion injury 1981 Volvo award in basic science. Spine. 1982;7(3):184–91.
116. Marshall LW, McGill SM. The role of axial torque in disc herniation. Clin Biomech (Bristol, Avon). 2010;25(1):6–9.

117. Simon J, McAuliffe M, Shamim F, Vuong N, Tahaei A. Discogenic low back pain. Phys Med Rehabil Clin N Am. 2014;25(2):305–17.
118. Ramadorai U, Hire J, DeVine JG, Brodt ED, Dettori JR. Incidental findings on magnetic resonance imaging of the spine in the asymptomatic pediatric population: a systematic review. Evid Based Spine Care J. 2014;5(2):95–100.
119. Petron DJ, Prideaux CC, Likness L. Interventional spine procedures in athletes. Curr Sports Med Rep. 2012;11(6):335–40.
120. Qaseem A, Wilt TJ, McLean RM, Forciea MA. Noninvasive treatments for acute, subacute, and chronic low back pain: a clinical practice guideline from the American College of Physicians. Ann Intern Med. 2017;166(7):514–30.
121. Delitto RS, Rose SJ. An electromyographic analysis of two techniques for squat lifting and lowering. Phys Ther. 1992;72(6):438–48.
122. Donelson R. Is your client's back pain "rapidly reversible"? Improving low back care at its foundation. Prof Case Manag. 2008;13(2):87–96.
123. VanGelder LH, Hoogenboom BJ, Vaughn DW. A phased rehabilitation protocol for athletes with lumbar intervertebral disc herniation. Int J Sports Phys Ther. 2013;8(4):482.
124. Vora AJ, Doerr KD, Wolfer LR. Functional anatomy and pathophysiology of axial low back pain: disc, posterior elements, sacroiliac joint, and associated pain generators. Phys Med Rehabil Clin N Am. 2010;21(4):679–709.
125. Purcell L, Micheli L. Low back pain in young athletes. Sports Health. 2009;1(3):212–22.
126. Beresford ZM, Kendall RW, Willick SE. Lumbar facet syndromes. Curr Sports Med Rep. 2010;9(1):50–6.
127. van Kleef M, Vanelderen P, Cohen SP, Lataster A, Van Zundert J, Mekhail N. 12. Pain originating from the lumbar facet joints. Pain Pract. 2010;10(5):459–69.
128. Willick SE, Kendall RW, Roberts ST, Morton K. An emerging imaging technology to assist in the localization of axial spine pain. PM R. 2009;1(1):89–92.
129. Lakadamyali H, Tarhan NC, Ergun T, Cakir B, Agildere AM. STIR sequence for depiction of degenerative changes in posterior stabilizing elements in patients with lower back pain. AJR Am J Roentgenol. 2008;191(4):973–9.
130. Winslow JJ, Jackson M, Getzin A, Costello M. Rehabilitation of a young athlete with extension-based low back pain addressing motor-control impairments and central sensitization. J Athl Train. 2018;53(2):168–73.
131. Lakemeier S, Lind M, Schultz W, Fuchs-Winkelmann S, Timmesfeld N, Foelsch C, et al. A comparison of intraarticular lumbar facet joint steroid injections and lumbar facet joint radiofrequency denervation in the treatment of low back pain: a randomized, controlled, double-blind trial. Anesth Analg. 2013;117(1):228–35.
132. Shuang F, Hou S-X, Zhu J-L, Liu Y, Zhou Y, Zhang C-L, et al. Clinical anatomy and measurement of the medial branch of the spinal dorsal ramus. Medicine. 2015;94(52):e2367.
133. Schleip R, Jager H, Klingler W. What is 'fascia'? A review of different nomenclatures. J Bodyw Mov Ther. 2012;16(4):496–502.
134. Tesarz J, Hoheisel U, Wiedenhofer B, Mense S. Sensory innervation of the thoracolumbar fascia in rats and humans. Neuroscience. 2011;194:302–8.
135. Yahia L, Rhalmi S, Newman N, Isler M. Sensory innervation of human thoracolumbar fascia. An immunohistochemical study. Acta Orthop Scand. 1992;63(2):195–7.
136. Tozzi P, Bongiorno D, Vitturini C. Fascial release effects on patients with non-specific cervical or lumbar pain. J Bodyw Mov Ther. 2011;15(4):405–16.
137. Vleeming A, Schuenke MD, Masi AT, Carreiro JE, Danneels L, Willard FH. The sacroiliac joint: an overview of its anatomy, function and potential clinical implications. J Anat. 2012;221(6):537–67.
138. Cohen SP, Chen Y, Neufeld NJ. Sacroiliac joint pain: a comprehensive review of epidemiology, diagnosis and treatment. Expert Rev Neurother. 2013;13(1):99–116.
139. Prather H. Sacroiliac joint pain: practical management. Clin J Sport Med. 2003;13(4):252–5.

140. Peebles R, Jonas CE. Sacroiliac joint dysfunction in the athlete: diagnosis and management. Curr Sports Med Rep. 2017;16(5):336–42.
141. Stoev I, Powers AK, Puglisi JA, Munro R, Leonard JR. Sacroiliac joint pain in the pediatric population. J Neurosurg Pediatr. 2012;9(6):602–7.
142. Saunders J, Cusi M, Robinson D, Van der Wall H. Sacroiliac joint dysfunction in the athlete: diagnosis and management. Curr Sports Med Rep. 2018;17(2):73–4.
143. Murakami E, Aizawa T, Kurosawa D, Noguchi K. Leg symptoms associated with sacroiliac joint disorder and related pain. Clin Neurol Neurosurg. 2017;157:55–8.
144. Slobodin G, Rimar D, Boulman N, Kaly L, Rozenbaum M, Rosner I, et al. Acute sacroiliitis. Clin Rheumatol. 2016;35(4):851–6.
145. van der Wurff P, Buijs EJ, Groen GJ. A multitest regimen of pain provocation tests as an aid to reduce unnecessary minimally invasive sacroiliac joint procedures. Arch Phys Med Rehabil. 2006;87(1):10–4.
146. Laslett M, Aprill CN, McDonald B, Young SB. Diagnosis of sacroiliac joint pain: validity of individual provocation tests and composites of tests. Man Ther. 2005;10(3):207–18.
147. Saunders J, Cusi M, Van der Wall H. What's old is new again: the sacroiliac joint as a cause of lateralizing low back pain. Tomography (Ann Arbor, Mich). 2018;4(2):72–7.
148. Murakami E, Tanaka Y, Aizawa T, Ishizuka M, Kokubun S. Effect of periarticular and intraarticular lidocaine injections for sacroiliac joint pain: prospective comparative study. J Orthop Sci. 2007;12(3):274–80.
149. Borowsky CD, Fagen G. Sources of sacroiliac region pain: insights gained from a study comparing standard intra-articular injection with a technique combining intra- and peri-articular injection. Arch Phys Med Rehabil. 2008;89(11):2048–56.
150. Hammer N, Mobius R, Schleifenbaum S, Hammer KH, Klima S, Lange JS, et al. Pelvic belt effects on health outcomes and functional parameters of patients with sacroiliac joint pain. PLoS One. 2015;10(8):e0136375.
151. Singla V, Batra YK, Bharti N, Goni VG, Marwaha N. Steroid vs. platelet-rich plasma in ultrasound-guided sacroiliac joint injection for chronic low back pain. Pain Pract. 2017;17(6):782–91.
152. Cusi M, Saunders J, Hungerford B, Wisbey-Roth T, Lucas P, Wilson S. The use of prolotherapy in the sacroiliac joint. Br J Sports Med. 2010;44(2):100–4.
153. Kim WM, Lee HG, Jeong CW, Kim CM, Yoon MH. A randomized controlled trial of intra-articular prolotherapy versus steroid injection for sacroiliac joint pain. J Altern Complement Medicine (New York, NY). 2010;16(12):1285–90.
154. Hoffman MD, Agnish V. Functional outcome from sacroiliac joint prolotherapy in patients with sacroiliac joint instability. Complement Ther Med. 2018;37:64–8.
155. Maas ET, Ostelo RW, Niemisto L, Jousimaa J, Hurri H, Malmivaara A, et al. Radiofrequency denervation for chronic low back pain. Cochrane Database Syst Rev. 2015;(10):Cd008572.
156. Zaidi HA, Montoure AJ, Dickman CA. Surgical and clinical efficacy of sacroiliac joint fusion: a systematic review of the literature. J Neurosurg Spine. 2015;23(1):59–66.
157. Bina RW, Hurlbert RJ. Sacroiliac fusion: another "magic bullet" destined for disrepute. Neurosurg Clin N Am. 2017;28(3):313–20.
158. Marinsek M. Basic landing characteristics and their application in artistic gymnastics. Sci Gymn J. 2010;2(2):59–67.
159. Sands WA, McNeal JR, Penitente G, Murray SR, Jemni M, Mizuguchi S, et al. Stretching the spines of gymnasts: a review. Sports Med (Auckland, NZ). 2016;46(3):315–27.
160. d'Hemecourt PA, Luke A. Sport-specific biomechanics of spinal injuries in aesthetic athletes (dancers, gymnasts, and figure skaters). Clin Sports Med. 2012;31(3):397–408.
161. Bergmark A. Stability of the lumbar spine. A study in mechanical engineering. Acta Orthop Scand Suppl. 1989;230:1–54.
162. Key J, Clift A, Condie F, Harley C. A model of movement dysfunction provides a classification system guiding diagnosis and therapeutic care in spinal pain and related musculoskeletal syndromes: a paradigm shift-Part 2. J Bodyw Mov Ther. 2008;12(2):105–20.

163. Willardson JM. Core stability training: applications to sports conditioning programs. J Strength Cond Res. 2007;21(3):979–85.
164. O'Sullivan PB, Burnett A, Floyd AN, Gadsdon K, Logiudice J, Miller D, et al. Lumbar repositioning deficit in a specific low back pain population. Spine. 2003;28(10):1074–9.
165. O'Sullivan P. Diagnosis and classification of chronic low back pain disorders: maladaptive movement and motor control impairments as underlying mechanism. Man Ther. 2005;10(4):242–55.
166. Mannion RJ, Woolf CJ. Pain mechanisms and management: a central perspective. Clin J Pain. 2000;16(3 Suppl):S144–56.
167. Puentedura EJ, Louw A. A neuroscience approach to managing athletes with low back pain. Phys Ther Sport. 2012;13(3):123–33.
168. Lee SW. Musculoskeletal injuries and conditions: assessment and management. New York: Demos Medical; 2017.

Chapter 9
Upper Extremity Injuries in Gymnasts

Leah G. Concannon, Melinda S. Loveless, and Sean T. Matsuwaka

9.1 Gymnastics and the Upper Extremity

The upper extremity is subjected to extreme forces in gymnasts. Unlike other sports, gymnastics requires weight-bearing on, landing on, and catching oneself with the upper extremities. Vaulting and tumbling involve explosive power and weight-bearing through the arms. High bar and uneven bars generate forces through swinging and catching, parallel bars adds static holds, while rings and pommel horse generate their own unique forces, with extremes of static holds and swinging maneuvers on rings, and extended upper extremity weight-bearing on pommel horse.

Most studies of injury epidemiology in gymnastics focus on artistic gymnastics, with very limited data regarding other disciplines [1]. Studies examining both the high school and NCAA injury surveillance systems have demonstrated that the overall upper extremity injury rate across all sports is approximately 20% [2–4]. That rate is significantly higher in gymnastics, and male gymnasts have a higher incidence of upper extremity injuries than females. In a 2019 systematic review, 42.8% of injuries in male gymnasts were to the upper extremity, compared to 30.8% for females [5]. In females, lower extremity injuries still predominate, at 51% of the total, while they represent only 33% of injuries to males [5]. Within the upper extremity, wrist injuries are most common in females, followed by elbow, while shoulder is most common in males, followed by wrist [6].

The differences in upper extremity injury frequency partially stem from the fact that the three unique events for men (pommel horse, rings, and parallel bars), as well as high bar, are all strictly "arm" events, whereas females only have one "arm" event, uneven bars. Certainly, upper extremity weight-bearing occurs quite significantly on vault, beam, and floor as well for females, but men also compete in vault and floor.

L. G. Concannon (✉) · M. S. Loveless · S. T. Matsuwaka
Department of Rehabilitation Medicine, University of Washington, Seattle, WA, USA
e-mail: mlovel@uw.edu; smatsuwa@uw.edu

9.1.1 Gymnastics Technique

There is some literature to support the concept that differences in technique of basic gymnastics elements may change forces through the upper extremity. Round-offs and back handsprings are some of the earliest skills learned by gymnasts and are repeated tens, if not hundreds, of times a day on beam and floor. With the rise in popularity of the Yurchenko vault, the number of repetitions of these skills has only increased. Additionally, the forces are larger on vault given the speed of the approach and generally less padding on the vault runway.

On a round-off, hand placement can occur in one of three ways: both hands parallel, fingers of initial contact limb pointing toward the second contact hand (reverse technique), or second hand pointing toward the initial hand (T-shape technique). The second contact limb tends to undergo greater forces [7]. Farana et al. have studied these hand placements extensively [7–10] and have found that the T-shape technique leads to lower peak ground reaction force, lower elbow and wrist axial compression forces, and lower elbow internal adduction moment than the other two techniques. It is thought, therefore, that the T-shape technique may lead to less overuse injuries, though this has yet to be studied. The difficulty is that many gymnasts learn these skills at a very young age when technique is not always of the highest priority. Changing an ingrained habit in an older gymnast may be challenging but could be considered in athletes with elbow or wrist pain or injury.

Hand placement in back handsprings has also been evaluated, though less rigorously. Again, there are three hand placements to choose from: fingers pointing out 45 degrees, hands parallel, and fingers pointing in 45 degrees. Turning the hands in decreases wrist hyperextension and also decreases the effects of carrying angle at the elbow [11]. Additionally, this position allows for easier elbow flexion, particularly important if the gymnast is "short" or under-rotated, which would otherwise cause even greater wrist extension, particularly in the parallel technique [11]. Poor shoulder flexibility, with limitations of full shoulder flexion, may also lead to increased hyperextension at the wrist [12]. If the shoulders collapse at impact into less than full flexion, this will also increase wrist extension angle [12]. Both of these errors are most typically seen in younger gymnasts who are still perfecting the skill. Wrist extension of 95 degrees was common when performing back handsprings in one study, as opposed to only 67 degrees during active range of motion testing [12]. This is important, as older research has suggested that greater than 95 degrees of hyperextension at the wrist may increase risk of scaphoid waist fracture [13]. Range of motion and neuromuscular control of the shoulder girdle can have significant influences on the biomechanics of the wrist during a back handspring and therefore can be targets for rehabilitation from wrist injuries as well [12].

Pommel horse places considerable strain through the wrists of male gymnasts, as the entire exercise, which may last up to 40 seconds, requires support on the hands.

Forces through the wrist range from 1.1 times body weight on circles to up to two times body weight on scissors and flairs [14]. This is a comparable load to that seen on heel strike in runners, yet the lower body is better adapted to weight-bearing than the upper extremity. In one study of 17 collegiate male gymnasts, 15 had wrist pain (13 of the gymnasts had bilateral pain), and all but one said pommel horse was the most painful event for them [14].

9.1.2 Evaluation

As with any injury, a thorough history of any upper extremity injury in gymnasts includes not only questions about the injury itself but also about surrounding circumstances. For gymnasts, it is important to gather if there have been any recent increases in training load. This can include starting to learn a new skill, as this can put new stresses on the body. In particular, Yurchenko-style vaults, pirouetting skills on uneven bars or high bar, and new strength moves on rings may all lead to new demands on the upper extremities of gymnasts. One should ascertain if the gymnast is in season or not, but it is important to remember that many gymnasts actually increase their hours in the summer or "off season," and this is often the time to focus on new skill acquisition, so it may be just as dangerous from an overuse injury perspective. It is important to know the dominant arm/hand for both tumbling and pirouetting skills. On physical exam, it is always important to evaluate the entire kinetic chain, including both strength and flexibility. Gymnasts may compensate for poor shoulder flexibility with increased movement through the spine, or vice versa. Limitations in proximal shoulder girdle strength and flexibility may affect technique and increase risk of more distal upper extremity injuries.

9.1.3 Treatment

Treatment of many upper extremity injuries begins with a period of rest. This may require complete rest from weight-bearing, which would then also include avoiding hanging from the bar or rings. The gymnast can focus on core, lower extremity, and proximal shoulder girdle strengthening during this time, as well as maintaining flexibility. After an adequate rest period, weight-bearing exercises should proceed gradually, adding unstable surfaces and plyometrics only after sufficient proximal strength in these positions is demonstrated. Only after the gymnast can successfully perform conditioning exercises should they be allowed to tumble and swing. Initial use of a Tumbl Trak, which is similar to a long trampoline, may help with the progression to full tumbling.

9.2 Shoulder

Due to the high load and range of motion required, most shoulder injuries in gymnasts are related to overuse. The unique weight-bearing puts significant stress on the glenohumeral joint and surrounding soft tissue structures, especially as the joint is not designed for weight-bearing with its shallow glenoid and loose capsule. Most of the stabilization in midrange is provided by surrounding musculature and tendons, putting them at high risk of injury given the need for dynamic stabilization during gymnastics.

Leather dowel grips, which improve grip strength on rings, uneven bars, and high bar, allow for higher velocity movements and thus increased stress on the shoulders [15]. Gymnasts also use various hand positions on the bars which involve supporting the moving body while the shoulder is in extremes of internal and external rotation. Forces on the shoulder while swinging on bars can be up to 3.1–3.6 times body weight [16]. All of this can contribute to various injuries in the shoulders of gymnasts.

The most commonly noted shoulder pathology includes rotator cuff tendonitis/tendinopathy or tears, labral and biceps tendon pathology, instability/subluxation, multidirectional instability (MDI), and sprain/strain injuries. Less common injuries include acromioclavicular (AC) joint sprain [17], Salter-Harris fractures of the proximal humeral physis [18], and stress fractures in the clavicles [19–21].

9.2.1 Clinical Approach

History In general, athletes with shoulder pathology will complain of pain in the shoulder girdle and often experience radiation of pain into the upper arm. Specific rotator cuff pathology may localize to the area of tendon insertion on the humeral head, whereas pathology of the labrum or capsule may be vague or described as deep within the shoulder. With overuse injuries, insidious onset of pain is common. A history of changes in training or new skills that are being learned should be ascertained to determine any contributing factors.

Exam A thorough evaluation of an athlete's shoulder involves more than just a detailed shoulder exam; it is important to perform a thorough evaluation of the athlete's neurologic system to rule out pathology of the cervical spine, brachial plexus, or peripheral nerves. Inspection of the shoulders is performed to evaluate posture, muscle bulk, and resting scapular position. A lax shoulder may appear squared off due to inferior subluxation of the humeral head. During active shoulder movements, scapular position is observed for scapular dyskinesis. Palpation of the shoulder girdle should include the AC joint, biceps tendon anteriorly, rotator cuff tendons around the humeral head, and the anterior and posterior glenohumeral joint. Passive and active shoulder range of motion (ROM) in all planes should be evaluated. Reduced active motion with intact passive motion may indicate a rotator cuff tear.

The deltoid should be tested in three positions to evaluate the anterior, middle, and posterior deltoid—flexion with thumb up, abduction with palm down, and extension with thumb down. There are many special tests that can test for specific pathology within the shoulder, and the exam can be tailored based on the differential diagnosis of the performing clinician.

Imaging In the absence of trauma, radiographs of the shoulder are likely to be unremarkable in most gymnasts. However, radiographs can be useful to evaluate for Hill-Sachs or bony Bankart lesions in the setting of prior dislocation injury and can also be used to evaluate for degenerative changes, especially at the AC joint, and for evidence of calcific tendonitis. Magnetic resonance imaging (MRI) or magnetic resonance arthrography (MRA) is recommended for persistent pain or if there is concern for pathology that may require surgical intervention. MRA has an advantage in superior visualization of labral and rotator cuff tears. MRA also provides improved ability to differentiate labral tears from normal anatomic variants of the labrum [22]. Ultrasound can be utilized in evaluation of the rotator cuff and biceps tendons, bursae, the AC joint, and more superficial portions of the labrum and glenohumeral joint.

Treatment Treatment of most shoulder problems begins with a period of rest to reduce pain, followed by rehabilitation. Modalities and analgesic medications can be used to reduce pain. In some cases, particularly in older athletes, injections of corticosteroid are used for pain relief; however, one must be cautious with use of steroid around tendon so as not to put the gymnast at risk of tendon rupture. While resting and rehabilitating shoulder injuries, it is important that the gymnast maintain lower extremity flexibility and lower extremity and core strength given their importance in the kinetic chain [23]. Gymnasts may be able to modify routines on the floor and balance beam to avoid use of the injured shoulder.

The rehabilitation program should target imbalances in strength and flexibility and correct any errors in technique which may contribute to injury. The program begins with range of motion exercises and scapular stabilization exercises [23, 24]. Initial strengthening exercises may be performed with weight training. However, this applies a distal load to the shoulder which is opposite of the usual proximal load (body) that is supported by the shoulder in gymnastics activities. Therefore, after initial strengthening, it is important to be able to progress through steps that mimic usual gymnastics activities with reduced load. After ROM and strengthening exercises, the gymnast begins a closed-chain weight-bearing progression. This involves activities such as wall push-ups, press-outs, dips, sitting press-ups, push-ups, pull-ups, elevated push-ups, and piked handstand push-ups with the gymnast's feet supported on an elevated surface. To increase shoulder stabilization, the gymnast can then progress to push-up exercises with the hands on a mini trampoline or wobble board which enhances balance and proprioception training. Plyometrics are the last phase and incorporate pushing off and landing on the hands while maintaining some lower extremity support, often in a push-up position [24, 25]. This helps to strengthen the rotator cuff for dynamic stabilization [26]. Lastly, the gymnast starts the return to gymnastics-specific activities including tumbling with progression to more difficulty as able. There should be no pain or worsening of symptoms throughout the progression of exercises, and if there is, then the athlete should return to prior level of rehabilitation exercises [25]. For return to play, strength and range of motion should be symmetric in both shoulders [24]. When training on the rings, use of a Herdos or similar device decreases forces on the shoulder by supporting the forearm and therefore reducing the lever arm of the upper extremity [27]. However, the muscle activation patterns are not quite the same as when training without the device so it may not completely prepare the shoulder for return to normal activity on the rings. Therefore, use of a belt attached to the rings by a pulley system, which likely simulates similar muscle activation, may represent a good next step to train the shoulder girdle muscles for return to the rings [28, 29].

After successful treatment of a shoulder problem, it is important to focus on prevention of future shoulder injuries. Gymnasts should maintain proper shoulder conditioning through a balance of strengthening shoulder girdle muscles and maintaining full range of motion through stretching. Chapters 11 and 12 have more detailed information on rehab and return to sport in gymnastics.

9.2.2 Impingement and Rotator Cuff

Gymnastics requires repetitive motion into extremes of movement and can lead to shoulder impingement. External impingement involves impingement of soft tissues including the long head biceps tendon, supraspinatus, and subacromial subdeltoid bursa under the bony coracoacromial arch. This occurs in positions of abduction, elevation, and external or internal rotation. Muscle fatigue, tendon overload, glenohumeral instability, and strength imbalances may contribute to this impingement. Internal impingement is often related to instability in the posterior glenohumeral joint and causes impingement of posterior soft tissues between the bony glenoid and humeral head. Impingement can lead to tendinopathy if gymnasts continue to train through pain and can lead to imbalances which predispose to further injury [15, 23, 30].

Gymnasts with impingement and rotator cuff injuries typically present with insidious onset of pain that progressively worsens. While pain is often diffuse, it is usually worst in the superolateral or posterior shoulder and is increased with overhead movements or activities reaching behind the back. The supraspinatus tendon is the most commonly injured, resulting in painful abduction, particularly between 70 and 120 degrees of abduction. In the setting of an acute rotator cuff tear, the athlete may describe weakness in the shoulder, but with chronic partial tears, he or she may not notice weakness [15, 30]. There may be limitation of abduction or internal rotation range of motion [30]. Strength of the deltoid and rotator cuff muscles should be evaluated and may be decreased. The supraspinatus is isolated with the Jobe (empty can) test, and with an injured supraspinatus tendon, there will generally be pain and sometimes weakness. Resisted external rotation should be performed in 0 and 90°

of abduction as well to evaluate the infraspinatus and teres minor. Subscapularis strength is tested with the lift off, belly press, or bear hug tests. Tests for impingement include the Neer sign and Hawkins-Kennedy sign [30].

Treatment of impingement and rotator cuff injury follows the course outlined above. With full tears of the rotator cuff, surgery can be pursued.

9.2.3 Labral Tears

While most labral tears in gymnasts are due to overuse, with repeated traction causing microtears, there can be traumatic injuries as well. A fall on an outstretched arm that is slightly flexed and abducted can produce compression and superior subluxation of the humeral head, which can also lead to labral injury. Either of these can lead to a specific type of labral tear, a SLAP tear (superior labrum from anterior to posterior). Another cause of a labral tear is anterior shoulder subluxation/instability caused by an external rotation and abduction force [22, 31]. Additionally, if the gymnast maintains grip on an apparatus to avoid improper dismount or other injury, there may be unexpected and increased stress on the shoulder in a loaded position. In addition to labral injuries, this mechanism can lead to injuries to ligaments, tendons, or muscles [32]. In female gymnasts, a common cause for a labral tear is moving from bar to bar on the uneven bars [33] while male gymnasts tend to have more injuries on rings and parallel bars [26]. On the rings, when moving from a handstand position to hanging position, there is a short period of time when muscle activity around the shoulders drops very quickly, yet the shoulders are still being exposed to a high load. This can lead to the long head biceps tendon pulling on the labrum and subsequent SLAP lesions, as the load on the stabilizing structures often exceeds the failure load [34]. The superior labrum at the biceps insertion is also at high risk for injury with gymnastics activities that involve rotating on a loaded shoulder, which commonly occurs on the rings, uneven bars, and high bar [23].

SLAP tears often present with pain and weakness in the shoulder, especially with abduction, internal rotation, and cross body movements. There can be mechanical symptoms such as popping, clicking, or catching as well.

There are many tests for labral pathology, including the active compression test (O'Brien) (Fig. 9.1). With the O'Brien test, it is important to clarify where the athlete experiences pain and with which position(s). Pain with the O'Brien test in both external and internal rotation that localizes to the superior shoulder can be related to AC joint pathology [35]. For the O'Brien test to indicate labral pathology, there should be pain in the internally rotated position (thumb down) that improves with the externally rotated position (palm-up). Other labral provocative maneuvers include Kibler dynamic labral shear (Fig. 9.2), crank test, and Kim biceps load test I and II. As individuals with labral tears often have other pathology, tests for rotator cuff pathology and instability may be positive in addition to labral tests [22, 31]. Additionally, biceps tendon pathology can be evaluated with the Speed and Yergason tests and may be positive in the setting of biceps tendon pathology or SLAP tear [35].

Fig. 9.1 Active compression test (O'Brien test) for labral pathology. The arm is forward flexed to 90 degrees with the elbow in extension, with 10–15 degrees of adduction, and internal rotation (thumb down). The examiner exerts downward force on the arm while the patient resists (**a**). This is then repeated with the arm in the palm-up position (**b**). Pain present in thumb down position, relieved with palm-up position, is a positive test

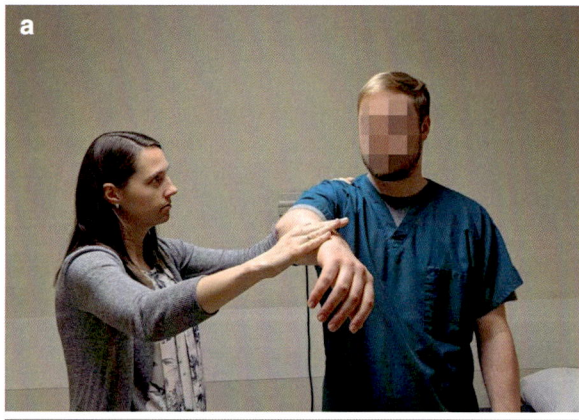

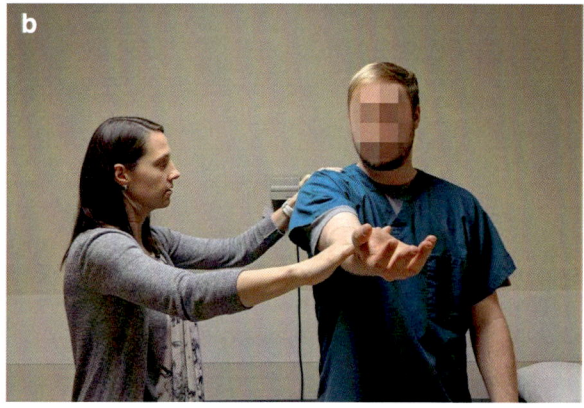

When there is labral or biceps tendon pathology, initial exercises should minimize activation of the biceps and then slowly add load to the biceps to strengthen as tolerated. Pull-ups and horizontal rows while supine are a good activity for biceps strengthening in gymnasts. While labral tears, biceps tendon pathology, and rotator cuff tears may do well with conservative management, many do require surgical intervention due to the risk of tear or injury progression and inability to return to prior level of performance [23]. For SLAP tears, surgery can involve resection or repair of the labrum and biceps tenotomy or tenodesis [31].

9.2.4 Multidirectional Instability (MDI)

In gymnasts, MDI is most likely due to repetitive microtrauma of the stabilizers of the glenohumeral joint that eventually leads to laxity in the capsule and ligaments. Congenital laxity may also be a contributor, but most gymnasts with MDI do not have a history of major trauma or joint dislocation. In the setting of

Fig. 9.2 Dynamic shear test for labral pathology. The examiner is behind the patient. The patient's arm is placed in 70 degrees of abduction and external rotation with the elbow flexed (**a**). An anterior force is applied to the posterior shoulder as the arm is moved to 120 degrees of abduction (**b**). Reproduction of pain in the posterior/superior shoulder is a positive test

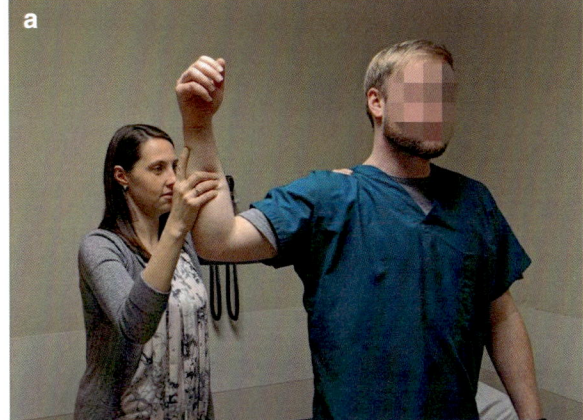

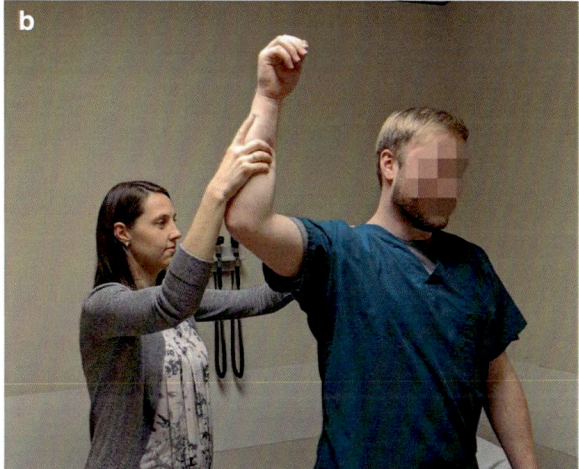

MDI, rotator cuff dysfunction and scapular dyskinesis may also contribute to pain and secondary injury [36–38].

Gymnasts with MDI may describe nonfocal shoulder pain, instability in the shoulder with a sense that the shoulder could dislocate, and/or frequent subluxations or dislocations. They may also experience intermittent neurologic symptoms with numbness or tingling in the arm. Dislocation/subluxation events may occur spontaneously or with activity. With MDI, the athlete is often able to self-reduce dislocations. Those with anterior instability generally have pain or instability with abduction, extension, and external rotation (e.g., overhead movements, throwing), while those with posterior instability may avoid positions of flexion, adduction, and internal rotation (e.g., push-ups, pushing doors open). Inferior instability can occur when carrying heavy items. Anteroinferior instability is most common in MDI [37, 38].

Glenohumeral laxity is evaluated in the anterior, posterior, and inferior directions. A diagnosis of MDI requires symptomatic laxity in at least two directions,

Fig. 9.3 Positive sulcus sign indicating inferior shoulder instability. With an inferior force placed on the arm, note the depression inferior to the acromion

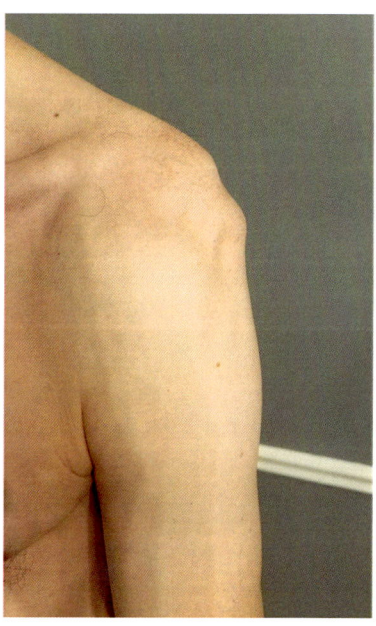

Table 9.1 Beighton criteria for generalized ligamentous laxity [40]

Passive hyperextension of the small finger metacarpophalangeal joint past 90 degrees	1 point each side
Passive opposition of the thumb to the volar forearm	1 point each side
Active hyperextension of the elbow past 10 degrees	1 point each side
Active hyperextension of the knee past 10 degrees	1 point each side
Ability to place palms on floor with knees extended	1 point

with one being inferior [37–39]. Inferior shoulder laxity is evaluated with the sulcus sign [38] (Fig. 9.3). Exam maneuvers for anterior glenohumeral laxity include the apprehension and relocation tests, load-and-shift test, and anterior drawer test; posterior glenohumeral laxity is evaluated with the posterior drawer test and the posterior jerk [38]. With these maneuvers, there should be reproduction of the patient's symptoms, not just instability, to diagnose MDI. Additionally, generalized ligamentous laxity is evaluated with the Beighton criteria [40] (Table 9.1). Those with a score of 4 or higher have generalized ligamentous laxity [35]; those with a score of at least 2 are at higher risk of glenohumeral instability but not necessarily MDI [41].

Treatment for MDI focuses on optimizing scapulothoracic motion, improving proprioception, and strengthening of the dynamic glenohumeral stabilizers including the rotator cuff, deltoid, and scapular stabilizers. If this is ineffective over a course of at least 3–6 months, then surgical stabilization of the glenohumeral joint can be considered. The more commonly utilized surgical techniques include open inferior capsular shift and arthroscopic capsular plication. After initial immobilization followed by gradual rehabilitation, return to sport occurs at least 6 months postoperatively [23, 37, 38].

9.3 Elbow

Injuries to the elbow in adolescent athletes tend to result from overuse. Acute injuries, such as dislocations, do occur but are less common. The epiphyseal plate and apophysis are the weakest links in the skeletally immature athlete, while ligamentous injuries become more common as athletes reach skeletal maturity. While detailed return to throwing protocols exist for pitchers, there is not a similar correlate in the literature for gymnasts. The treatment of many elbow pathologies begins with full rest from upper extremity weight-bearing exercises, before progressing through a slow return to play.

9.3.1 Medial Elbow

The medial epicondylar physis is susceptible to traction injuries in the younger athlete, as is the insertion of the ulnar collateral ligament (UCL) on the sublime tubercle of the ulna. As the athlete ages and the physis closes, the UCL itself and the common flexor tendon insertion are more vulnerable [42].

Little League Elbow The most well-known adolescent injury about the elbow is likely Little League elbow. Classically, Little League elbow refers to injury of the medial epicondylar growth plate (apophysitis or avulsion fracture) due to repetitive tension overload. It may begin as simply irritation of the flexor-pronator mass before it progresses. It may include injuries to the UCL, particularly in the older athlete as they reach skeletal maturity and the physis closes. There can often be a spectrum of disorders; in addition to the medial elbow pathology, there can be lateral (from compression overload) and posterior elbow pathology associated with it. As the name implies, much of the literature is focused on young baseball players, particularly pitchers. However, the pathology can also be seen in other overhead sports, including gymnastics.

Athletes with Little League elbow typically present with slow onset of pain and possibly swelling over the medial epicondyle, generally without instability or locking [43]. A small flexion contracture may also be seen [44]. Radiographs may be normal early on in the disease process but can also demonstrate asymmetric widening of the medial epicondylar physis, separation, and eventual fragmentation [43, 45]. Complete rest for at least 4–6 weeks is the initial treatment, with slow return to play over another 6 weeks if pain has resolved [43].

Medial Epicondyle Avulsion Fractures Avulsion fractures of the medial epicondyle can be seen after a discrete injury in older athletes, and stress fractures can also be seen from chronic overuse. Fractures of the medial epicondyle can also be seen with elbow dislocation. These are generally managed nonoperatively, with a long arm cast in 90 degrees of flexion for 2–4 weeks. Nonunion is common, though not often symptomatic. In part because of the risk of nonunion and a risk of developing instability later, surgery is more often used in the throwing or overhead athlete, including gymnasts [46], especially if there is instability on exam, excessive displacement (greater than 5–15 mm), or incarceration of the avulsed fragment [43, 44]. Displacement may be best measured using the distal humerus axial view on x-ray [47, 48].

Ulnar Collateral Ligament Injury Injuries to the UCL tend to occur in more skeletally mature athletes, and are also most commonly reported in baseball pitchers, but can be seen in other overhead athletes, including gymnasts. The UCL is composed of three bands (anterior, posterior, transverse), and the anterior band is the primary stabilizer against valgus forces [49]. Gymnasts are less likely to have the extensive valgus loads that are seen in throwing athletes; however, they can stress the UCL with repetitive axial loading, often in extension [50]. One small case series on female gymnasts reported that, in contrast to pitchers who generally have chronic overuse injuries with midsubstance tears, the gymnasts all had acute injuries with tear at the origin of the UCL or at its distal insertion. A bail transition from high bar to low (which requires a half twist in the air and catching in handstand) caused the most injuries in this study [50].

Onset of UCL injury can be acute or chronic. There is typically focal tenderness on exam, and there may be instability with valgus stress [43]. Palpation should be performed with the elbow at 50–70 degrees of flexion, to move the muscle mass anterior to the UCL [49]. Valgus stress test is performed at 30 degrees of flexion while palpating the medial joint line. The milking maneuver is done with the shoulder in 70–90 degrees of abduction, externally rotated, elbow at 70 degrees of flexion. The provider should palpate the medial elbow while fully supinating the forearm and then pull on the patient's thumb to produce a valgus force at the elbow. Pain, apprehension, or instability are all positive tests [49].

Radiographs should evaluate for avulsion and loose bodies and also examine the lateral and posterior elbow for associated injuries. Medial joint opening that is greater than a 0.5 mm difference compared to the asymptomatic side, or greater than 2 mm on stress valgus views, is consistent with instability of the UCL [45, 49]. However, asymmetries have been found in asymptomatic baseball players, so advanced imaging is generally recommended. MRI is very sensitive for full thickness tears, but MR arthrography has greater sensitivity for partial thickness tears [45, 49]. Stress ultrasound has also been used to assess for stability [43].

For patients with partial tears, conservative care for pitchers initially includes complete rest, often with bracing for 4–6 weeks, followed by gradual return to sport over 3–6 months [43, 49]. A similar approach seems reasonable in gymnasts with overuse injuries.

Surgical repair of a completely torn UCL has a generally favorable outcome, though there is scant literature related to gymnasts. The literature that is available demonstrates a generally favorable return to sport [51, 52], though in one study the gymnasts took, on average, 2 more months to return to sport than the pitchers (12 months vs 10 months) [53].

9.3.2 Lateral Elbow

Injuries to the lateral elbow include Panner disease and osteochondritis dissecans (OCD), most often of the capitellum. Many believe that Panner disease and OCD exist on a continuum of disordered endochondral ossification [54], with age at presentation determining the differences (Table 9.2). Panner disease is typically seen in athletes 10 years old and younger, though it can occur up to 12 years, while OCD lesions tend to occur in athletes 12 and older [42, 55].

In baseball players, the valgus stress seen during the late cocking and early acceleration phase of throwing results in lateral compressive forces, while in gymnasts the repetitive axial load in extension is thought to be the cause of lateral elbow pathologies [54, 56].

Panner Disease Panner disease is an osteochondrosis of the capitellum; it is a developmental disorder of the epiphysis and its secondary ossification centers. It tends to affect the dominant arm and is more common in males than females when all sports are taken together [54].

The etiology of osteochondroses is poorly understood [42]. Panner disease can be thought of similarly to Legg-Calve-Perthes disease, which tends to be better known by practitioners. Athletes usually are 10 years old or younger and generally complain of dull ache and stiffness in the elbow that develops over time. On exam, athletes complain of tenderness over the capitellum. They may demonstrate a loss of full extension and even a loss of pronation when the disease is advanced [54, 55].

Radiographs will initially show demineralization, progressing to sclerosis and volume loss, and then irregularity, fissuring, or fragmentation of the capitellum [42, 57]. Comparison images of the asymptomatic side may be helpful. MRI demonstrates low T1 signal, with low or high T2 signal depending on the viability of

Table 9.2 Key differences between Panner disease and osteochondritis dissecans (OCD) of the elbow

	Panner disease	OCD
Age (years)	7–12 (though generally <10)	12–15
History/exam	Pain; no mechanical symptoms	Pain, locking, catching, limited motion
Imaging	No loose body	May have loose body
Treatment	Rest	Depends on stability of lesion
Prognosis	Favorable	Guarded

underlying tissue [42]. With resolution of symptoms, reossification occurs, though a persistent flattening of the capitellum may occur in some patients [54].

Treatment is generally rest until pain-free, with gradual return to activities. The duration of rest is variable, anywhere from 2 months to a year or more, depending on the patient's response [58, 59]. Immobilization for 1–3 weeks may be needed initially if pain is severe [60]. The prognosis is favorable for full recovery.

Osteochondritis Dissecans Osteochondritis dissecans (OCD) is an avascular necrosis of the articular cartilage and subchondral bone and is typically seen in athletes 13–15 years of age. OCDs are relatively common in gymnasts; in one small study, OCD lesions were seen in one third of gymnasts, as compared to 10% of control athletes (swimmers, track and field), though in both groups some of these were asymptomatic [61]. The true etiology of OCDs is likely multifactorial, though repetitive microtrauma likely plays a role in their development. In the elbow, OCD is most common in the capitellum but can also be seen in the trochlea, olecranon, and radial head. Unlike Panner disease that has a favorable prognosis, OCD lesions in the elbow may be career ending for gymnasts [61, 62].

Athletes may have a loss of full extension on exam (up to 20 degrees) and lateral elbow swelling. They may complain of locking, which is not seen in Panner disease. More advanced cases may have some loss of pronation range of motion and crepitus with passive pronation and supination [54, 62]. There is some literature to support an increased carrying angle on the affected side [54]. The radiocapitellar compression test is positive if there is increased pain when performing active pronation/supination in full extension, while the examiner provides an axial load, and can be indicative of an OCD lesion [63].

Anteroposterior (AP), lateral, and oblique x-ray views of the elbow should be performed if an OCD is suspected. Imaging may be normal initially or may demonstrate a lucency in the subchondral bone of the anterior aspect of the capitellum (Fig. 9.4). Sclerosis and a crescent sign may be present in older lesions [54, 57]. Fragmentation of the capitellum can occur, and loose bodies may be present, which are not seen in Panner disease [45]. AP x-ray views with 45 degrees of elbow flexion may be helpful [57]; however, one study indicates that this view is better for detecting lesions in baseball players, which tend to be more anterior and proximal than those of gymnasts [56]. Lesions can be broken into three groups on radiographs: Grade I has localized flattening or radiolucency, Grade II is a nondisplaced fragment, and Grade III is a displaced or detached fragment [64].

On MRI, similar to Panner disease, the OCD lesion will have low signal on T1 and variable signal on T2-weighted images [42]. MR arthrogram is recommended to evaluate the articular cartilage and the stability of any loose bodies seen [45]. Stable lesions have intact articular cartilage and stable subchondral bone [54]. Unstable lesions will have a peripheral ring of high signal on T2-weighted images, or a fluid-filled cyst, with impending or true collapse of the subchondral bone, tear of the articular cartilage, or loose fragments within the joint [54, 63]. MRI is 100% sensitive for detecting instability only if all three of the following are present: fluid interface/peripheral rim of high T2 signal, tear of articular cartilage, and cysts at the

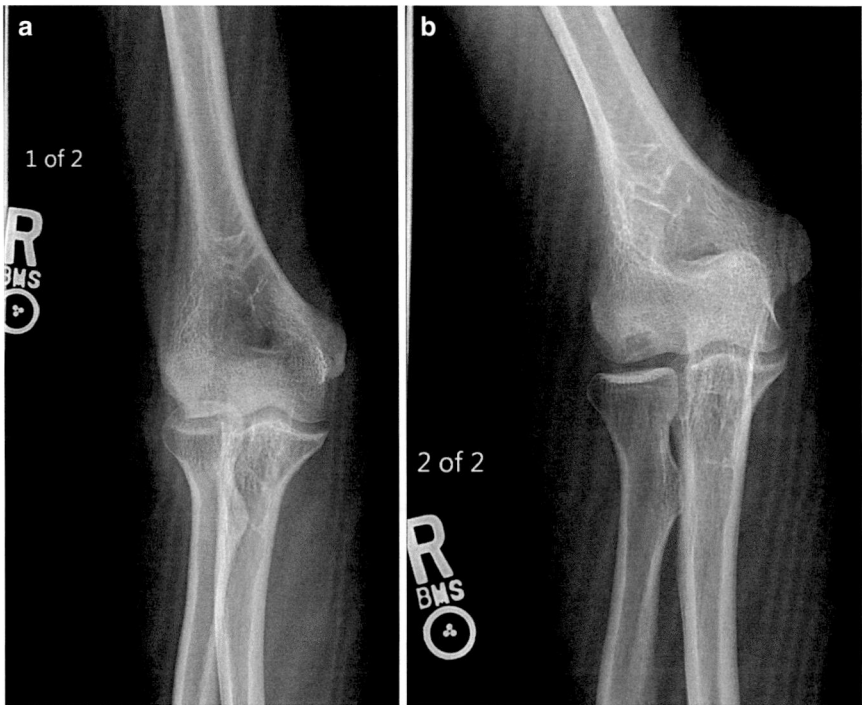

Fig. 9.4 OCD of the elbow. Notice the lucency in the capitellum. Elbow AP (**a**) and elbow AP oblique lateral (external) rotation (**b**) views

donor site. Disruption of the articular cartilage is the most sensitive for instability when occurring in isolation [42]. If the cartilage is intact, this will also dictate the approach of any surgical drilling procedures, to avoid disrupting normal cartilage. In addition, ligamentous structures should be evaluated on MRI, particularly of the medial elbow, as in some athletes it is the high valgus load that contributes to the lateral compressive forces [42]. Care must be taken to identify the normal anatomic sulcus between the capitellum and lateral condyle, a so-called pseudodefect [45, 54, 57]. This pseudodefect is located posteriorly, as opposed to true lesions which are generally anterior, as mentioned above. Ultrasound can also be used to visualize the capitellum and note any articular defects or even displaced fragments [42, 54], though it must be used in experienced hands.

Treatment of OCD depends on appropriately classifying the lesion as stable or unstable [55]. Stable, nondisplaced lesions in a gymnast with open physes can generally be managed conservatively. Even in this category, however, athletes who continue to stress the elbow have worse outcomes [64]. Rest is generally recommended for at least 3–6 months, with slow return to sport beginning after that [58, 63–66]. However, in one study of 24 patients that had conservative care, at 5-year follow-up, only 17% were pain-free, and over half had pain with everyday activities [67], indicating that close follow-up is necessary to ensure improvement in symptoms. Some have suggested follow-up imaging before allowing return to play, with repeat x-rays every 4–6 weeks to ensure the lesion is healing. Progression of the lesion despite rest may be an indication for operative management [63, 65, 68]. MRI may also be repeated at 6 months before allowing full return to play [63].

Surgery is performed for those with persistent symptoms, despite conservative care, loose bodies with mechanical symptoms, or an unstable lesion [54, 63]. Takahara [64] classifies an unstable lesion as having one of the following: a mature capitellum with a closed growth plate, fragmentation (a Grade II or III lesion on radiographs), or a loss of elbow extension greater than or equal to 20 degrees. All of these athletes should be referred for surgery.

Not all athletes will return to prior level of competition even with surgery, and degenerative arthritis may present later in life [45, 54]. In athletes with a closed physis, less than half may return to prior level of competition [64]. Results of surgery in gymnasts are poor, but this is in older studies [69, 70]. Newer techniques may provide better outcomes. In a systematic review of 492 athletes (35 gymnasts), 86% returned to sports at a mean of 5.6 months after surgery [71]. The highest return to sport was found with osteochondral autograft (94%), followed by debridement and marrow stimulation (71%) and finally OCD fixation (64%). Reoperation was required in less than 5% of patients, for repeat debridement or loose body removal.

9.3.3 Posterior Elbow

Olecranon Apophysitis/Stress Fracture Forceful triceps contraction can cause traction forces across the olecranon physis. This is often seen in throwers but can also be seen in other sports, including gymnastics [70, 72]. If the physis is open, it can result in an apophysitis or stress fracture if the physis is closed. Pain is often a vague posterior or posteromedial pain, and there may be associated swelling. The snapping extension test (a forceful extension of the elbow) and the arm bar test may be positive (Fig. 9.5) [43]. Radiographs may show widening of the physis, with or without fragmentation or sclerosis, though advanced imaging may be needed to detect stress fracture. Apophysitis and stress fractures can generally be managed conservatively with rest [43, 70]. Surgery may be indicated after failure of 3–6 months of conservative care [60].

9.3.4 Elbow Dislocation

After the shoulder, the elbow is the second most frequently dislocated joint in the general population [73] and the most frequently dislocated joint in the pediatric population [74]. In a study of collegiate athletes in all sports, elbow dislocations and subluxations together accounted for 3% of all elbow injuries [75]. Interestingly, in

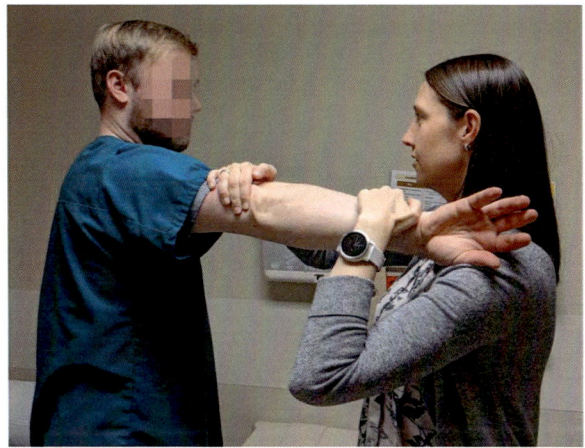

Fig. 9.5 Arm bar test for posterior elbow pathology. The patient places their hand on the examiner's shoulder with the elbow extended and the arm in maximum internal rotation. A downward force is then applied to the olecranon to force maximum extension. Reproduction of pain is a positive test

this 5-year study, the only sports to report elbow dislocations were women's gymnastics, wrestling, football, and women's volleyball. In high school athletes, the rate has been reported as high as 9% of all elbow injuries [73].

In other sports, player-to-player contact is the most likely cause [75], but in gymnastics dislocations can result after a fall on an outstretched hand, with full or near full extension and supination [57].

Dislocations are described based on the relationship of the ulna and radius to the humerus, with posterior dislocation being the most common [74]. Nerve injury, most frequently to the ulnar nerve, can occur, and therefore careful neurological assessment is required [74]. Due to the traumatic nature of the injury, the remainder of the arm should also be assessed for injury.

Initial AP and lateral radiographs are usually sufficient for evaluation. The medial epicondyle can become entrapped in the joint and should also be evaluated with radiographs [57]. CT can be performed if fracture is suspected but not appreciated on x-ray. Postreduction radiographs should also be performed to confirm relocation. A "drop sign" on lateral elbow radiographs indicates a high likelihood of repeat instability. This is positive when the ulnohumeral distance is equal to or greater than 4 mm [76]. Relocation generally requires conscious sedation. Stability of the joint should be assessed while the patient is still sedated. Repeat neurovascular exam should be completed after reduction and once the patient can participate.

As long as the elbow is stable, immobilization in a sling for less than a week is all that is required before simple range of motion exercises can begin [74]. Longer immobilization is more likely to lead to loss of full extension, which is the most common complication [73]. Surgical repair is performed if the elbow remains unstable after relocation. Return to sport occurs over several weeks [73–75]. Persistent instability may manifest as posterolateral rotatory instability, with symptoms ranging from lateral elbow pain, occasional snapping, or frank instability. This often requires surgical management [44].

9.4 Wrist and Hand Injuries

The wrist and hand are commonly injured in all levels of gymnastics due to frequent upper extremity weight-bearing, high loads of force, and excess ranges of motion that are required in various events [77–79]. The wrist is at risk of both acute and overuse injuries that can eventually lead to degenerative changes as gymnasts age [79–82]. The young gymnast with open physes is at especially high risk of long-term pain and disability resulting from the well-documented phenomenon of "gymnast's wrist" or distal radial physis injury. As in the elbow, for most wrist injuries, often a period of full rest from weight-bearing activities is required. Physical therapy can strengthen forearm musculature to dissipate forces through the wrist, improve range of motion and biomechanics, and provide proprioceptive training [80, 83, 84]. Preventative measures include wrist splints, such as Lion Paws, Tiger Paws, or Gibson braces, to reduce wrist extension and provide palm padding, though evidence for this is limited [79, 82, 83].

9.4.1 Distal Radial Physis Injury

Injury to the distal radial physis is the most well-studied wrist injury in gymnasts and is commonly known as "gymnast's wrist" [45, 57, 77, 81, 82]. This occurs due to repetitive loading of the joint in skeletally immature gymnasts with open physes. The physis closes between 13–15 years in females and 15–17 years in males. Typical gymnastics activities result in forces at the wrist between 2 and 16 times body weight [45, 79, 81, 83, 85–87]. The radius bears 80% of these axial forces through the wrist, while the ulna bears only 20%. This repetitive axial loading in extension is thought to cause ischemia to the radial metaphysis and epiphysis, resulting in inhibition of ossification.

Clinically, athletes complain of dorsal wrist pain with weight-bearing activities, relieved with rest. Examination reveals tenderness and swelling over the distal radius and pain with wrist extension and axial loading. Range of motion may be normal or mildly reduced, and grip strength may be diminished due to pain [80–83].

Imaging findings include haziness and widening of the distal radial physis and an irregular and sclerotic metaphysis [45, 57, 79, 85]. This can usually be seen on radiographs (Fig. 9.6) and can be further evaluated with MRI. Comparison views of the asymptomatic side may be helpful.

Treatment includes decreasing upper extremity weight-bearing, and, in more severe cases, immobilization with bracing or casting [45, 81, 83]. Reevaluation can be performed after 6–12 weeks of rest, depending on the severity of symptoms and imaging findings. Positive ulnar variance compared to the uninjured wrist, radial-sided physeal widening, or radial-sided early physis closure, indicates a greater severity of injury and will generally require longer rest periods [79, 82, 83, 88]. Return to gymnastics can occur before resolution of radiographic abnormalities, which often lags behind improvement of clinical symptoms. In more severe cases,

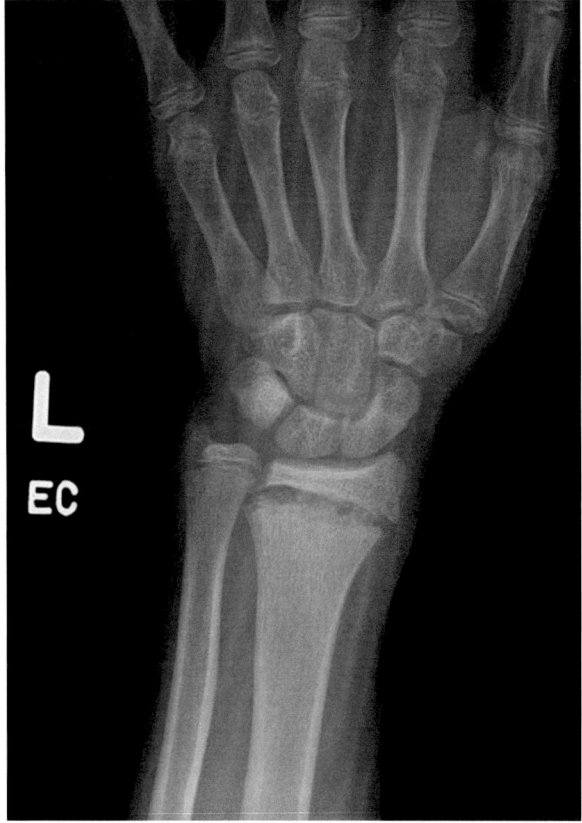

Fig. 9.6 Distal radial physis injury. PA wrist. Note the widening of the radial physis and bony resorption at the distal metaphysis

however, providers may consider reimaging the wrist for up to a year after diagnosis, in part to assess for premature closure of the physis [45, 82]. When returning to sport, especially in severe cases with early radial physis closure, positive ulnar variance may occur as the ulnar physis remains open and continues to grow causing a relative length discrepancy [77, 79, 82, 85]. This leads to excessive forces through the ulnar side of the wrist with weight-bearing and results in ulnar impaction (described below) which can cause triangular fibrocartilage complex (TFCC) tears or degenerative changes to carpal bones [57, 77, 82, 85]. In these instances of radial physeal arrest and positive ulnar variance, surgical intervention can be considered, such as ulnar shortening osteotomy with or without distal ulna epiphysiodesis. The goal is to prevent long-term injuries to the TFCC or carpal bones and ligaments [45, 83].

9.4.2 Ulnar Impaction Syndrome

Positive ulnar variance can result from a variety of causes, including genetic factors, trauma, and early closure of the radial physis. This causes the ulna to bear excessive amounts of weight when loading the wrist in extension and causes increased

Fig. 9.7 Positive ulnar variance on clenched fist view

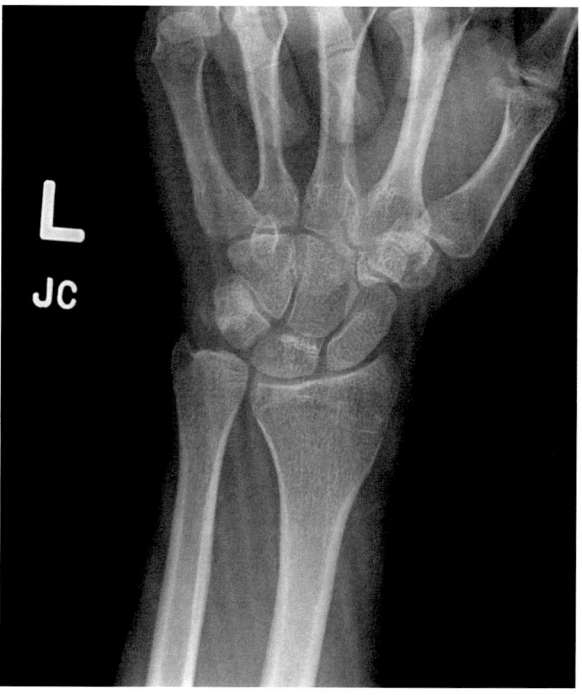

compression of the TFCC and carpal bones, primarily the lunate and triquetrum [80, 82, 83, 87, 89]. This is termed ulnar impaction syndrome or ulnar abutment, and athletes often describe insidious onset of ulnar-sided wrist pain with wrist extension and loading [82, 83, 89]. Examination is notable for tenderness to palpation at the dorsal ulnar styloid, lunate, or triquetrum, and pain with wrist extension, ulnar deviation, and axial loading [80, 82, 83, 89]. Injury to the distal radioulnar joint (DRUJ) can present similarly to this condition but is more likely if pain on exam results from compression of the radius and ulna together while performing pronation and supination [83].

Radiographs for ulnar impaction syndrome demonstrate positive ulnar variance with the forearm in neutral position or positive ulnar variance that may only be visualized with forearm pronation and a clenched fist (Fig. 9.7). In more advanced cases, radiographs can demonstrate cystic changes and sclerosis to the ulna, lunate, and triquetrum [82, 83]. MRI can detect marrow edema, chondromalacia, TFCC tears, and intercarpal ligamentous injuries that result from ulnar impaction [79, 80, 83, 87]. Occasionally, athletes may have neutral or negative ulnar variance on imaging but still experience dynamic impaction causing pain [89].

Treatment of ulnar impaction includes rest from weight-bearing activities. For more severe and chronic symptoms, intraarticular steroid injections can be utilized judiciously but avoided in younger athletes [80, 83]. If conservative measures fail, surgical interventions may include debridement or repair of TFCC tears, and in skeletally mature patients, ulnar recession, wafer resection, or shortening osteotomy to reduce ulnar variance [80, 82, 83].

9.4.3 Triangular Fibrocartilage Complex (TFCC) Injuries

The TFCC consists of multiple structures: central disc, meniscus homolog, extensor carpi ulnaris tendon sheath, and multiple superficial ligaments of the radius, ulna, and carpal bones [82, 83, 90, 91]. It functions to stabilize the ulnar wrist by supporting the DRUJ and provides shock absorption at the ulnocarpal joint [82]. TFCC injuries can occur as an isolated event or due to overuse, such as in ulnar impaction or extensor carpi ulnaris subluxation [83]. Central tears are more commonly chronic injuries and are due to repetitive axial loading with ulnar deviation. Peripheral tears are more often acute injuries that occur from forced extension, such as a fall onto an outstretched hand, or repetitive twisting of the wrist [82, 83, 89, 91]. Both acute and chronic TFCC injuries occur frequently in gymnasts [82].

Symptoms include ulnar-sided wrist pain which is worse with ulnar deviation, wrist extension, or gripping, as well as clicking and popping with pronation and supination [83, 91]. Examination reveals tenderness with deep palpation between the flexor carpi ulnaris and the ulnar styloid, and pain with wrist pronation, extension, and ulnar deviation [80, 82] (Fig. 9.8). The "press test" is highly sensitive for TFCC tears and involves having the patient push-up off a chair from a seated position (Fig. 9.9). A positive result is ulnar-sided pain [92].

The TFCC is not visualized on x-ray, but positive ulnar variance may be seen, which is a risk factor for TFCC injury [91]. MRI or MRI arthrogram can demon-

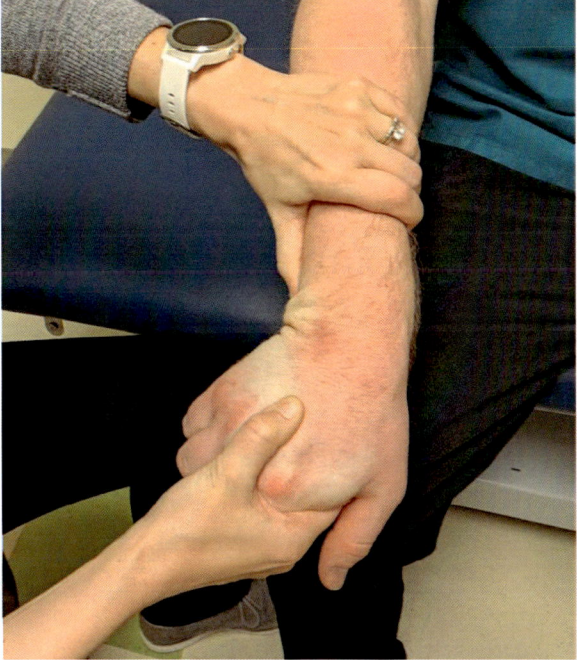

Fig. 9.8 Test for TFCC pathology. The examiner places the patient's wrist in slight extension and ulnar deviation. An axial load is then applied. Reproduction of pain is a positive test

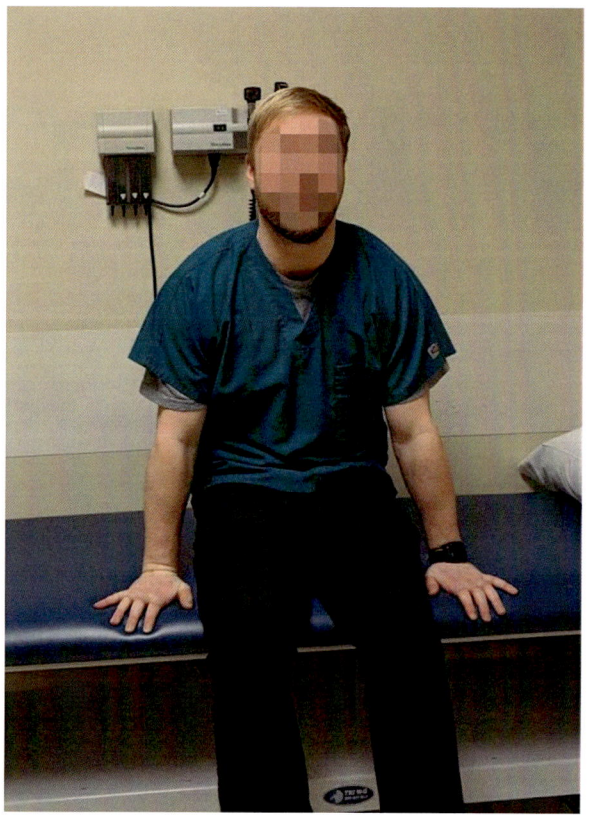

Fig. 9.9 Press test for TFCC pathology. The patient attempts to lift themselves up from a chair or exam table using their hands. Reproduction of pain is a positive test

strate cartilage changes and tears, but sensitivity is only 60%, while specificity is 90% [82, 93]. The gold standard for diagnosis is surgical arthroscopy [83]. Because of the TFCC's role in stabilizing the DRUJ, athletes with suspected TFCC tears should also be evaluated for DRUJ instability [82, 91]. As mentioned previously, with DRUJ instability, pain occurs on exam when compressing the radius and ulna together while performing pronation and supination [83, 94]. Other maneuvers include the "piano key sign," which involves pressing the palm on a table and noting exaggerated dorsal-palmar translation compared to the other side [80, 91, 94].

Initial management of suspected TFCC injury includes 4–6 weeks of rest with consideration of immobilization for more severe tears [80, 82, 91]. Physical therapy can strengthen forearm musculature and correct biomechanical loading issues to reduce excessive impact to the TFCC [83]. Steroid injections into the ulnocarpal joint can be considered in chronic injuries in older gymnasts [83]. Surgical intervention can be performed if athletes fail conservative treatment, have DRUJ instability, or are elite competitors who require faster symptom resolution [82, 91]. Debridement rather than repair is usually performed for central tears because they are poorly vascularized, while peripheral tears can be repaired as they have better vascularization. Both treatments have good outcomes [80, 82, 83, 91]. For athletes with positive ulnar variance, ulnar shortening procedures can be performed simultaneously [83]. Debridement requires a period of at least 2 weeks of immobilization, while arthroscopic repair requires at least 6–12 weeks before gradual return to sport [83, 91].

9.4.4 Scaphoid Injuries

The scaphoid is the most frequently fractured carpal bone [84, 91, 94]. Fractures and impaction can occur in gymnasts due to repetitive axial loading of the wrist in extension and radial deviation [82, 83, 91]. Impaction involves the dorsal rim of the scaphoid contacting the dorsal lip of the radius [80]. Gymnasts are especially vulnerable to stress fractures when rapidly increasing their amount of training [83]. Acute fractures typically occur due to a fall onto an outstretched hand [57]. The scaphoid waist is often the site of fracture due to maximal torsional load of the scaphoid in this area [83], but young athletes also commonly have fractures distal to the scaphoid waist [57].

Presenting symptoms for scaphoid impaction and fractures include chronic or acute radial-sided wrist pain, worse with the aforementioned loading activities [81]. Examination is significant for tenderness over the anatomic snuffbox, reduced range of motion, and weak grip strength [80, 83, 94]. X-rays, including a scaphoid view with the wrist in ulnar deviation, may be negative at initial presentation, or fractures may be seen as an area of sclerosis, typically at the scaphoid waist [57, 83, 84, 91] (Fig. 9.10). Gymnasts with scaphoid impaction may have an ossicle or hypertrophic

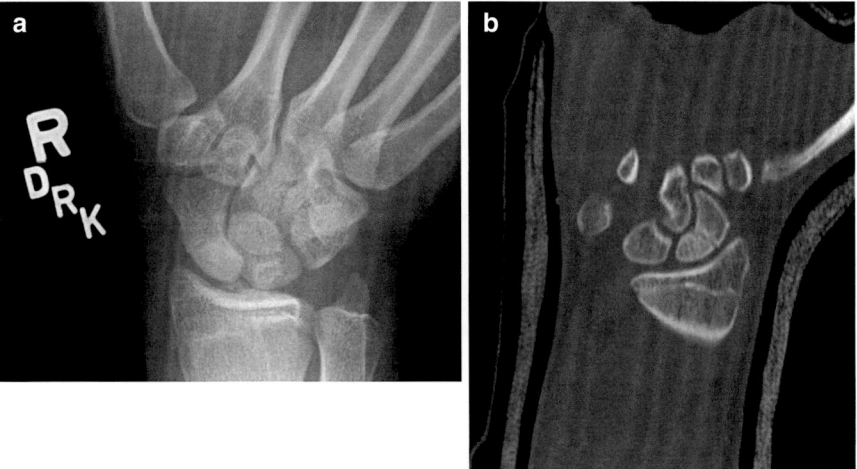

Fig. 9.10 Scaphoid fracture (waist). PA wrist with ulnar deviation (**a**) and coronal CT (**b**). This is a healing fracture with bony remodeling

ridge along the dorsal scaphoid rim on x-ray. MRI is the gold standard to assess for scaphoid fractures and will show scaphoid edema with or without a definitive fracture line [82, 83]. A negative MRI has a 100% negative predictive value for scaphoid injury [95].

Management includes either a long or short arm thumb spica cast for at least 8–12 weeks, depending on location of the fracture. Given that blood normally travels in a retrograde fashion from the distal to proximal scaphoid, proximal fractures may require up to 6 months to heal [82, 83, 91, 96]. Scaphoid fractures should be high on the differential diagnosis of dorsal radial wrist pain due to high risk for nonunion and avascular necrosis if not recognized and treated early and must be followed closely until healing is complete [83, 84]. Therefore, in acute wrist injuries with suspected scaphoid fractures without x-ray findings, the wrist should be immobilized via casting or splinting and x-rays repeated in 10–14 days [97]. Healing of documented fractures should be confirmed with CT or MRI, with resolution of tenderness at the anatomical snuffbox before a gymnast can gradually return to activities [83]. Physical therapy can strengthen forearm musculature and improve range of motion at the wrist after immobilization. Bracing is usually recommended when returning to sport. In other sports, this is often a rigid brace, but as this is not practical in gymnastics, braces such as Lion Paws or Tiger Paws can be used [80, 81, 91]. Surgery with open reduction and internal fixation may be necessary for both acute fractures and stress fractures if casting fails, the fracture appears displaced, or the fracture occurs to the proximal pole of the scaphoid [80, 82, 94]. Surgery may also be considered for faster return to sport [83, 84]. Scaphoid impaction syndrome that fails conservative measures can be treated surgically with a cheilectomy of the hypertrophic dorsal ridge [80, 98].

9.4.5 Scapholunate Ligament Injury/Dissociation

The scapholunate ligament is important in providing stability to the carpal bones of the wrist and is the most commonly injured wrist ligament in gymnasts [80, 82, 99]. Injuries occur often due to falls on an outstretched hand or loading the wrist with extension and ulnar deviation, causing the capitate to drive between the scaphoid and lunate [80, 82, 83, 91, 99]. Pain is usually chronic in nature and located over the dorsal radial wrist in association with swelling, clicking, or popping, decreased wrist range of motion, and weakened grip strength [82, 91, 99, 100]. Watson's test involves the examiner placing pressure over the volar proximal scaphoid and moving the wrist from extension with ulnar deviation to flexion with radial deviation. This movement will elicit a palpable clunk as the scaphoid subluxes, which indicates complete ligament tear and scapholunate instability [80, 82, 91].

Radiographs are often normal, but complete tears or chronic partial tears may demonstrate dissociation between the scaphoid and lunate that measures 3 mm or greater, or increased scapholunate or radiolunate angle [80, 82, 99–101]. Dynamic instability due to scapholunate ligament injury may be present only on stress views, which require fist clenching or ulnar deviation of the wrist [80, 82, 99]. MRI arthrogram can reliably visualize complete ligament tears, but not partial tears, and can demonstrate bony edema, but arthroscopy is the gold standard for assessment [80, 82, 91, 99]. Ultrasound has also been used but has variable sensitivity for detecting tears and instability [102, 103].

For management of incomplete ligament injuries, conservative measures include avoiding activities that cause excessive wrist extension, and wrist immobilization with splinting or bracing. This is followed by physical therapy and gradual return to activities over the course of 3 months [91, 99]. Surgical measures, including debridement or wire pin fixation, can be considered if nonoperative management fails or if return to sport must occur quickly [82]. Treatment for complete tears or dissociation on imaging involves surgical repair [82, 91, 100]. Chronically untreated ligament tears can result in scapholunate advanced collapse and can require carpal fusion, carpectomy, or wrist reconstruction, which can be career ending for gymnasts [82].

9.4.6 Ganglion Cysts

Ganglion cysts are benign fluid-filled cysts that typically measure 1–2 centimeters in size and occur commonly in the wrist. The most common location is over the dorsal scapholunate joint, but they can also occur dorsally over the radiocarpal joint, scaphotrapezial joint, or flexor carpi ulnaris tendon [91, 104, 105]. They may be asymptomatic, but can be a cause of chronic wrist pain in gymnasts [79, 80]. Ganglia can be primary occurrences or result from pathology, such as degenerative or traumatic tears to the underlying joint capsule or tendon sheath due to repetitive dorsal wrist stress from gymnastic activities [80, 91]. Symptoms include pain with wrist extension, which impinges the ganglia, or with wrist flexion, reduced range of motion, and decreased grip strength. Examination reveals a palpable firm, rubbery, fixed nodule which may or may not be tender, and transilluminates with light [105]. Imaging to identify occult ganglia can include ultrasound or MRI, with ultrasound being more cost-effective [106]. However, MRI allows for closer assessment of underlying ligamentous injuries [91].

Treatment involves immobilization with wrist splinting, pain control with oral medications, and possibly aspiration with or without steroid injection. If these measures fail, surgical excision can be considered. Treatment with aspiration or surgical excision has high rates of reoccurrence and has similar rates of resolution compared to conservative treatment, unless the stalk is identified and surgically removed [91, 104–107].

9.4.7 Dorsal Wrist Impingement

Dorsal wrist impingement is characterized by dorsal wrist pain associated with repetitive wrist extension and axial loading [80, 82]. It is a diagnosis of exclusion after other etiologies of dorsal wrist pain, such as scaphoid fracture or impaction syndrome, TFCC injury, DRUJ instability, and gymnast's wrist, are ruled out [79, 108]. Various etiologies have been proposed, including radiocarpal capsulitis and capsular impingement between the extensor carpi radialis brevis and scaphoid [109], thickening of the extensor retinaculum and synovitis of the extensor tendons creating tendon impingement [78, 110], or radiocarpal or midcarpal subcapsular soft tissue impingement [108]. Dorsal wrist ganglia may also be present. Diagnosis is made clinically based on symptoms and tenderness and swelling along the distal dorsal wrist, with imaging that excludes the aforementioned causes [79, 82, 108, 110]. Chronic cases may demonstrate osteophytes on the dorsal distal radius, scaphoid, or lunate on x-ray [80, 82, 111]. Treatment includes several weeks to months of rest from upper extremity weight-bearing, wrist splinting in neutral position, and physical therapy to correct biomechanics, strengthen forearm musculature, and improve range of motion. Steroid injections can be considered in older athletes with chronic symptoms. In cases that fail conservative management, surgical excision of the affected capsule, soft tissue, or retinaculum is performed, sometimes with posterior interosseous neurectomy [80, 82].

9.4.8 Grip Lock

Grip lock injuries occur to gymnasts who use leather dowel grips to reduce friction and improve grip while performing routines on the high bar or uneven bars. The injury occurs when a grip becomes worn and stretched out and overlaps around the bar, causing it to catch or lock in place. This immobilizes the gymnast's hand and wrist while the gymnast's body continues to rotate and results in a wrist sprain, extensor tendon injury, or forearm fracture [81, 83, 112, 113]. Injuries have only been reported in men, possibly due to having larger hands and higher repetitive forces on grips [113] as well as the relatively smaller size of the high bar in relation to the uneven bars. Anecdotally, however, the authors have known one female gymnast with grip lock with resulting forearm fracture requiring surgery. If the grip lock is severe, extricating the gymnast from the bar may be difficult and should be undertaken with care. Radiographic evaluation should include x-rays to assess for fracture, and MRI should be considered to evaluate ligament or tendon injuries. Management of grip lock injuries is dependent on what is injured and can include a range of nonconservative management to surgical fixation of fractures. Residual deficits of decreased wrist range of motion and pain may persist, but most gymnasts return to sport [83, 113]. Prevention of grip lock injuries includes regular checks of grips for stretching out over time and ensuring that they are not long enough to overlap around the bar before a routine. Worn or stretched out grips should be replaced, and athletes should not borrow other gymnasts' grips [81, 114, 115].

Fig. 9.11 Rips due to friction from swinging on bars

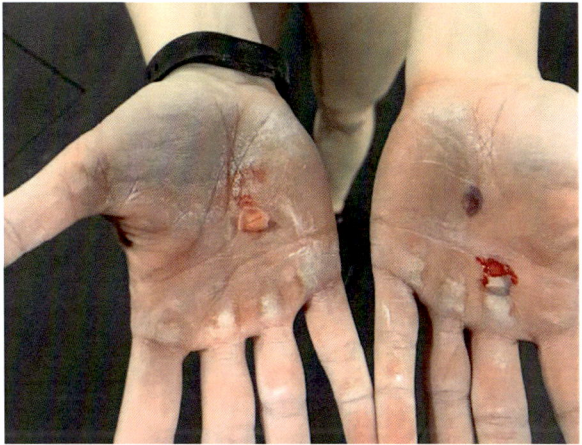

9.4.9 Rips

Rips, calluses, and blisters are common injuries in gymnasts who need to grip an apparatus while hanging, swinging, or supporting themselves (Fig. 9.11). High levels of friction between the hands and apparatus occur and can lead to skin blisters and eventually tearing, referred to as "rips" [81, 114]. These can also occur on the wrist and forearm from leather grips themselves. Treatment of rips should include trimming away excess torn skin, cleaning the exposed area, and cleaning the equipment if blood is present. The injured area should be covered with padded dressings to prevent further ripping, infection, and transmission of infection. Providers should note that the blisters, rips, or the dressings on them may reduce gripping ability and thereby place the gymnast at higher risk of other injuries [81, 114]. Practically, many gymnasts simply train with rips without any extra protection. While this does leave them vulnerable to secondary infection, this is rarely seen. Prevention of rips and blisters includes reducing friction using grips or chalk, ensuring appropriate fit of grips, and shaving down calluses to prevent rips.

References

1. Edouard P, Steffen K, Junge A, Leglise M, Soligard T, Engebretsen L. Gymnastics injury incidence during the 2008, 2012 and 2016 Olympic Games: analysis of prospectively collected surveillance data from 963 registered gymnasts during Olympic Games. Br J Sports Med. 2018;52(7):475–81.
2. Hootman JM, Dick R, Agel J. Epidemiology of collegiate injuries for 15 Sports: prevention initiatives. J Athl Train. 2007;42(2):311–9.
3. Kay MC, Register-Mihalik JK, Gray AD, Djoko A, Dompier TP, Kerr ZY. The epidemiology of severe injuries sustained by National Collegiate Athletic Association student-athletes, 2009–2010 through 2014–2015. J Athl Train. 2017;52(2):117–28.

4. Roos KG, Marshall SW, Kerr ZY, Golightly YM, Kucera KL, Myers JB, et al. Epidemiology of overuse injuries in collegiate and high school athletics in the United States. Am J Sports Med. 2015;43(7):1790–7.
5. Thomas RE, Thomas BC. A systematic review of injuries in gymnastics. Phys Sportsmed. 2019;47(1):96–112.
6. Caine D, Nassar L. Gymnastics injuries. In: Caine D, Mafulli N, editors. Epidemiology of pediatric sports injuries individual sports. Basel: KARGER; 2005. p. 18–58.
7. Farana R, Jandacka D, Uchytil J, Zahradnik D, Irwin G. Technique selection "the coaches challenge" influencing injury risk during the first contact hand of the round off skill in female gymnastics. J Hum Kinet. 2017;56(1):51–9.
8. Farana R, Jandacka D, Uchytil J, Zahradnik D, Irwin G. Musculoskeletal loading during the round-off in female gymnastics: the effect of hand position. Sport Biomech. 2014;13(2): 123–34.
9. Farana R, Jandacka D, Uchytil J, Zahradnik D, Irwin G. The influence of hand positions on biomechanical injury risk factors at the wrist joint during the round-off skills in female gymnastics. J Sports Sci. 2017;35(2):124–9.
10. Farana R, Exell T, Strutzenberger G, Irwin G. Technique selection in young female gymnasts: elbow and wrist joint loading during the cartwheel and round-off. Eur J Sport Sci. 2018;18(3):423–30.
11. Sands W, McNeal J. Hand position in a back handspring. Technique [Internet]. 2006;8–9. [Cited 2018 Nov 25]. Available from: http://www.usagymlegacy.org/library/decade/2000s/
12. McLaren K, Byrd E, Herzog M, Polikandriotis JA, Willimon SC. Impact shoulder angles correlate with impact wrist angles in standing back handsprings in preadolescent and adolescent female gymnasts. Int J Sports Phys Ther. 2015;10(3):341–6.
13. Weber ER, Chao EY. An experimental approach to the mechanism of scaphoid waist fractures. J Hand Surg Am. 1978;3(2):142–8.
14. Markolf KL, Shapiro MS, Mandelbaum BR, Teurlings L. Wrist loading patterns during pommel horse exercises. J Biomech. 1990;23(10):1001–11.
15. Aronen JG. Problems of the upper extremity in gymnasts. Clin Sports Med. 1985;4(1): 61–71.
16. Sands WA. Injury prevention in women's gymnastics. Sport Med. 2000;30(5):359–73.
17. Saluan P, Styron J, Freeland Ackley J, Prinzbach A, Billow D. Injury types and incidence rates in precollegiate female gymnasts: a 21-year experience at a single training facility. Orthop J Sport Med. 2015;3(4):2325967115577596.
18. Kosnik M, Paulseth S, Abzug A. Salter-Harris fracture of the proximal humerus in an adolescent gymnast. J Orthop Sport Phys Ther. 2018;48(9):729.
19. Carson JT, McCambridge TM, Carrino JA, McFarland EG. Case report: bilateral proximal epiphyseal clavicular stress-related lesions in a male gymnast. Clin Orthop Relat Res. 2012;470(1):307–11.
20. Fallon KE, Fricker PA. Stress fracture of the clavicle in a young female gymnast. Br J Sports Med. 2001;35:448–9.
21. Fujioka H, Nishikawa T, Koyama S, Yamashita M, Takagi Y, Oi T, et al. Stress fractures of bilateral clavicles in an adolescent gymnast. J Shoulder Elb Surg. 2014;23:e88–90.
22. Chang D, Mohana-Borges A, Borso M, Chung CB. SLAP lesions: anatomy, clinical presentation, MR imaging diagnosis and characterization. Eur J Radiol. 2008;68(1):72–87.
23. Aldridge S, Willems WJ. Treatment and rehabilitation of common upper extremity injuries. In: Caine DJ, Russell K, Lim L, editors. Handbook of sports medicine and science: gymnastics. Oxford: Wiley-Blackwell; 2013. p. 125–36.
24. Cools AM, Borms D, Castelein B, Vanderstukken F, Johansson FR. Evidence-based rehabilitation of athletes with glenohumeral instability. Knee Surg Sport Traumatol Arthrosc. 2016;24(2):382–9.
25. Nassar L, Sands W. The artistic gymnast's shoulder. In: Wilk KE, Reinold MM, Andrews JR, editors. The athlete's shoulder. 2nd ed. Philadelphia: Churchill Livingstone; 2009. p. 491–506.

26. Goulart NBA, Lunardi M, Waltrick JF, Link A, Garcias L, Melo de O, et al. Injuries prevalence in elite male artistic gymnasts. Rev Bras Educ Física e Esporte. 2016;30(1):79–85.
27. Dunlavy JK, Sands WA, McNeal JR, Stone MH, Smith SL, Jemni M, et al. Strength performance assessment in a simulated men's gymnastics still rings cross. J Sport Sci Med. 2007;6(1):93–7.
28. Bernasconi S, Tordi N, Parratte B, Rouillon J-D, Monnier G. Surface electromyography of nine shoulder muscles in two iron cross conditions in gymnastics. J Sports Med Phys Fitness. 2004;44(3):240–5.
29. Bernasconi SM, Tordi NR, Parratte BM, Rouillon J-DR, Monnier GG. Effects of two devices on the surface electromyography responses of eleven shoulder muscles during azarian in gymanstics. J Strength Cond Res. 2006;20(1):53–7.
30. Patel DR, Breisach S. Evaluation and management of shoulder pain in skeletally immature athletes. Transl Pediatr. 2017;6(3):181–9.
31. Brockmeyer M, Tompkins M, Kohn DM, Lorbach O. SLAP lesions: a treatment algorithm. Knee Surg Sport Traumatol Arthrosc. 2016;24(2):447–55.
32. Bak K, Kalms SB, Olesen S, Jørgensen U. Epidemiology of injuries in gymnastics. Scand J Med Sci Sports. 1994;4(2):148–54.
33. Wadley GH, Albright JP. Women's intercollegiate gymnastics: injury patterns and "permanent" medical disability. Am J Sports Med. 1993;21(2):314–20.
34. Caraffa A, Cerulli G, Rizzo A, Buompadre V, Appoggetti S, Fortuna M. An arthroscopic and electromyographic study of painful shoulders in elite gymnasts. Knee Surg Sport Traumatol Arthrosc. 1996;4:39–42.
35. Haley CA. History and physical examination for shoulder instability. Sports Med Arthrosc. 2017;25(3):150–5.
36. Caplan J, Julien TP, Michelson J, Neviaser RJ. Multidirectional instability of the shoulder in elite female gymnasts. Am J Orthop. 2007;36(12):660–5.
37. Best MJ, Tanaka MJ. Multidirectional instability of the shoulder: treatment options and considerations. Sports Med Arthrosc. 2018;26(3):113–9.
38. Cody EA, Strickland SM. Multidirectional instability in the female athlete. Oper Tech Sports Med. 2014;22(1):34–43.
39. Neer CS, Foster CR. Inferior capsular shift for involuntary inferior and multidirectional instability of the shoulder. A preliminary report. J Bone Joint Surg Am. 1980;62(6):897–908.
40. Beighton P, Horan F. Orthopaedic aspects of the Ehlers-Danlos syndrome. J Bone Joint Surg Br. 1969;51(3):444–53.
41. Cameron KL, Duffey ML, DeBerardino TM, Stoneman PD, Jones CJ, Owens BD. Association of generalized joint hypermobility with a history of glenohumeral joint instability. J Athl Train. 2010;45(3):253–8.
42. Dwek JR. A segmental approach to imaging of sports-related injuries of the pediatric elbow. Sports Health. 2012;4(5):442–52.
43. Makhni EC, Jegede KA, Ahmad CS. Pediatric elbow injuries in athletes. Sports Med Arthrosc Rev. 2014;22(3):e16–24.
44. Smucny M, Kolmodin J, Saluan P. Shoulder and elbow injuries in the adolescent athlete. Sports Med Arthrosc Rev. 2016;24(4):188–94.
45. Paz DA, Chang GH, Yetto JM, Dwek JR, Chung CB. Upper extremity overuse injuries in pediatric athletes: clinical presentation, imaging findings, and treatment. Clin Imaging. 2015;39(6):954–64.
46. Beck JJ, Bowen RE, Silva M. What's new in pediatric medial epicondyle fractures? J Pediatr Orthop. 2018;38(4):e202–6.
47. Cao J, Smetana BS, Carry P, Peck KM, Merrell GA. A pediatric medial epicondyle fracture cadaveric study comparing standard AP radiographic view with the distal humerus axial view. J Pediatr Orthop. 2018;39(3):e205–9.
48. Farnsworth CL, Souder CD, Bomar JD, Edmonds EW, McNeil NP. The distal humerus axial view. J Pediatr Orthop. 2014;35(5):449–54.

49. Dugas J, Chronister J, Cain EL, Andrews JR. Ulnar collateral ligament in the overhead athlete: a current review. Sports Med Arthrosc Rev. 2014;22(3):169–82.
50. Nicolette GW, Gravlee JR. Ulnar collateral ligament injuries of the elbow in female division I collegiate gymnasts: a report of five cases. Open Access J Sport Med. 2018;9(2018 Sep 7):183–9.
51. Argo D, Trenhaile SW, Savoie FH, Field LD. Operative treatment of ulnar collateral ligament insufficiency of the elbow in female athletes. Am J Sports Med. 2006;34(3):431–7.
52. Kodde IF, Rahusen FTG, Eygendaal D. Long-term results after ulnar collateral ligament reconstruction of the elbow in European athletes with interference screw technique and triceps fascia autograft. J Shoulder Elb Surg. 2012;21(12):1656–63.
53. Jones KJ, Dines JS, Rebolledo BJ, Weeks KD, Williams RJ, Dines DM, et al. Operative management of ulnar collateral ligament insufficiency in adolescent athletes. Am J Sports Med. 2014;42:117–21.
54. Kobayashi K, Burton KJ, Rodner C, Smith B, Caputo AE. Lateral compression injuries in the pediatric elbow: Panner's disease and osteochondritis dissecans of the capitellum. J Am Acad Orthop Surg. 2004;12(4):246–54.
55. Ellington MD, Edmonds EW. Pediatric elbow and wrist pathology related to sports participation. Orthop Clin North Am. 2016;47(4):743–8.
56. Kajiyama S, Muroi S, Sugaya H, Takahashi N, Matsuki K, Kawai N, et al. Osteochondritis dissecans of the humeral capitellum in young athletes: comparison between baseball players and gymnasts. Orthop J Sport Med. 2017;5(3):1–5.
57. Delgado J, Jaramillo D, Chauvin NA. Imaging the injured pediatric athlete: upper extremity. Radiographics. 2016;36(6):1672–87.
58. Bojanić I, Levaj I, Dimnjaković D, Smoljanović T. Osteochondritis dissecans of the elbow. Paediatr Croat. 2018;62(3):111–20.
59. Sakata R, Fujioka H, Tomatsuri M, Kokubu T, Mifune Y, Inui A, et al. Treatment and diagnosis of Panner's disease. A report of three cases. Kobe J Med Sci. 2015;61(2):E36–9.
60. Greiwe RM, Saifi C, Ahmad CS. Pediatric sports elbow injuries. Clin Sports Med. 2010;29(4):677–703.
61. Dexel J, Marschner K, Beck H, Platzek I, Wasnik S, Schuler M, et al. Comparative study of elbow disorders in young high-performance gymnasts. Int J Sport Phys Ther Sport Med. 2014;35(11):960–5.
62. Pengel KB. Common overuse injuries in the young athlete. Pediatr Ann. 2014;43(12):e297–308.
63. Baker CL 3rd, Romeo AA, Baker CL Jr. Osteochondritis dissecans of the capitellum. Am J Sports Med. 2010;38(9):1917–28.
64. Takahara M, Mura N, Sasaki J, Harada M, Ogino T. Classification, treatment, and outcome of osteochondritis dissecans of the humeral capitellum. J Bone Joint Surg. 2007;89(6):1205–14.
65. Matsuura T, Kashiwaguchi S, Iwase T, Takeda Y, Yasui N. Conservative treatment for osteochondrosis of the humeral capitellum. Am J Sports Med. 2008;36(5):868–72.
66. Mihara K, Tsutsui H, Nishinaka N, Yamaguchi K. Nonoperative treatment for osteochondritis dissecans of the capitellum. Am J Sports Med. 2009;37(2):298–304.
67. Takahara M, Ogino T, Fukushima S. Nonoperative treatment of osteochondritis dissecans of the humeral capitellum. Am J Sports Med. 1999;27(6):728–32.
68. Maruyama M, Takahara M, Satake H. Diagnosis and treatment of osteochondritis dissecans of the humeral capitellum. J Orthop Sci. 2018;23(2):213–9.
69. Jackson DW, Silvino N, Reiman P. Osteochondritis in the female gymnast's elbow. Arthroscopy. 1989;5(2):129–36.
70. Maffulli N, Chan D, Aldridge MJ. Overuse injuries of the olecranon in young gymnasts. J Bone Joint Surg Br. 1992;74(2):305–8.
71. Westermann RW, Hancock KJ, Buckwalter JA, Kopp B, Glass N, Wolf BR. Return to sport after operative management of osteochondritis dissecans of the capitellum: a systematic review and meta-analysis. Orthop J Sport Med. 2016;4(6):online 1–8.

72. Chan D, Albridge M, Maffulli N, Davies M. Chronic stress injuries of the elbow in young gymnasts. Br J Radiol. 1991;64(768):1113–8.
73. Dizdarevic I, Low S, Currie DW, Comstock RD, Hammoud S, Atanda A. Epidemiology of elbow dislocations in high school athletes. Am J Sports Med. 2016;44(1):202–8.
74. Parsons BO, Ramsey ML. Acute elbow dislocations in athletes. Clin Sports Med. 2010;29(4):599–609.
75. Goodman AD, Twomey-Kozak J, DeFroda SF, Owens BD. Epidemiology of shoulder and elbow injuries in National Collegiate Athletic Association wrestlers, 2009-2010 through 2013-2014. Phys Sportsmed. 2018;46(3):361–6.
76. Coonrad RW, Roush TF, Major NM, Basamania CJ. The drop sign, a radiographic warning sign of elbow instability. J Shoulder Elb Surg. 2005;14(3):312–7.
77. Overlin AJF, Chima B, Erickson S. Update on artistic gymnastics. Curr Sports Med Rep. 2011;10(5):304–9.
78. Wilson SM, Dubert T, Rozenblat M. Extensor tendon impingement in a gymnast. J Hand Surg Am. 2006;31(1):66–7.
79. DiFiori JP, Caine DJ, Malina RM. Wrist pain, distal radial physeal injury, and ulnar variance in the young gymnast. Am J Sports Med. 2006;34(5):840–9.
80. Webb B, Rettig L. Gymnastic wrist injuries. Clin Sport Med. 1998;17(3):611–21.
81. Overlin AJF. Gymnastics. In: Madden C, Putukian M, McCarty E, Young C, editors. Netter's sports medicine. 2nd ed. Philadelphia: Elsevier; 2018. p. 682–8.
82. Benjamin HJ, Engel SC, Chudzik D. Wrist pain in gymnasts. Curr Sports Med Rep. 2017;16(5):322–9.
83. Wolf MR, Avery D, Wolf JM. Upper extremity injuries in gymnasts. Hand Clin. 2017;33(1):187–97.
84. Nakamoto JC, Saito M, Medina G, Schor B. Scaphoid stress fracture in high-level gymnast: a case report. Case Rep Orthop. 2011;2011:1–3.
85. Keller MS. Gymnastics injuries and imaging in children. Pediatr Radiol. 2009;39(12):1299–306.
86. DiFiori JP, Puffer JC, Aish B, Dorey F. Wrist pain in young gymnasts: frequency and effects upon training over 1 year. Clin J Sport Med. 2002;12(6):348–53.
87. Tolat AR, Sanderson PL, De Smet L, Stanley JK. The gymnast's wrist: acquired positive variance following chronic. J Hand Surg Am. 1992;17(6):678–81.
88. Difiori JP, Puffer JC, Aish B, Dorey F. Wrist pain, distal radial physeal injury, and ulnar variance in young gymnasts: does a relationship exist? Am J Sports Med. 2002;30(6):879–85.
89. Jarrett CD, Baratz ME. The management of ulnocarpal abutment and degenerative triangular fibrocartilage complex tears in the competitive athlete. Hand Clin. 2012;28(3):329–37.
90. Taljanovic M, Sheppard J, Jones M, Switlick D, Hunter T, Roger L. Sonography and sonoarthrography of the scapholunate and lunotriquetral ligaments and triangular fibrocartilage disk: initial experience and correlation with arthrography and magnetic resonance arthrography. Ultrasound Med. 2008;27:179–91.
91. Parmelee-Peters K, Eathorne SW. The wrist: common injuries and management. Prim Care. 2005;32(1):35–70.
92. Lester B, Halbrecht J, Levy I, Gaudinez R. "Press test" for office diagnosis of triangular fibrocartilage complex tears of the wrist. Ann Plast Surg. 1995;35(1):41–5.
93. De Smet L. Magnetic resonance imaging for diagnosing lesions of the triangular fibrocartilage complex. Acta Orthop Belg. 2005;71(4):396–8.
94. Rettig AC. Athletic injuries of the wrist and hand (part I): traumatic injuries of the wrist. Sport Med. 2003;31(6):1038–48.
95. Cook PA, Yu JS, Wiand W, Cook AJ, Coleman CR, Cook AJ. Suspected scaphoid fractures in skeletally immature patients: application of MRI. J Comput Assist Tomogr. 21(4):511–5.
96. Slade JF, Milewski MD. Management of carpal instability in athletes. Hand Clin. 2009;25(3):395–408.
97. Baldassarre RL, Hughes TH. Investigating suspected scaphoid fracture. BMJ. 2013;346:f1370.
98. Linscheid R, Dobyns J. Athletic injuries of the wrist. Clin Orthop Relat Res. 1985:141–51.

99. Snider MG, Alsaleh KA, Mah JY. Scapholunate interosseus ligament tears in elite gymnasts. Can J Surg. 2006;49(4):290–1.
100. Manuel J, Moran SL. The diagnosis and treatment of scapholunate instability. Hand Clin. 2010;26(1):129–44.
101. Kocher MS, Waters PM, Micheli LJ. Upper extremity injuries in the paediatric athlete. Sport Med. 2000;30(2):117–35.
102. Dao KD, Solomon DJ, Shin AY, Puckett ML. The efficacy of ultrasound in the evaluation of dynamic scapholunate ligamentous instability. J Bone Joint Surg. 2004;86(7):1473–8.
103. Finlay F, Lee R, Friedman L. Ultrasound of intrinsic wrist ligament and triangular fibrocartilage injuries. Skelet Radiol. 2004;33(2):85–90.
104. Head L, Gencarelli JR, Allen M, Boyd KU. Wrist ganglion treatment: systematic review and meta-analysis. J Hand Surg Am. 2015;40(3):546–553.e8.
105. Meena S, Gupta A. Dorsal wrist ganglion: current review of literature. J Clin Orthop Trauma. 2014;5(2):59–64.
106. Gant J, Ruff M, Janz BA. Wrist ganglions. J Hand Surg Am. 2011;36(3):510–2.
107. Dias J, Buch K. Palmar wrist ganglion: does intervention improve outcome patient-reported treatment outcomes. Hand Surg. 2003;28B(2):172–6.
108. Terng SCA, Kuypers KC, Koch AR. Inter-carpal soft tissue entrapment. A possible explanation for chronic dorsal wrist pain. J Hand Surg Am. 2006;31(1):41–6.
109. Henry M. Arthroscopic management of dorsal wrist impingement. J Hand Surg Am. 2008;33(7):1201–4.
110. VanHeest AE, Luger NM, House JH, Vener M. Extensor retinaculum impingement in the athlete: a new diagnosis. Am J Sports Med. 2007;35(12):2126–30.
111. Rettig AC. Athletic injuries of the wrist and hand. Part II: overuse injuries of the wrist and traumatic injuries to the hand. Am J Sports Med. 2004;32(1):262–73.
112. Sathyendra V, Payatakes A. Grip lock injury resulting in extensor tendon pseudorupture: case report. J Hand Surg Am. 2013;38(12):2335–8.
113. Bezek EM, VanHeest AE, Hutchinson DT. Grip lock injury in male gymnasts. Sports Health. 2009;1(6):518–21.
114. Hecht SS, Burton MS. Medical coverage of gymnastics competitions. Curr Sports Med Rep. 2009;8(3):113–8.
115. Updegrove GF, Aiyer AA, Fortuna KL. Segmental forearm fracture due to grip-lock injury in male gymnast. JBJS Case Connect. 2015;5(2):1–5.

Chapter 10
Lower Extremity Injuries in Gymnasts

Nicole B. Katz, Ellen Casey, Alexia G. Gagliardi, and Jay C. Albright

10.1 Lower Extremity Introduction

The physical demands of gymnastics place extreme loads on many regions of a gymnast's body. Prior research demonstrates a higher prevalence of lower limb injuries (54.1–70.2%) compared to upper limb injuries (17.1–25.0%) in gymnasts [1–17]. This trend was observed during the last three Olympic Games (2008, 2012, and 2016), where the majority of gymnastic injuries were in the lower limbs (63%) compared to the trunk (23%) or upper limbs (14%) [18]. This trend is also seen in subelite, collegiate, and adolescent gymnasts; injuries to the lower limbs were found to be the most common, followed by injuries to the upper limbs, spine, and trunk [19–21]. Moreover, a recent study assessing all reported injuries in NCAA women's gymnastics between 2009 and 2014 revealed that half were to the lower limbs [22]. For these reasons, a complete understanding of the most common lower limb injuries and the best course of treatment is necessary to provide the optimal medical care.

N. Katz
Lewis School of Medicine at Temple University, Philadelphia, PA, USA
e-mail: Nicole.Katz@Temple.edu

E. Casey (✉)
Department of Physiatry, Hospital for Special Surgery, New York, NY, USA
e-mail: caseye@hss.edu

A. G. Gagliardi
Children's Hospital Colorado, Aurora, CO, USA
e-mail: Alexia.Gagliardi@childrenscolorado.org

J. C. Albright
University of Colorado School of Medicine, Children's Hospital Colorado, Aurora, CO, USA
e-mail: Jay.Albright@childrenscolorado.org

10.1.1 Lower Extremity Injury Epidemiology

The *lower limb* or extremity refers to the hip and the anatomic structures distal to it. Among gymnasts, the most commonly injured lower limb joints are the ankle (10–46% of all injuries) and the knee (5.1–26.2% of all injuries) [1, 8–17, 23]. However, the most recent analysis of NCAA women's gymnastics injuries (2009–2014) found the most commonly injured regions to be the ankle (17.9%), Achilles tendon (13.6%), trunk (13.4%), and foot (12.4%) [22]. To better understand the ankle and foot injury rates in gymnastics, Hunt et al. [24] evaluated all foot and ankle injuries in 1076 elite athletes participating in 37 sports at an NCAA Division 1 institution between 2010 and 2012. This study revealed that gymnastics has the highest rate of ankle and foot injuries overall and the most missed time due to these injuries. This study also reported that ankle and lower leg/Achilles tendon injuries were the most likely to be recurrent issues.

With the exception of one study, sprains accounted for the majority of gymnastics ankle injuries [19–22]. Hudash et al. [6] found the most common ankle injury to be talotibial joint impingement (55.6%) followed by sprains/strains (44.4%). Ankle sprains were the most commonly reported injury by gymnasts participating in the 2002–2004 USA Gymnastics National Women's Artistic Championships [25] as well as the 2008, 2012, and 2016 Olympics [18]. In a study assessing injuries in collegiate gymnasts over 5 years, of the 47 ankle sprains reported, 66.0% included the lateral ligament complex, and 25.5% included the deltoid ligament. Ankle sprains have been shown to affect gymnasts 3 years post injury [6], so this high incidence rate is significant in the careers of gymnasts. O'Kane et al. [7] determined that ankle fractures comprise 22.6% of ankle injuries in gymnasts. Finally, damage to the tibiotalar cartilage is also found to be a pain generator in gymnasts [26].

The knee joint is also a commonly injured joint in gymnasts. Hudash et al. [6] reported patellofemoral pain (22.7%), followed by synovitis (18.1%), tendinitis (13.6%), and sprains (13.6%) to be the most common knee injuries. The knee has the largest proportion of severe injuries (30.2%) and injuries requiring surgery (20.9%) [22]. Internal derangements (ACL ruptures, meniscal tears, and osteochondritis dissecans) composed the largest proportion of severe knee injuries (47.1%) and knee injuries requiring surgery (41.2%) [22]. Unfortunately, the two most common lower extremity injuries—ankle sprains and knee internal derangements—were also determined to have the highest percentage of time loss in gymnastics [20]. A greater appreciation of these injuries is needed to aid in preventing excessive time lost. Although ankle and knee injuries are the most common among gymnasts, other anatomical regions of the lower extremity are also at risk. Among collegiate gymnasts, lower leg/Achilles tendon (13.6% of all injuries) and hip and thigh injuries (6.9% of all injuries) are also quite common [22]. Additionally, lower limb fractures (including both stress fractures and true fractures) are common, with 32% of all fractures occurring in the feet [8].

Although the ankle and knee are the most commonly injured joints in gymnasts overall, injury type, location, and rates vary by age and sex. Research on gymnasts

6–17 years of age revealed that as age increased, so did the frequency of lower extremity injuries [21]. Specifically, in gymnasts 6–11 years of age, upper extremity injuries were more common than lower extremity injuries, whereas in gymnasts 12–17 years of age, lower extremity injuries were most common than upper extremity injuries [21]. Westermann et al. [27] found that though male and female collegiate gymnasts had similar injury rates overall, the anatomic region injured differed based on sex. Male gymnasts obtain more injuries to the upper extremities (53.4%) than lower extremities (32.8%) [8, 27], while female gymnasts obtain more injuries to the lower extremities than upper extremities [1, 8–17, 27]. But, even for males who suffer more upper limb injuries overall, the lower limb body parts most often injured are the ankles (30%) and knees (23%) [8]. Additionally, the sites of chronic and acute injuries are different between men and women in this population. Most chronic injuries occur at the ankles and knees in men but at the feet and knees in women. Acute injuries more often occur at the ankles and feet in men but at the ankles and knees in women [8]. Besides sustaining more lower limb injuries overall (1.7:1 female/male ratio), female gymnasts obtain more acute (1.42:1) and chronic (2.5:1) lower limb injuries compared to males [8].

The discrepancy in injury rates between male and female gymnasts may be attributed to the different events in which they compete [14, 28, 29]. Males compete in floor exercise, pommel horse, still rings, vault, parallel bars, and horizontal (high) bar events, while females compete in vault, uneven bars, balance beam, and floor exercise. The high bar is associated with significant hand and wrist injuries in male gymnasts [28, 30], and though not studied exclusively, the pommel horse is believed to be as well [27]. Floor exercise [20], balance beam [9, 14], and vault [20] have been shown to commonly result in injuries to female gymnasts. Participation in these events may increase the risk of lower limb injury and will be discussed later in this chapter.

It is important to consider how the specific physical demands of the sport contribute to common injuries among gymnasts. Nearly every event requires a takeoff and landing, subjecting the tibiotalar and talonavicular joints to high loads [26, 31]. The forces at the ankle during tumbling takeoffs and landings range from 5 to 23 times that of a gymnast's body weight [31, 32]. This stress on the ankle joints likely contributes to the high incidence and severity of ankle injuries.

Besides the anatomical stress present during takeoff and landing, the mechanics of the sport predispose gymnasts to injury. Vault takeoffs, backward tumbling, and landings require repeated hyperdorsiflexion of the ankle joint, which can result in chronic irritation to the soft tissues and articular surfaces [6]. The emphasis placed on landing without taking any steps, or "sticking the landing," has been linked to injury. Harringe et al. [26] reported that 52% of injuries obtained by collegiate gymnasts occur during landing. Furthermore, McNitt-Gray [33] found that recreational gymnasts less concerned with landing scores, compared to elite gymnasts, altered their landing strategy to dissipate the impact forces over a longer period while velocity increased. The difference in landing mechanics combined with the fact that elite gymnast are performing skills with more height, twists, and flips explains the finding that the more highly competitive gymnasts have higher injury rates compared to the noncompetitive or less competitive gymnasts [3, 4, 34]. Given the evidence that supports landings as the riskiest exercise phase in gymnastics [26], it is unsurprising that acute injuries occur most often during the landing from dismounts [6] or during tumbling in the floor exercise event [4, 6].

Although floor routines last only 90 seconds, this is the longest event performed by gymnasts; in addition, the floor exercise is responsible for a third of competition injuries [20], the greatest percentage of all acute injuries [4, 7, 14], and the highest rate of knee and ankle injuries [35]. Though this event consists of a wide variety of movements, it is the landing phase that contributes to most injuries. Because floor exercise routines consist of many acrobatic skills in a series, any small mistake can affect the ankle during the landing phase [26] and result in joint compression and rotation which may lead to injury [4, 5, 7, 9, 12, 14, 26, 34, 36]. In competitive gymnasts, 49% of all injuries (acute and overuse) occurred while landing in a floor exercise routine [7].

Just as in the floor exercise, the landings after dismounting the other apparatuses are also associated with injury [20]. The majority of the ankle sprains obtained from the balance beam and vault were a result of the dismount [22]. Landing from the vault contributes to more than 25% of all gymnastic injuries, primarily involving the ankle and knee [20]. In a study conducted by Hunter and Torgan [37], 83.3% of the major knee injuries reported were attributed to dismounts, with 63.6% involving a twisting dismount. Similar to landing a tumbling pass, in dismounting from an apparatus, the gymnast is coming in contact with the ground from a significant height. A dismount from the upper uneven bar is a distance of over 8 feet and from the vault is over 4 feet.

Several studies have compared types and rates of injury in practice versus competition. A study of the National Collegiate Athletic Association between the years 1988 and 2004 revealed that lower limb injuries were common in both competition and practice [20]. Since the majority of injuries obtained during competitions (70.7%) were from landings, [20] the lack of assistance by coaches, harder landing surfaces (loose foam pits and more cushioned mats are often used in practice), and increased pressure to "stick the landing" in competition may also contribute. In practice, the most common injury site was the ankle, and the second most common body part was the knee [20]. In competition, the knee was the most commonly injured body part followed by the ankle [20, 22]. Overall, gymnasts are 3–9.95 times more likely to sustain an ankle ligament sprain [20, 22] and 5.43–6 times more likely to sustain a knee injury in competitions than in practices [20, 22].

10.1.2 Clinical Approach

The clinical evaluation of a gymnast with a lower limb injury is similar to that of any other athlete; however, it should include specific questions and physical exam maneuvers to determine the exact cause and optimal rehabilitation strategy to enable the gymnast's complete return to sport. Because reinjury is a common problem in gymnastics (the reinjury rate is 33% in highly competitive female gymnasts) [14], early detection and proper management are imperative to prevent the recurrence of these injuries.

When taking a gymnast's history, it is important to ask about pain with both daily activities and gymnastics movements. Specific questions like, "are you or your coach modifying your training because of this pain? If so, is it helping?" can help identify the severity of the pain as well as provide insight into how much education should be provided to the gymnast, coach, and family. In addition, questions about recent changes to training as well as prior injuries are important. With regard to training, questions should address recent changes to practice sessions (duration, frequency, time of day, different order of events), coaching (new technique in spotting, new practice structure), equipment (different landing surfaces, new equipment, addition/subtraction of tape or an orthosis), and physical demands (learning a new skill, different sequences of skills, new competition level). Understanding the athlete's goals is also a key component in devising an individualized medical plan, so questions about gymnast's aspirations and significant upcoming competitions should be asked.

The following sections will review the most commonly seen lower limb injuries, diagnostic tests, and treatment options in order to provide a guide for medical providers who evaluate and treat gymnasts.

10.2 Hip and Thigh

Gymnastics requires a balance between extensive hip range of motion and control [38], and a lack of balance between the two can contribute to hip and thigh injuries. Hip pain in a gymnast may be due to intra- and extra-articular factors. Many of the causes of hip pain in gymnasts will be reviewed in this section.

10.2.1 Impingement, Hip Dysplasia, and Labral Tears of the Hip

Intra-articular causes of hip pain include femoroacetabular impingement (FAI), hip dysplasia, and labral tears. FAI describes increased contact between the femoral head and acetabulum due to abnormal bony morphology in the hip joint. This can be due to increased bone growth on the femoral head (Cam-type FAI) or increased bone around the acetabular rim (Pincer-type FAI). Both types of FAI are associated with the development of labral tears [39]. Hip dysplasia, the undercoverage of the acetabulum of the femoral head, is another intra-articular hip problem seen in gymnasts. Since hip dysplasia is more common in females [40] and associated with an increased range of motion (ROM) [41], this hip shape may enable the gymnast to attain the desired hip motion and flexibility demanded for gymnastics participation. However, the sport's demand for a large ROM may lead to compensatory soft tissue laxity [42–44] and exacerbate hip dysplasia [45, 46]. Though the greater ROM may be seen as a benefit, if it is secondary to an unstable hip joint, it can lead to joint subluxation and labral tears. Both the instability of the hip joint from hip dysplasia and the reduced joint space from intra-articular FAI can cause damage to the labrum [47, 48]. Cadaveric studies have shown increased labral loads in the presence of increased hip abduction and external rotation, hip movements that are common in gymnastics [47].

Impingement of the hip may also be due to extra-articular causes. Subspine impingement involves contact between the anterior inferior iliac spine (AIIS) and the distal anterior femoral neck during flexion of the hip [49, 50]; trochanteric–pelvic impingement (TPI) occurs with contact between the greater trochanter and the ilium during hip abduction in extension [49]; and iliopsoas impingement is due to traction between the iliopsoas tendon and the capsule–labrum complex of the hip [51]. Although the joint morphology and anatomy contributing to extra-articular impingement are likely congenital, the excessive hip ROM and repetitive maneuvers requiring end-range motions may contribute to the development of symptomatic hip impingement in gymnasts [42–44, 47, 52].

Hip diagnostic maneuvers should mimic the multiplanar motions of gymnastics. The physical examination for intra- and extra-articular hip injuries should involve five examination positions: standing, seated, supine, lateral, and prone [53]. Pain with end-range hip flexion and rotation can occur in both dysplasia and FAI with or without labral pathology. Extra-articular hip injuries can be differentiated from intra-articular pathology by their clinical presentation. Subspine and iliopsoas impingement both present with anterior hip pain in flexion, but patients with iliopsoas impingement will also often report a snapping sensation when actively flexing the hip. Conversely, TPI presents with both lateral hip and groin pain during active hip abduction and extension. With this impingement, patients often report feeling that the hip gets stuck and the ROM in the abducted and extended position is decreased [54]. While radiographs should be used to confirm an FAI or hip dysplasia diagnosis, MRI should be used to better visualize the labrum. Labral tears have a classic pathology in which the labrum appears hypertrophic and torn and can result in an intrasubstance ganglion cyst formation [41, 55, 56]. Conservative treatment, including physical therapy and movement modification, is often the best course of treatment for the aforementioned hip injuries. However, if this approach proves unsuccessful, hip arthroscopy to address FAI, hip dysplasia, and labral tears may be indicated. To our knowledge, there are no studies investigating return-to-gymnastics after hip arthroscopy, but rates of return-to-play in all athletes range from 50% to 80% [57–59].

10.2.2 Stress Fractures of the Hip and Thigh

Gymnasts are at risk for a variety of stress fractures, including those of the femoral neck and the femoral shaft. The etiology of stress fractures is complex and likely includes repeated stress placed on the bone during tumbling and landing, often in the setting of reduced bone density and quality. The Female Athlete Triad (low energy availability, amenorrhea/oligomenorrhea, and decreased bone mineral density) [60] is often seen in athletes participating in sports that emphasize leanness [61], and therefore, likely a contributing factor to bone stress injuries in gymnasts. The low energy availability (derived from an inadequate intake of calories) can lead to hormonal adaptations that adversely affect the menstrual cycle as well as bone metabolism [62]. With decreased bone density, gymnasts are more vulnerable to bone stress injuries. Chapter 6 describes the Female Athlete Triad in more detail.

Femoral stress fractures present clinically as hip or groin pain that is exacerbated with weight-bearing and internal rotation. Radiographs may show evidence of stress fractures, but these injuries are best visualized with MRI [63]. Femoral neck stress fractures are divided into two types: compression and tension types. A compression-type stress fracture occurs in the inferior-medial femoral neck, whereas a tension-side stress fracture occurs in the superior-lateral aspect of the femoral neck. The diagnosis of a femoral neck stress fracture should be followed with a break in the athlete's training to allow the fracture to heal and prevent fracture progression. Most femoral neck and shaft stress fractures can be managed conservatively with rest, activity modification, and protected weight-bearing. However, gymnasts with a tension-type femoral neck stress fracture may result in a complete femoral neck fracture [63]. Therefore, athletes with tension-type femoral neck stress fractures, low bone mineral density, and delayed healing may require surgical treatment such as an intramedullary nail [63, 64]. Clinically indicated lab tests as well as a DEXA scan should be ordered, and the clinician should evaluate for other aspects of the Female Athlete Triad. If they are present, nutritional and sports psychology counseling may aid the patient in increasing energy intake to prevent future bone stress injuries. Full diagnostic criteria and treatment of gymnasts with The Female Athlete Triad can be found in Chap. 6.

10.2.3 Apophysitis and Avulsion Fractures

Growth plate injuries, including apophysitis and apophyseal avulsion fractures of the hip and pelvis, can occur in gymnasts. Apophysitis is irritation at the growth plate caused by the pull of the inserting tendon. Chronic inflammation occurs when the apophysis undergoes the ossification of fibrocartilage to hyaline cartilage, thereby increasing susceptibility to an avulsion fracture. Since most ossification centers fuse by 17 years of age (except the ischial apophysis and anterior superior iliac spine that fuse by 35 years of age), these injuries occur in skeletally immature athletes—adolescents between 13 and 17 years of age [65–69]. The high prevalence of these injuries among gymnasts may be attributed to intensive training in young athletes with open apophyses.

The most common sites of avulsion injuries in pediatric and adolescent athletes are the ischial tuberosity (IT), anterior inferior iliac spine (AIIS), and the anterior superior iliac spine (ASIS). Though less common, apophysitis and avulsion fractures can also occur at the iliac crest [67, 68, 70–72]. The IT is the origin of the hamstring muscles, and irritation of this attachment site can be caused by powerful flexion of the hip with extension at the knee joint [42]. The AIIS is the origin of one of the heads of the rectus femoris which may be strained with vigorous hip hyperextension and knee flexion [73, 74]. The ASIS is the origin of the sartorius and the tensor fasciae latae, and injury can occur during sudden straining or twisting [74]. The iliac crest is the attachment site of the abdominal muscles and may be injured during forceful twisting or lateral flexion.

Physical examination of a gymnast with apophysitis or an avulsion fracture may reveal swelling and tenderness of the area as well as possible weakness in the affected muscle groups. Additionally, passive stretch of the injured muscle groups often reproduces the pain [73]. The bone fragmentation associated with apophysitis or avulsion fractures can be visualized with radiographs; however, normal X-rays have been reported among patients with these diagnoses, and therefore, advanced imaging might be warranted [75]. Apophysitis should be treated with a brief period of rest followed by physical therapy. Avulsion fractures are treated more intensely with a period of rest involving protected weight-bearing, physical therapy, and then return to play in usually 6–8 weeks. The Definitive decision on when the gymnast is able to appropriately return to full activity is dependent on the radiographic signs of healing and clinical examination [73]. Avulsion fractures occasionally require surgery if the fracture is significantly displaced or there is chronic pain associated with nonunion [70, 71, 76–79].

10.2.4 Tendon Injuries

The soft tissues of the upper leg of gymnasts are also at risk of injury. Hamstring injuries may result from sudden hip abduction or flexion which often occur in leaps or straddle jumps [6]. Considering that most muscle strains were found to occur during the first hour of gymnastics practice [12], insufficient warm-ups might be a contributing factor to strains, including hamstring strains. High hamstring tendinopathy, also known as proximal hamstring tendinopathy, can be especially debilitating and is a main cause of underperformance in athletes [80]. Iliopsoas tendinopathy and bursitis are injuries less reported in the literature but seen clinically in gymnasts. The iliopsoas is involved in decelerating the hip and energy transfer during running [81]. Mild injuries to the hip and thigh have also been reported from direct and forceful contact with the uneven parallel bars [82].

Patients with tendinopathy or bursitis will often report that the pain began insidiously, but they may also be able to identify a specific mechanism of injury [80]. Tendinopathy, bursitis, and strains are often diagnosed through palpation and strength testing, but ultrasound imaging or MRI may be required to determine the severity of the injury [83, 84]. Treatment of these upper leg injuries can vary from conservative to invasive. Conservative management will almost always include some type of activity modification. Ideally, the physician should provide specific guidelines for what movements, events, and training the gymnast may participate in during the rehabilitation and recovery process. The gymnast should be provided with an estimated timeline for return to gymnastics and the necessary parameters for full return, including resolution of injury on imaging, reduction in pain, and improvement in strength. Additionally, in most cases, gymnasts should be referred to a physical therapist who has expertise in treating this type of athlete and injury. Goals of physical therapy for hip and pelvic injuries often include improvements in strength and neuromuscular control of the lumbopelvic-hip muscles to enhance core stability.

10.3 Knee

Gymnasts are at risk for acute and overuse knee injuries. Acute injuries often occur during landing and may cause ligamentous injuries, meniscus tears, or patellar subluxations or dislocations. Overuse injuries to the knee are especially common in growing gymnasts. Patellofemoral pain syndrome, apophysitis, tendonitis, and osteochondritis dissecans are common causes of chronic pain in these athletes.

10.3.1 Ligamentous and Meniscus Tears

The most common knee injuries reported in the gymnastics literature are ligament tears. Gymnasts are at risk for anterior cruciate ligament (ACL) tears (Fig. 10.1) [85, 86] from landing with their knees in a hyperextended position [6] or in a valgus or varus load. This valgus or varus landing position often occurs when they attempt to land a twisting skill without fully completing the rotation [87]. Tears to the medial collateral ligament (MCL), lateral collateral ligament (LCL), and meniscus (Fig. 10.2) have also been associated with gymnastics [88].

The mechanism of injury combined with the clinical presentation focuses the clinician's physical examination. For example, ~65% of patients presenting with an acute knee injury and a significant effusion have an ACL injury [89]. Clinically, the Lachman's, anterior drawer, and pivot shift tests should be included to assess for anterior cruciate ligament injury. Varus and valgus stress testing at full extension and at 30 degrees of flexion should be used to examine the medial and lateral collateral ligaments [90]. The posterior drawer test should be used to assess the posterior cruciate ligament. The integrity of the menisci should be assessed with a combination of McMurray's, Thessaly's, and Apley's tests. X-ray should be used to evaluate for associated fracture and may show a Segond fracture, which is indicative of an ACL tear (Fig. 10.3). MRI should be performed if ligament or meniscus tear is suspected.

When determining the best course of treatment, physicians should consider the nature of the injury, the patient's desired activity level, and level of skeletal maturity. Treatment for ligament injuries may include a combination of activity modification,

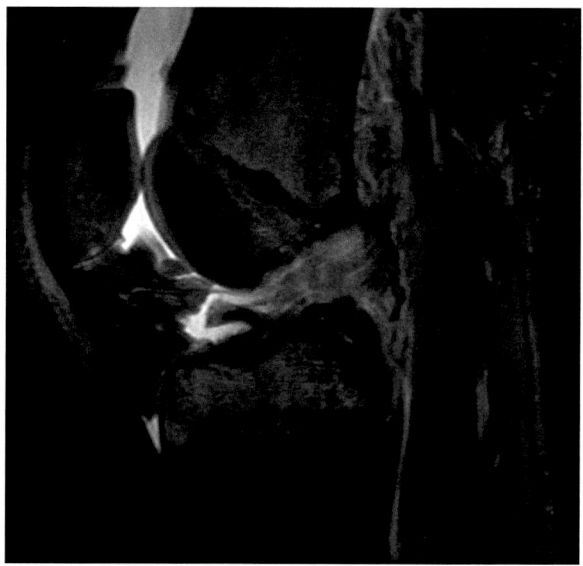

Fig. 10.1 MRI demonstrating a complete midsubstance anterior cruciate ligament (ACL) rupture

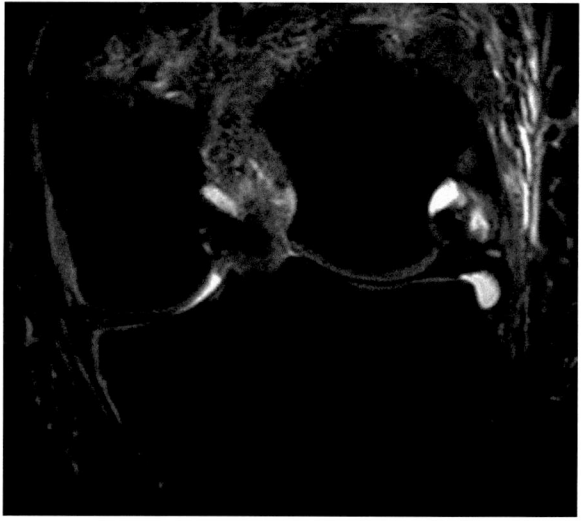

Fig. 10.2 Complex tear of the posterior body and posterior horn of the medial meniscus on coronal image of MRI

bracing, physical therapy, and/or surgery. Low-grade MCL and LCL tears may be treated nonoperatively with anti-inflammatories and rest. High-grade tears to the collateral ligaments, particularly the LCL, may require surgical management. A complete tear of the PCL is more likely to need to be managed surgically among gymnasts wishing to return to high levels of activity. ACL reconstruction is recommended for gymnasts who wish to return to their sport as the surgery likely lowers the risk of further cartilage and/or meniscal injury [91]. Around 65% of athletes that undergo ACL reconstruction return to their sport at the same level as before the injury, despite the possibility of ongoing symptoms in the years following surgery [6, 92].

Fig. 10.3 X-ray demonstrating a Segond fracture which indicates ACL rupture

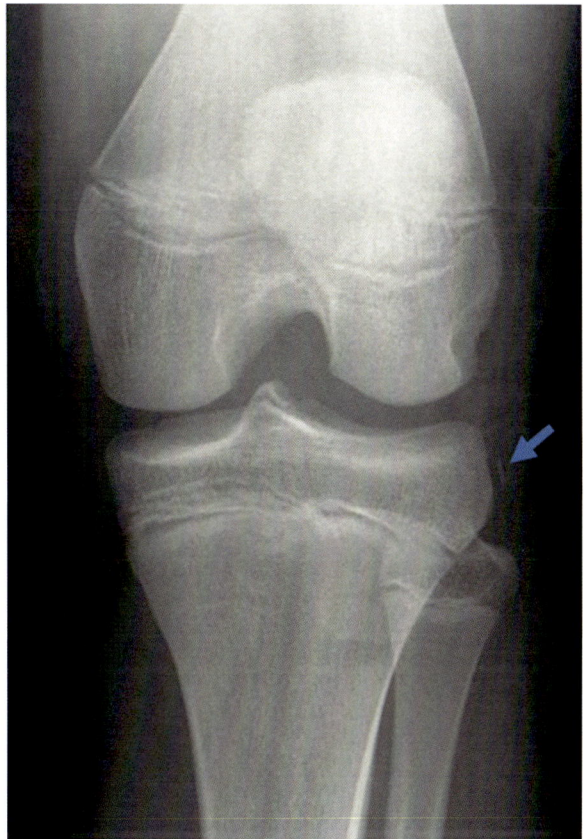

10.3.2 Patellar Instability

Patellar instability is the dislocation or subluxation of the patella out of the trochlear groove. Patellar instability may be due to an acute injury and can become a chronic instability pattern that may even lead to difficulty with activities of daily living. Anatomical risk factors for patellar instability include a shallow trochlear groove, a lateral insertion of the quadriceps tendon on the patella (a high Quadriceps Angle), genu valgum, patella alta (a high riding patella in the trochlear groove), femoral anteversion, external tibial torsion, and tight lateral structures including the IT band or vastus lateralis. The medial patellofemoral ligament (MPFL) and/or the medial retinaculum is likely injured in an acute injury and may lead to recurrent patellar instability. Patellar instability may lead to pain, osteochondral damage, and accelerated patellofemoral arthritis even at the initial instability event; however, this is more likely with chronic instability [85, 93, 94]. The pathology or damage caused by patellar instability should be diagnosed with a thorough patient history and clinical examination looking for any of the anatomical risk factors mentioned above, including the presence of a J-sign or patellar apprehension. Radiographs, including AP, lateral, and merchant (sunrise) views, should be performed to assess for obvious osteochondral fractures. MRI may be necessary to assess the integrity of the articular cartilage, MPFL, and trochlear groove, particularly in patients that present with a large knee effusion even without obvious abnormality on radiographs. Treatment of the initial dislocation or instability event, without osteochondral fracture or loose body, is typically accomplished with a short period of immobilization, physical therapy, activity modification, and bracing in a patellar stabilizer. Surgical treatment, such as an MPFL reconstruction or trochleoplasty, may be necessary but is typically reserved for cases in which an osteochondral loose body is present, in the chronic setting where conservative measures have failed, or when there is significant deformity that is likely to prevent conservative measures from working.

10.3.3 Anterior Knee Pain

Anterior knee pain is common in gymnasts, and like other athletes, it can be due to a variety of injuries. In younger gymnasts with open physes, repetitive jumping and landing can cause apophysitis at the lower margin of the patella origin (Sinding–Larsen–Johansson syndrome) or the tibial tubercle insertion (Osgood–Schlatter disease). Gymnasts with closed physes are more likely to develop patellar tendinopathy (jumpers' knee). Although patellofemoral pain (PFP) is more common in running athletes than gymnasts, it presents similarly in gymnasts with peripatellar pain and crepitus, often in the setting of weak hip abductors and excessive femoral adduction and internal rotation with landings.

Assessing gymnasts with anterior knee pain should include examination of the patella (patellar mobility, apprehension, J-sign) as well as a kinetic chain evaluation to investigate for proximal and distal factors that can contribute to knee pain. Radiographs may be used to determine the cause of anterior knee pain and evaluate for growth plate injury and patella or trochlear dysplasia. For gymnasts with abnormalities of the tibial tubercle or inferior pole of the patella, apophysitis must be distinguished from an avulsion fracture. Typically, athletes with an avulsion fracture will have had an acute injury to initiate the pain and will be unable to perform a straight leg raise. In addition, they typically have more swelling than athletes with apophysitis. Musculoskeletal ultrasound is a useful tool to assess the patellar tendon and extra-articular tissues of interest; MRI is rarely indicated for anterior knee pain.

The pathologies causing anterior knee pain are predominantly due to overuse, so a combination of pain control (ice, anti-inflammatory medications, bracing, or taping), activity modification, and physical therapy may be sufficient to alleviate pain.

Fig. 10.4 MRI demonstrating an unstable osteochondritis dissecans (OCD) lesion of the knee (A)

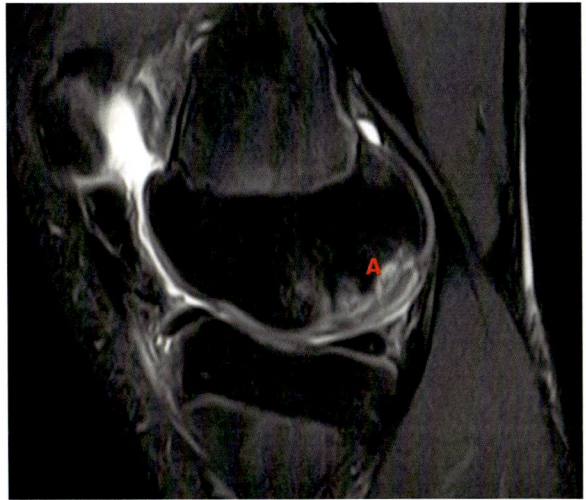

10.3.4 Osteochondritis Dissecans

Osteochondritis dissecans (OCD) of the knee is a common cause of knee pain in gymnasts. Patients typically have insidious onset of knee pain and may complain of instability, locking, or other functional impairments (Fig. 10.4). Typically, these lesions occur at the lateral aspect of the medial femoral condyle but may also be seen on the lateral femoral condyle or patella. Radiographs are used to diagnose these lesions, and MRI is used to determine if the lesion is stable or unstable. For stable/low-risk lesions, nonoperative management is the standard of care and typically includes activity modification, bracing, and protected weight-bearing [95]. When nonoperative treatment fails to alleviate knee pain or allow healing of the lesion, surgery may be necessary. For unstable/high-risk defects, or in the case of failed healing after 3–6 months of nonoperative management, surgery may be necessary. There are a multitude of surgical procedures used to treat unstable OCD lesions, all of which have the goal of preserving articular cartilage.

10.4 Lower Leg, Ankle, and Foot

The lower legs, ankles, and feet of gymnasts are prone to both traumatic and overuse injuries. Muscle strains, ankle sprains, fractures, Achilles tendon injuries, ankle impingement, and apophysitis are all common lower leg injuries seen in gymnasts.

10.4.1 Shin and Calf Injuries

Medial tibial stress syndrome (MTSS), tibial stress fractures, and calf muscle strains are common lower leg injuries for gymnasts. MTSS is sometimes referred to as shin splints. It is particularly common in female gymnasts [86–88] and may be due to the excessive foot pronation seen in gymnasts [89]. Stress fractures result from the repetitive forces applied to the tibia from running, jumping, and landing from a significant height [6] and are more common if the gymnast has other components of the Female Athlete Triad, as previously discussed. Calf strains can be caused by the constant high demand placed on the gastrocnemius, soleus, and plantaris muscles to support and propel the gymnast. As with upper leg strains, these too occur mostly during the first hour of practice [12], which suggests insufficient warm-ups might be a contributing factor. Overall, the majority of lower leg injuries in gymnasts were found to be mild and particularly aggravated by the running approach during vault [82].

Diagnosis of MTSS is made by the presence of diffuse pain and tenderness along the posteromedial border of the distal third of the tibia. This pain may be reproduced with heel raises and resisted plantar flexion. Additionally, slight swelling may be detected with palpation [90]. Radiographic imaging can be ordered to solidify the diagnosis, but it is important to know that though some X-rays may show signs of thickening along the affected area (posterior cortex of the tibia), often radiographs are normal. If the X-rays appear normal, MRI may aid in confirming the diagnosis and guiding the treatment. When assessing the MRI of a patient suspected of having MTSS, the Fredericson grading system may be used. This validated scale correlates the extent of bone morphological changes with the patient's clinical symptoms to provide an estimate for expected healing time, and consequently, return to gymnastics [91, 92].

A tibial stress fracture may present similar to MTSS, although the pain is often more focal with a stress fracture [82]. Due to the poor sensitivity of radiographs for tibial stress fractures, MRI should be obtained if suspicion is high [90]. Identifying the exact location of the tibial stress fracture (anterior vs. posterior medial) is essential since blood supply, and therefore, treatment and prognosis vary. Lab tests and bone density testing may be indicated for patients with stress fractures who are also at risk for The Female Athlete Triad.

Similar to a hamstring strain, the diagnosis of calf strain is made predominantly based on the history and by palpation and strength testing, but MRI or ultrasound imaging may be used to obtain a more complete understanding of the injury.

Treatment of shin and calf injuries varies based on severity of the injury. Unlike a tibial stress fracture that requires immediate cessation of painful sport participation, gymnasts with MTSS may be able to continue to train. Treatment of MTSS involves activity modification (e.g., use soft landing surfaces, focus on bars over other events), pain relief (ice, taping, compression sleeve, soft tissue manipulation), and physical therapy (calf stretching, strengthening of the ankle plantar flexors as well as foot intrinsic muscles). Of note, recurrence of "shin splints" is common [90].

Tibial stress fractures should be managed similar to other stress fractures; however, if the stress fracture is in the anterior aspect of the tibia where there is increased tension and reduced blood perfusion, a greater recovery period should be expected [95, 96]. Often gymnasts need to use crutches or be placed in a cast or boot for pain-free ambulation for a minimum of 2 weeks. The period of NWB will be longer for higher-grade stress fractures (based on X-ray or MRI findings) or if located in the anterior tibia, due to the risk of delayed healing or nonunion. Prolonged healing of greater than 9 months often requires a surgical treatment [97, 98]. Although occasionally used as part of the treatment in gymnasts, bone stimulators have not been shown to have a significant effect on healing [99–101]. Once the gymnast is pain-free with ambulation and radiographs show signs of healing, he/she should start physical therapy focusing on improving strength in the lower limb and foot musculature, optimizing the kinetic chain and core stability, and gradually returning to gymnastics. Specifically for patients with The Female Athlete Triad, nutritional and sports psychology counseling should be suggested to aid them in decreasing their energy deficit and preventing future bone stress injuries.

Calf strains are treated similar to MTSS with activity modification (limited jumping and plantar flexion, use of soft landings, focus on bar work), pain relief (ice, limited use of NSAIDs, heel lift or boot), physical therapy (calf stretching, strengthening of the ankle plantar flexors with transition from isometric to concentric to eccentric strengthening), and gradual return to gymnastics.

10.4.2 Ankle Sprains

As previously discussed, ankle sprains are the most common gymnastics injury [19–22] and are typically caused by falls and landings from dismounts and tumbling. Ankle sprains account for the largest proportion of injuries on the balance beam (16.7% of all injuries that occurred on the balance beam), floor exercise (16.4% of all injuries that occurred during floor exercise), and vault (12.8% of all injuries that occurred on the vault) [22]. Ankle sprains are frequently caused by trauma as well as by contact with immobile objects such as the apparatus/ground [18]. The mechanisms of ankle sprains may include inversion or eversion placement when landing due improper technique, stepping off the mat, or landing with the foot in the seams of the mat. Specifically, under-rotation in a tumbling pass can result in landing with significant forces on the ankle in an acute angle with the floor and/or in a hyper-dorsiflexed position. These high impact positions force the ligaments to stretch further than anatomically designed and can cause a tear either acutely or from repetitive stress [22, 102].

Athletes with ankle sprains may present with an inability to bear weight on the ankle, limited ankle ROM, and swelling and tenderness around the ankle joint. Generally, ankle sprains are diagnosed without imaging, but the Ottawa ankle rules (validated guidelines to aid the physician in determining if radiographic examination is necessary) should be applied [103, 104]. MRI might be ordered in the setting of an ankle sprain, if additional injuries are suspected such as osteochondral defect of the medial talar dome or a syndesmotic sprain.

Since ankle sprains were found to affect gymnasts up to 3 years post injury, [6] the focus of treatment should include prevention strategies in addition to treatment of the current sprain. The extent of immobilization and physical therapy necessary will differ based on the severity of the sprain, but early mobilization is encouraged. Athletes with ankle sprains may also benefit from bracing their ankles during training and competitions in efforts to decrease the reinjury rates [105] while rehabilitating their ankle back to its preinjury strength.

10.4.3 Fractures

Salter–Harris fractures, which are fractures of the epiphyseal plate, may occur in the distal tibia or fibula in this population if skeletally immature. Gymnasts are particularly at risk for this type of fracture because intense, high impact training occurs while many are skeletally immature. In young athletes who are still growing, the epiphyseal plates are two to five times weaker than the surrounding fibrous tissue [106, 107]. Since the ligaments in adolescents are stronger than the cartilage and bone to which they are attached and the epiphyseal cartilage in adolescents is less resistant to repetitive stress than the articular cartilage in adults, younger gymnasts are more vulnerable to growth plate fractures [108–110]. Therefore, increased involvement and difficulty of skills practiced from an early age have been suggested to predispose these athletes to growth plate injuries [111].

Fractures of the foot may be acute, traumatic fractures, or stress fractures. Of all bony injuries in gymnasts' feet, 42% are stress fractures [8]. In a study assessing injuries in female club gymnasts, 31.3% of all stress fractures were in the foot, most commonly located in the metatarsals [7]. As previously discussed, the young age of gymnasts and the Female Athlete Triad, in combination with the high impact of the sport, may be contributing factors to these injuries.

Similar to gymnasts with ankle sprains, athletes with Salter–Harris fractures may be unable to bear weight, have limited ankle ROM, as well as have swelling and bony tenderness. Salter–Harris fractures are usually diagnosed with radiographs and clinical examination. Patients with metatarsal stress fractures may present with focal pain, swelling, and decreased ability to bear weight or hop. Radiographic imaging and possibly MRI should be used to diagnose a stress fracture.

Salter–Harris fracture treatment differs based on the type and whether the tibia or fibula is affected. Typically, Salter–Harris types 1 and 2 are often treated with immobilization, while types 3–5 may necessitate surgery [112]. Fibula fractures often require immobilization in a boot; however, fractures of the tibia tend to require casting and often a period of nonweight-bearing. Foot fractures typically require immobilization with a boot or cast until there is clinical and radiographic healing. Physical therapy to address abnormal movement patterns and weakness is typically helpful in order to progress gymnasts back to sport.

10.4.4 Achilles Tendon Injuries

The Achilles tendon is another structure at risk of injury in gymnastics. The mechanics of the sport predispose gymnasts to tendinopathy because of the repetitive jumping, landing, and plantar flexion. These athletes apply constant high loads and stress on their Achilles tendons throughout training sessions and competition events [90]. Gymnasts are susceptible to Achilles tendon ruptures for the same reasons. Ruptures are more common in athletes between 20 and 40 years of age, but younger athletes are also at risk [90]—specifically during the takeoff and landing phase of tumbling when the Achilles musculotendinous complex can be suddenly overloaded [113, 114]. Kerr et al. [22] reported that lower leg and Achilles tendon injuries were responsible for a larger proportion of injuries in the floor exercise event than in any other event.

Achilles tendinopathy presents with pain and/or tenderness over the Achilles tendon 2–6 cm proximal to the calcaneus and may be accompanied by localized swelling and/or crepitus [115]. Conversely, an Achilles tendon rupture will present with significant pain and the inability of the athlete to actively plantar flex his/her foot. A palpable defect will also be present, and the Thompson test can be used to confirm the rupture with high accuracy [114]. Musculoskeletal ultrasound or MRI can confirm the diagnosis of both Achilles tendinopathy and rupture and provide information about severity and associated injury.

Treatment of Achilles tendinopathy should be conservative and include activity modification (avoid repetitive plantar flexion, use soft landings), pain relief with taping and ice, and physical therapy (plantar flexor stretching, slow concentric and eccentric plantar flexor strengthening) [116, 117]. Immobilizing the tendon in a boot may be beneficial for acute, yet severe, symptoms [116]. In most cases, gymnasts who wish to return to gymnastics after an Achilles rupture elect to undergo surgical repair [118, 119]. After surgery, the average return to sport at preinjury level is 4 months and 94% of athletes return to their preinjury functional level in their given sport by 6 months [118]. Fortunately, the re-rupture rate is low [120].

10.4.5 Apophysitis

Both Sever's and Iselin's diseases involve inflammation of the apophysis at the calcaneus and the fifth metatarsal, respectively. It is important to differentiate calcaneal apophysitis from a calcaneal fracture or contusion, which can occur acutely from one poor landing or hitting the heel on an apparatus [82, 108, 121]. Radiographs of Sever's and Iselin's may be normal or show sclerosis at the apophysis. Treatment for Sever's includes heel cups and stretching. In addition, wearing a heel cup brace may be beneficial for gymnasts with Sever's. Gymnasts with Iselin's may need to implement activity modification or have a brief period of immobilization if the pain is severe.

References

1. Bak K, Kalms SB, Olesen S, Jargensen U. Epidemiology of injuries in gymnastics. Scand J Med Sci Sports. 1994;4(2):148–54.
2. Harringe ML, Lindblad S, Werner S. Do team gymnasts compete in spite of symptoms from an injury? Br J Sports Med. 2004;38(4):398–401.
3. Snook GA. Injuries in women's gymnastics. A 5-year study. Am J Sports Med. 1979;7(4):242–4.
4. Pettrone FA, Ricciardelli E. Gymnastic injuries: the Virginia experience 1982–1983. Am J Sports Med. 1987;15(1):59–62.
5. Meeusen R, Borms J. Gymnastic injuries. Sports Med. 1992;13(5):337–56.
6. Hudash GW, Albright JP. Women's intercollegiate gymnastics injury patterns and permanent medical disability. Am J Sports Med. 1993;21:314–20.
7. O'Kane JW, Levy MR, Pietila KE, Caine DJ, Schiff MA. Survey of injuries in Seattle area levels 4 to 10 female club gymnasts. Clin J Sport Med. 2011;21(6):486–92.
8. Dixon M, Fricker P. Injuries to elite gymnasts over 10 yr. Med Sci Sports Exerc. 1993;25(12):1322–9.
9. Garrick JG, Requa RK. Epidemiology of women's gymnastics injuries. Am J Sports Med. 1980;8(4):261–4.
10. Weiker GG. Injuries in club gymnastics. Phys Sports Med. 1985;13(4):63–6.
11. Caine D, Knutzen K, Howe W, Keeler L, Sheppard L, Henrichs D, et al. A three-year epidemiological study of injuries affecting young female gymnasts. Phys Therap Sport. 2003;4:10–23.
12. Lindner KJ, Caine DJ. Injury patterns of female competitive club gymnasts. Can J Sport Sci. 1990;15(4):254–61.
13. Kolt GS, Kirkby RJ. Epidemiology of injury in elite and subelite female gymnasts: a comparison of retrospective and prospective findings. Br J Sports Med. 1999;33(5):312–8.
14. Caine D, Cochrane B, Caine C, Zemper E. An epidemiologic investigation of injuries affecting young competitive female gymnasts. Am J Sports Med. 1989;17(6):811–20.
15. Steele VA, White JA. Injury amongst female gymnasts. Proceedings of the Society of Sports Sciences: Sport and Science Conference; Liverpool, School of Physical Education and Recreation; 1983.
16. Kolt GS, Kirkby RJ. Epidemiology of injury in Australian female gymnasts. Sports Med Train Rehabil. 1995;6(3):223–31.
17. Kerr G, Minden H. Psychological factors related to the occurrence of athletic injuries. J Sport Exerc Psychol. 1988;10(2):167–73.
18. Edouard P, Steffen K, Junge A, Leglise M, Soligard T, Engebretsen L. Gymnastics injury incidence during the 2008, 2012 and 2016 Olympic Games: analysis of prospectively collected surveillance data from 963 registered gymnasts during Olympic Games. Br J Sports Med. 2018;52(7):475–81.
19. Cupisti A, D'Alessandro C, Evangelisti I, Umbri C, Rossi M, Galetta F, et al. Injury survey in competitive sub-elite rhythmic gymnasts: results from a prospective controlled study. J Sports Med Phys Fitness. 2007;47(2):203–7.
20. Marshall SW, Covassin T, Dick R, Nassar LG, Agel J. Descriptive epidemiology of collegiate women's gymnastics injuries: National Collegiate Athletic Association Injury Surveillance System, 1988–1989 through 2003–2004. J Athl Train. 2007;42(2):234–40.
21. Singh S, Smith GA, Fields SK, McKenzie LB. Gymnastics-related injuries to children treated in emergency departments in the United States, 1990–2005. Pediatrics. 2008;121(4):e954–e60.
22. Kerr ZY, Hayden R, Barr M, Klossner DA, Dompier TP. Epidemiology of National Collegiate Athletic Association Women's Gymnastics Injuries, 2009–2010 Through 2013–2014. J Athl Train. 2015;50(8):870–8.
23. Kirialanis P, Malliou P, Beneka A, Gourgoulis V, Giofstidou A, Godolias G. Injuries in artistic gymnastic elite adolescent male and female athletes. J Back Musculoskelet Rehabil. 2002;16(4):145–51.

24. Hunt KJ, Hurwit D, Robell K, Gatewood C, Botser IB, Matheson G. Incidence and epidemiology of foot and ankle injuries in elite collegiate athletes. Am J Sports Med. 2017;45(2):426–33.
25. Caine DJ, Nassar L. Gymnastics injuries. Med Sport Sci. 2005;48:18–58.
26. Harringe ML, Renstrom P, Werner S. Injury incidence, mechanism and diagnosis in top-level teamgym: a prospective study conducted over one season. Scand J Med Sci Sports. 2007;17(2):115–9.
27. Westermann RW, Giblin M, Vaske A, Grosso K, Wolf BR. Evaluation of men's and women's gymnastics injuries: a 10-year observational study. Sports Health. 2015;7(2):161–5.
28. Bezek EM, Vanheest AE, Hutchinson DT. Grip lock injury in male gymnasts. Sports Health. 2009;1(6):518–21.
29. Lanese RR, Strauss RH, Leizman DJ, Rotondi AM. Injury and disability in matched men's and women's intercollegiate sports. Am J Public Health. 1990;90:1459–62.
30. Samuelson M, Reider B, Weiss D. Grip lock injuries to the forearm in male gymnasts. Am J Sports Med. 1996;24(1):15–8.
31. Brüggemann GP. Biomechanics of gymnastic techniques. Sports Sci Rev. 1994;3(2):79–120.
32. McNitt-Gray J, editor. The influence of joint flexion, impact velocity, rotation, and surface characteristics on the forces and torques experienced during gymnastics landings. Federation International de Gymnastics Scientific/Medical Symposium Proceedings; 1991; Indianapolis, IN: USA Gymnastics.
33. McNitt-Gray JL. Kinematics and impulse characteristics of drop landings from three heights. Int J Sport Biomech. 1991;7(2):201–24.
34. Lowry CB, Leveau BF. A retrospective study of gymnastics injuries to competitors and non-competitors in private clubs. Am J Sports Med. 1982;10(4):237–9.
35. Kirialanis P, Malliou P, Beneka A, Giannakopoulos K. Occurrence of acute lower limb injuries in artistic gymnasts in relation to event and exercise phase. Br J Sports Med. 2003;37(2):137–9.
36. Sands WA, Shultz BB, Newman AP. Women's gymnastics injuries. A 5-year study. Am J Sports Med. 1993;21(2):271–6.
37. Hunter LY, Torgan C. Dismounts in gymnastics: should scoring be reevaluated? Am J Sports Med. 1983;11(4):208–10.
38. Gittoes MJR, Irwin G, Kerwin D. Kinematic landing strategy transference in backward rotating gymnastics dismounts. J Appl Biochem. 2013;29(253–260).
39. Kappe T, Kocak T, Bieger R, Reichel H, Fraitzl CR. Radiographic risk factors for labral lesions in femoroacetabular impingement. Clin Orthop Relat Res. 2011;469(11):3241–7.
40. Mladenov K, Dora C, Wicart P, Seringe R. Natural history of hips with borderline acetabular index and acetabular dysplasia in infants. J Pediatr Orthop. 2002;2002(22):607–12.
41. Leunig M, Podeszwa D, Beck M, Werlen S, Ganz R. Magnetic resonance arthrography of labral disorders in hips with dysplasia and impingement. Clin Orthop Relat Res. 2004;418:74–80.
42. Duthon VB, Charbonnier C, Kolo FC, Magnenat-Thalmann N, Becker CD, Bouvet C, et al. Correlation of clinical and magnetic resonance imaging findings in hips of elite female ballet dancers. Arthroscopy. 2013;29(3):411–9.
43. Hamilton WG, Hamilton LH, Marshall P, Molnar M. A profile of the musculoskeletal characteristics of elite professional ballet dancers. Am J Sports Med. 1992;20(3):267–73.
44. Steinberg N, Hershkovitz I, Peleg S, Dar G, Masharawi Y, Heim M, et al. Range of joint movement in female dancers and nondancers aged 8 to 16 years: anatomical and clinical implications. Am J Sports Med. 2006;34(5):814–23.
45. Mangat G, Dieppe P. Hypermobility, arthritis and congenital hip dislocation. Br J Rheumatol. 1990;29(1):77.
46. Wynne-Davies R. Acetabular dysplasia and familial joint laxity: two etiological factors in congenital dislocation of the hip. A review of 589 patients and their families. J Bone Joint Surg. 1970;52(4):704–16.
47. Dy CJ, Thompson MT, Crawford MJ, Alexander JW, McCarthy JC, Noble PC. Tensile strain in the anterior part of the acetabular labrum during provocative maneuvering of the normal hip. J Bone Joint Surg Am. 2008;90(1):1464–72.

48. Wassilew GI, Janz V, Heller MO, Tohtz S, Rogalla P, Hein P, et al. Real time visualization of femoroacetabular impingement and subluxation using 320-slice computed tomography. J Orthop Res. 2013;31(2):275–81.
49. Bardakos NV. Hip impingement: beyond femoroacetabular. J Hip Preserv Surg. 2015;2(3):206–23.
50. Hetsroni I, Larson CM, Dela Torre K, Zbeda RM, Magennis E, Kelly BT. Anterior inferior iliac spine deformity as an extra-articular source for hip impingement: a series of 10 patients treated with arthroscopic decompression. Arthroscopy. 2012;28(11):1644–53.
51. Domb BG, Shindle MK, McArthur B, Voos JE, Magennis EM, Kelly BT. Iliopsoas impingement: a newly identified cause of labral pathology in the hip. HSS J. 2011;7(2):145–50.
52. Charbonnier C, Kolo FC, Duthon VB, Magnenat-Thalmann N, Becker CD, Hoffmeyer P, et al. Assessment of congruence and impingement of the hip joint in professional ballet dancers: a motion capture study. Am J Sports Med. 2011;39(3):557–66.
53. Martin HD, Kelly BT, Leunig M, Philippon MJ, Clohisy JC, Martin RL, et al. The pattern and technique in the clinical evaluation of the adult hip: the common physical examination tests of hip specialists. Arthroscopy. 2010;26(2):161–72.
54. Cheatham SW. Extra-articular hip impingement: a narrative review of the literature. J Can Chiropr Assoc. 2016;60(1):47–56.
55. Ross JR, Zaltz I, Nepple JJ, Schoenecker PL, Clohisy JC. Arthroscopic disease classification and interventions as an adjunct in the treatment of acetabular dysplasia. Am J Sports Med. 2011;39 Suppl:72s–8s.
56. Klaue K, Durnin CW, Ganz R. The acetabular rim syndrome. A clinical presentation of dysplasia of the hip. J Bone Joint Surg. 1991;73(3):423–9.
57. Ishøi L, Thorborg K, Kraemer O, Hölmich P. Return to sport and performance after hip arthroscopy for femoroacetabular impingement in 18- to 30-year-old athletes: a cross-sectional cohort study of 189 athletes. Am J Sports Med. 2018;26(11):2578–97.
58. Casartelli NC, Leunig M, Maffiuletti NA, Bizzini M. Return to sport after hip surgery for femoroacetabular impingement: a systematic review. Br J Sports Med. 2015;49(12):819–24.
59. Perets I, Hartigan DE, Chaharbakhshi EO, Ashberg L, Ortiz-Declet V, Domb BG. Outcomes of hip arthroscopy in competitive athletes. Arthroscopy. 2017;33(8):1521–9.
60. De Souza MJ, Nattiv A, Joy E, Misra M, Williams NI, Mallinson RJ, et al. 2014 female athlete triad coalition consensus statement on treatment and return to play of the female athlete triad: 1st International Conference held in San Francisco, California, May 2012 and 2nd International Conference held in Indianapolis, Indiana, May 2013. Br J Sports Med. 2014;48(4):289.
61. Torstveit MK, Sundgot-Borgen J. The female athlete triad: are elite athletes at increased risk? Med Sci Sports Exerc. 2005;37(2):184–93.
62. Nattiv A, Loucks AB, Manore MM, Sanborn CF, Sundgot-Borgen J, Warren MP. American College of Sports Medicine position stand. The female athlete triad. Med Sci Sports Exerc. 2007;39(10):1867–82.
63. Kiel J, Kaiser K. Stress reaction and fractures. Treasure Island, FL: StatPearls Publishing; 2018.
64. Słowiński JJ, Kudłacik K. Analysis of the impact of configuration of the stabilisation system for femoral diaphyseal fractures on the state of stresses and displacements. Appl Bionics Biomech. 2018;2018:8150568. eCollection.
65. O'Dell MC, Jaramillo D, Bancroft L, Varich L, Logsdon G, Servaes S. Imaging of sports-related injuries of the lower extremity in pediatric patients. Radiographics. 2016;36(6):1807–27.
66. Ogden JA. Radiology of postnatal skeletal development. X. Patella and tibial tuberosity. Skelet Radiol. 1984;11(4):246–57.
67. Rossi F, Dragoni S. Acute avulsion fractures of the pelvis in adolescent competitive athletes: prevalence, location and sports distribution of 203 cases collected. Skelet Radiol. 2001;30(3):127–31.
68. Metzmaker JN, Pappas AM. Avulsion fractures of the pelvis. Am J Sports Med. 1985;13(5):349–58.

69. Beaty J, Kasser J. Rockwood and Wilkins' fractures in children. 6th ed. Philadelphia, PA: Lippincott Williams & Wilkins; 2005.
70. Schuett DJ, Bomar JD, Pennock AT. Pelvic apophyseal avulsion fractures: a retrospective review of 228 cases. J Pediatr Orthop. 2015;35(6):617–23.
71. Fernbach SK, Wilkinson RH. Avulsion injuries of the pelvis and proximal femur. AJR Am J Roentgenol. 1981;137(3):581–4.
72. Sundar M, Carty H. Avulsion fractures of the pelvis in children: a report of 32 fractures and their outcome. Skelet Radiol. 1994;23(2):85–90.
73. Schiller J, DeFroda S, Blood T. Lower extremity avulsion fractures in the pediatric and adolescent athlete. J Am Acad Orthop Surg. 2017;25(4):251–9.
74. Sangal RB, Waryasz GR, Schiller JR. Femoroacetabular impingement: a review of current concepts. R I Med. 2013;97(11):33–8.
75. Arnaiz J, Piedra T, de Lucas EM, Arnaiz AM, Pelaz M, Gomez-Dermit V, et al. Imaging findings of lower limb apophysitis. AJR Am J Roentgenol. 2011;196(3):W316–25.
76. Gidwani S, Jagiello J, Bircher M. Avulsion fracture of the ischial tuberosity in adolescents: an easily missed diagnosis. BMJ. 2004;329(7457):99–100.
77. Biedert RM. Surgical management of traumatic avulsion of the ischial tuberosity in young athletes. Clin J Sport Med. 2015;25(1):67–72.
78. Ferlic PW, Sadoghi P, Singer G, Kraus T, Eberl R. Treatment for ischial tuberosity avulsion fractures in adolescent athletes. Knee Surg Sports Traumatol Arthrosc. 2014;22(4):893–7.
79. Veselko M, Smrkolj V. Avulsion of the anterior-superior iliac spine in athletes: case reports. J Trauma. 1994;36(3):444–6.
80. Lempainen L, Johansson K, Banke IJ, Ranne J, Mäkelä K, Sarimo J, et al. Expert opinion: diagnosis and treatment of proximal hamstring tendinopathy. Muscles Ligaments Tendons J. 2015;5(1):23–8.
81. Rauseo C. The rehabilitation of a runner with iliopsoas tendinopathy using an eccentric-biased exercise- a case report. Int J Sports Phys Ther. 2017;12(7):1150–62.
82. Kirby RL, Simms FC, Symington VJ, Garner JB. Flexibility and musculoskeletal symptomatology in female gymnasts and age-matched controls. Am J Sports Med. 1981;9(3):160–4.
83. Connell DA, Schneider-Kolsky ME, Hoving JL, Malara F, Buchbinder R, Koulouris G, et al. Longitudinal study comparing sonographic and MRI assessments of acute and healing hamstring injuries. AJR Am J Roentgenol. 2004;183(4):975–84.
84. Huwart A, Garrigues F, Jousse-Joulin S, Marhadour T, Guellec D, Cornec D, et al. Ultrasonography and magnetic resonance imaging changes in patients with polymyalgia rheumatica treated by tocilizumab. Arthritis Res Ther. 2018;20(1):11.
85. Grelsamer RP, Dejour D, Gould J. The pathophysiology of patellofemoral arthritis. Orthop Clin North Am. 2008;39(3):269–74, v.
86. Detmer DE. Chronic shin splints. Classification and management of medial tibial stress syndrome. Sports Med. 1986;3(6):436–46.
87. Andrish JT, Bergfeld JA, Walheim J. A prospective study on the management of shin splints. J Bone Joint Surg Am. 1974;56(8):1697–700.
88. Mubarak SJ, Gould RN, Lee YF, Schmidt DA, Hargens AR. The medial tibial stress syndrome. A cause of shin splints. Am J Sports Med. 1982;10(4):201–5.
89. Thacker SB, Gilchrist J, Stroup DF, Kimsey CD. The prevention of shin splints in sports: a systematic review of literature. Med Sci Sports Exerc. 2002;34(1):32–40.
90. Jones G, Wolf B. Evaluation and management of gymnastic injuries. Sports Med Update. 2008;January/February:2–9.
91. Fredericson M, Bergman AG, Hoffman KL, Dillingham MS. Tibial stress reaction in runners. Correlation of clinical symptoms and scintigraphy with a new magnetic resonance imaging grading system. Am J Sports Med. 1995;23(4):472–81.
92. Kijowski R, Choi J, Shinki K, Del Rio AM, De Smet A. Validation of MRI classification system for tibial stress injuries. AJR Am J Roentgenol. 2012;198(4):878–84.

93. Fithian DC, Paxton EW, Stone ML, Silva P, Davis DK, Elias DA, et al. Epidemiology and natural history of acute patellar dislocation. Am J Sports Med. 2004;32(5):1114–21.
94. Alaia MJ, Cohn RM, Strauss EJ. Patellar instability. Bull Hosp Jt Dis (2013). 2014;72(1):6–17.
95. Bahney CS, Hu DP, Miclau TR, Marcucio RS. The multifaceted role of the vasculature in endochondral fracture repair. Front Endocrinol (Lausanne). 2015;6(4)
96. Hulkko A, Orava S. Stress fractures in athletes. Int J Sports Med. 1987;8(3):221–6.
97. Zbeda RM, Sculco PK, Urch EY, Lazaro LE, Borens O, Williams RJ, et al. Tension band plating for chronic anterior tibial stress fractures in high-performance athletes. Am J Sports Med. 2015;43(7):1712–8.
98. Robertson GA, Wood AM. Return to sports after stress fractures of the tibial diaphysis: a systematic review. Br Med Bull. 2015;114(1):95–111.
99. Rue JP, Armstrong DW, Frassica FJ, Deafenbaugh M, Wilckens JH. The effect of pulsed ultrasound in the treatment of tibial stress fractures. Orthopedics. 2004;27(11):1192–5.
100. Beck BR, Matheson GO, Bergman G, Norling T, Fredericson M, Hoffman AR, et al. Do capacitively coupled electric fields accelerate tibial stress fracture healing? A randomized controlled trial. Am J Sports Med. 2007;36(3):545–53.
101. Mollon B, da Silva V, Busse JW, Einhorn TA, Bhandari M. Electrical stimulation for long-bone fracture-healing: a meta-analysis of randomized controlled trials. J Bone Joint Surg Am. 2008;90(11):2322–30.
102. Hecht SS, Burton MS. Medical coverage of gymnastics competitions. Curr Sports Med Rep. 2009;8(3):113–8.
103. Stiell IG, Greenberg GH, McKnight RD, Nair RC, McDowell I, Worthington JR. A study to develop clinical decision rules for the use of radiography in acute ankle injuries. Ann Emerg Med. 1992;21(4):384–90.
104. Plint AC, Bulloch B, Osmond MH, Stiell I, Dunlap H, Reed M, et al. Validation of the Ottawa Ankle Rules in children with ankle injuries. Acad Emerg Med. 1999;6(10):10005–9.
105. Olmsted LC, Vela LI, Denegar CR, Hertel J. Prophylactic ankle taping and bracing: a numbers-needed-to-treat and cost-benefit analysis. J Athl Train. 2004;39:95–100.
106. Schwab SA. Epiphyseal injuries in the growing athlete. Can Med Assoc J. 1977;117(6):626–30.
107. Salter RB, Harris WR. Injuries involving the epiphyseal plate. J Bone Joint Surg Am. 1963;45(587–622)
108. Hecht S. Gymnastics. In: Melion MB, Walsh WM, Madden C, Putukian M, Shelton GL, editors. Team physician's handbook. 3rd ed. Philadelphia: Hanley & Belfus Inc; 2002. p. 667–8.
109. Caine DJ, Lindner KJ. Overuse injuries of growing bones: the young female gymnast at risk? Phys Sports Med. 1985;13(12):51–64.
110. Caine DJ. Growth plate injury and bone growth: an update. Pediatr Exerc Sci. 1990;2(3):209–29.
111. Meeuwisse WH. Assessing causation in sport injury: a multifactorial model. Clin J Sport Med. 1994;4(3):166–70.
112. Foris LA, Waseem M. Fracture, Salter Harris. Treasure Island, FL: StatPearls Publishing; 2017. Available from: https://www.ncbi.nlm.nih.gov/books/NBK430688/.
113. Kannus P, Natri A. Etiology and pathophysiology of tendon ruptures in sports. Scand J Med Sci Sports. 1997;7(2):107–12.
114. Thompson TC, Doherty JH. Spontaneous rupture of tendon of Achilles: a new clinical diagnostic test. J Trauma. 1962;2:126–9.
115. Clement DB, Taunton JE, Smart GW. Achilles tendinitis and peritendinitis: etiology and treatment. Am J Sports Med. 1984;12(3):179–84.
116. Leach RE, James S, Wasilewski S. Achilles tendinitis. Am J Sports Med. 1981;9(2):93–8.
117. Lowdon A, Bader DL, Mowat AG. The effect of heel pads on the treatment of Achilles tendinitis: a double blind trial. Am J Sports Med. 1984;12(6):431–5.
118. Mandelbaum BR, Myerson MS, Forster R. Achilles tendon ruptures. A new method of repair, early range of motion, and functional rehabilitation. Am J Sports Med. 1995;23(4):392–5.

119. Wong J, Barrass V, Maffulli N. Quantitative review of operative and nonoperative management of Achilles tendon ruptures. Am J Sports Med. 2002;30(4):565–75.
120. Rettig AC, Liotta FJ, Klootwyk TE, Porter DA, Mieling P. Potential risk of rerupture in primary Achilles tendon repair in athletes younger than 30 years of age. Am J Sports Med. 2005;33(1):119–23.
121. Chilvers M, Donahue M, Nassar L, Manoli A 2nd. Foot and ankle injuries in elite female gymnasts. Foot Ankle Int. 2007;28(2):214–8.

Chapter 11
Rehabilitation of Gymnasts

David Tilley and David A. James

11.1 Introduction

The sport of gymnastics is one of the most impressive and demanding displays of athleticism. It requires gymnasts to possess a unique blend of sport qualities including strength, explosive power, flexibility, coordination, balance, and metabolic capacity that is unlike any other sport [1]. Alongside the large physical demands, it also requires an extraordinary amount of mental toughness, emotional capacity, and discipline. This is due to the high-risk nature of the skills trained, the presence of young children being exposed to high-level skills, and the large time commitment required over many years to achieve progress.

Due to this mosaic of factors, the rehabilitation process for gymnasts is often seen as an enigma to the medical field. The combination of high forces, extreme ranges of motion, high repetition, and high training workloads in young athletes who have not fully matured, all present a significant challenge. As discussed in previous chapters, there is a growing body of research and literature regarding injury incidence and common injury patterns within the sport. However, there is a paucity of research and peer-reviewed literature regarding the best methods of rehabilitation, return to sport, and injury prevention, although recent papers have begun the process of creating formalized protocols [2]. Due to the lack of available peer-reviewed literature, it is necessary to utilize a combination of anatomy, physiology, and movement science literature from other fields as a base. From here, the current gymnastics biomechanical and epidemiology data can be layered on top of rehabilitation principles to extrapolate best practices.

D. Tilley (✉)
Champion Physical Therapy and Performance, Waltham, MA, USA
e-mail: davetilley@champ.pt

D. A. James
University of Colorado School of Medicine, Physical Therapy Program, Aurora, CO, USA
e-mail: David.james@ucdenver.edu

A large chasm in the continuum of care exists within gymnastics sports medicine in that gymnasts often do not receive the sports-specific rehabilitation needed to return safely to training. When a lack of advanced rehabilitation is combined with a lack of systematic and validated return to sport progressions, gymnasts are often left stuck in the "gap" between traditional rehabilitation and sport training, frequently yielding high rates of reinjury and ongoing pain [3]. This often leads to the stacking of multiple injuries early in one's career, chronic reinjury, and mental health burden. Due to this, far too many gymnasts may not reach their full athletic potential, may continue to accumulate injuries, or may quit the sport as a result.

A recent review determined that injury rates in gymnastics range from 1.08 to 50.3 occurrences per 1000 hours of exposure, and are most common in the lower extremity (ankle sprains and internal knee derangements in particular, with the exception of male artistic gymnasts suffering more shoulder injuries) [4]. Of particular importance, the rehabilitation professional must take note of lumbar spine injuries in female gymnasts, shoulder and wrist injuries in male gymnasts, and lower body impact injuries in both genders, as these continue to be issues that plague gymnasts worldwide [3]. These areas of the body require additional attention due to their prevalence, as well as their potentially deleterious effects on long-term health and performance.

11.1.1 The Challenge of Skill and Force Variability in Gymnastics

As has been noted in previous chapters, gymnasts participate in a variety of different apparatuses based on their discipline and gender. Within those individual events, they perform hundreds of skills that have separate movement categories. Wide differences in skill movements exist for women's artistic, men's artistic, rhythmic, acrobatic, trampoline, tumbling, and other disciplines. For the training of these skills, a variety of drills, surfaces, and equipment are used, all of which produce different forces on a gymnast's body. The sport is also unique in that it places extremely high body weight forces repetitively on the upper extremity, which is not structurally evolved to handle these large forces. The upper extremity may encounter compressive forces of up to 8 times body weight during front handspring vaulting [5], while compressive forces at the wrist during a back handspring have been reported at 2.37 times body weight [6]. Most impressively, male gymnasts have recorded reaction forces of 7 times body weight at their hands during a high-bar giant swing [7].

Gymnastics is primarily a jumping and landing sport, requiring athletes to land hundreds of times per week under massive forces. In the lower body, peak ground reaction forces during tumbling have been recorded between 8.8 and 14.2 times body weight [8] and 15 times body weight in laboratory settings [9]. Peak forces at the Achilles tendon have been measured at 15 times body weight, and the forces at the tibiotalar joint up to 23 times body weight [7].

To make matters worse, many gymnasts have been trained to land in positions that significantly increase joint reaction forces and may leave them more susceptible to lower body injury. It is claimed that this landing position was taught to gymnasts because it was deemed to be more aesthetically pleasing from subjective evaluations. This concerning landing position is one with a more upright torso, the legs adducted together, limited angular displacement of the hips or knees shown during deceleration, and a more "quad-dominant" landing strategy. Failure to land within these arbitrarily set standards often results in scoring deduction within the judging system, serving as an ongoing barrier to cultural change. This less biomechanically efficient landing strategy has been suggested in research to drastically increase lower body injury risk, most notably for ACL tears [10, 11].

A more biomechanically sound landing technique is suggested in the literature for use, as it more optimally assists in dissipating high forces. Although individual anatomy must be considered for variability, the athlete should generally be taught to land with the feet hip width apart, the trunk and tibial angle more in parallel, and adequate angular displacement of the knees and hips upon landing [12]. It is worth noting that this landing technique is different than the sport-specific skill of 'bounding', often seen during tumbling, impacting the vaulting springboard, and other skills. The concept of bounding involves a high degree of body tension and stiffness, which allows the gymnast to tune the equipment, reduce the energy leakage during body shape changes, and maximally produce power for skills. This plyometric skill is different than that of a landing strategy which is typically seen during high force dismounts, vault landings, and final impacts of tumbling passes. Medical providers must be aware that mastery of both bounding technique and landing technique is crucial for injury risk reduction and gymnastics performance. As will be covered later in the lower extremity section, it is paramount that during the rehabilitation process both the quantity of landing (via surface and repetition) and the quality of landing (via neuromuscular training, strength training, and feedback) are prioritized for gymnasts. This more biomechanically efficient landing pattern is recommended regardless of the culture and scoring system of gymnastics that may be resistant to change in the present or future. The sport of gymnastics must continue to overcome the barriers to changing this landing technique, and it is the author's suggestion that the landing technique suggested in research be taught to gymnasts from a very young age so that their movement engrams are solidified prior to exposure to high impact skills.

Lastly, the spine of a gymnast endures astronomical forces during skills and landings [1, 13]. As noted by Sands in *The Science of Gymnastics*, compression forces on the spine of 11 times body weight were calculated during landing of

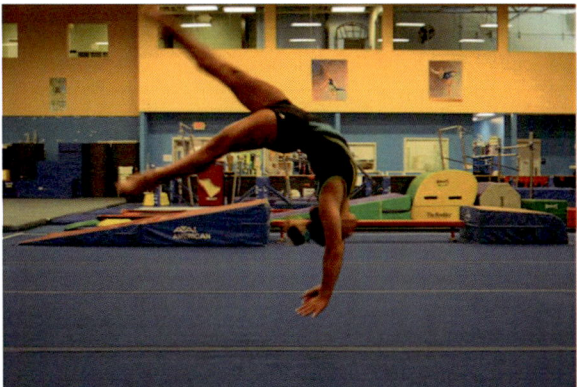

Fig. 11.1 Layout step-out

forward saltos, and compression forces of 7 times body weight were calculated during landing of backward saltos (see Fig. 11.1). It is critical that rehabilitation specialists understand the various movement pattern categories (flexion, extension, rotation, compression, traction) that are provocative for pain and create rehabilitation programs, as well as return to sport programs, according to these categories.

It is worth noting that the biomechanical research done on the many gymnastics skills are not considered the highest difficulty seen within the sport. The highest force skills can include multiple twists, rotations, and instances of suboptimal landing or re-gripping movements. Although not all of these conditions have been studied to make data available, it is likely that the forces of gymnastics are even higher than have been outlined in the available literature.

To complicate things even further, many athletes who suffer injuries are of a very young age and have specialized in the sport early [1]. It is not uncommon for a gymnast to begin training at 3–5 years of age and be exposed to extremely high force skills by the ages of 8–12. The culture of gymnastics has been sculpted to promote year-round training with no off-season or specific periodization formats required, despite a growing body of evidence that raises concerns for this as it relates to an increased risk of overuse injury, stalled athletic performance, burnout, and high attrition rates in young athletes [14–17].

The sport has also been resistant to the implementation of formalized strength and conditioning programs that include a balance of general physical preparation (GPP) and specific physical preparation (SPP). Many coaches and athletes in gymnastics are not open to considering more traditional strength and conditioning models that utilize external loading that are well supported across multiple youth sports in both medical and exercise physiology literature [17–19]. These factors further complicate the rehabilitation process for gymnasts, as many times the ability to restore an athlete's physiological loading tolerance and level of robustness is cut short by cultural friction, disagreement from gymnastics coaches, insurance coverage limitations, and a lack of communication between gymnastics professionals, medical professionals, gymnasts, and parents.

Despite these challenges, it has been exciting to see large changes occurring in the last 5 years to address these problems. As biomechanical and medical literature emerges for the science of gymnastics, and as members of interdisciplinary teams explore cultural change, new frontiers are being created for athlete-centered models of care. These models embrace a well-rounded and collaborative approach to rehabilitation. As more scientific literature is discussed and applied in training, many of the myths and misunderstandings surrounding these concepts are being transcended. The best traditional practices are being taken alongside valid coaching expertise and blended into the newest emerging science offered by medical and strength professionals.

This chapter aims to present the most current general and specific concepts regarding the rehabilitation of common gymnastics injuries. It also attempts to present the most current blend of gymnastics sports medicine research, strength and conditioning research, workload science, pathomechanical knowledge, stress neuroendocrinology, and gymnastics-specific rehabilitation techniques as it relates to the sport. It is beyond the scope of this chapter to outline every specific injury pattern or rehabilitation protocol, but specific examples will be offered when applicable. The authors hope that by presenting this information, it will open up new collaborative models for gymnastics sports medicine and rehabilitation.

11.2 General Rehabilitation Principles

Before exploring the specifics of common gymnastics injuries, it is important for the reader to understand a few pillar concepts that must be applied to all injuries. Specifically, the concepts of workload ratios, the five-stage rehabilitation process, and the crucial role of sports psychology (see Chap. 5 for a more detailed discussion of psychology in gymnastics).

11.2.1 Workload Ratios

The concept of workloads has been popularized by Tim Gabbett and many other researchers working in elite sports [20, 21]. The basic concept refers to the amount of work that is being performed in a given amount of time or the amount of work being performed in relation to the amount of recovery that is being allotted between bouts of training. The goal is to discover the amount of fitness that is being developed in relation to the amount of fatigue using objective data that is specific to the sport, so that injury risk can be seen in relation to exposure [20]. This research, along with literature on physeal growth plate injuries [22] and youth athlete injury risk [17], has been extremely helpful to understand new perspectives in overuse and acute injury risk. It has also been useful in assessing the early signs of nonfunctional overreaching or allostatic overload, which is when training stimuli are so high they produce maladaptive physiological results.

Much literature has been presented on the role of workloads in injury risk, although there is still debate on the exact applications to certain sports [23–25]. It is beyond the scope of this chapter to review this body of work relative to this topic. Instead, our focus will relate to how this body of evidence can be incorporated into the rehabilitation process. This is in an effort to ensure gymnasts appropriately rebuild their physiological capacity and fitness levels to tolerate high forces and training loads.

11.2.1.1 Acute to Chronic Workload Ratios and Rolling Averages

The majority of research on workloads centers around a concept known as the "acute to chronic workload ratio" [20]. This typically refers to comparing the workloads prescribed in a short window of training (usually between 3–7 days) of training compared to the previous 3 weeks. The purpose of this ratio is to track sudden changes in training volume and also monitor overall cumulative volume (chronic load). An emerging concept in the research has been "decay rates" which account for varying intensities of days, as is often seen in periodization models of sport training [26]. Decay rates provide objective guidance to the common understanding that more intense days of training with higher workloads have a bigger physiological impact on the following day's training, and also require more recovery time when compared to lighter days that have lower training loads.

It is essential that all of these concepts be utilized when designing a program for the rehabilitation of an injured gymnast. Understanding the steady progression of workload during exercise prescription must be observed to not only respect biological tissue healing, but also to administer the proper dosage of stress to elicit tissue adaptation [27, 28]. It is also crucial to understand the previous level of chronic workload the athlete was achieving. This information is helpful to rebuild their capacity for training, but also to be a guideline for what level of workload may have been concerning and contributed to certain injuries (overuse, fatigue based).

Clinicians are advised to compare the weekly average of workloads in relation to the previous 3 weeks when building programs. This refers to both the sets and repetitions of rehabilitation exercises, the exercise intensity, the neurological demand placed on athletes, and the total volume prescribed over the course of a week. When used in the return to sport phase, variables such as the force per skill, the force per surface or equipment, and the total force across an entire week's workload must be considered. The goal of this approach is to balance the development of fitness in relation to fatigue, which can be looked at by measuring both external and internal workloads as will be covered below. This allows the clinician to compare data and see the ratio of increasing stress on the athlete through their rehabilitation.

Errors can occur on either end of the loading spectrum, in the forms of both under - and overdosage [29]. Without the appropriate rise of exercise stress and the progression of athletes through advanced strength and conditioning programs (i.e., underdosage), concern for premature return to sports and reinjury risk may remain high [30]. This is speculated to be because the athlete did not fully restore their chronic load tolerance to the level that gymnastics requires. Athletes must be pushed appropriately, yet safely, in the rehabilitation process to regain the capacity to handle such loads.

The rate of progression must also not be too fast as to risk a disruption in tissue homeostasis and recovery (i.e., overdosage). The "sweet spot" of acute to chronic loading progression should be the intended target [20], and communication with athletes should be regular to monitor internal training load. Readers are encouraged to read the applications of workloads and periodization presented by Lorenz and Morrison for more specific rehabilitation guidelines [28].

11.2.1.2 The Inverted U Curve and Fitness Being Protective

One of the crucial concepts to emerge from the research on workloads is that there appears to be a "U curve" between low and high bouts of acute training [21, 29]. There is a common misconception that high volumes of training are always dangerous, while in reality this may be misguided. It seems that the extremes of the curve, both excessive undertraining and excessive overtraining, may lead to deleterious effects on performance and injury risk.

Excessively high chronic training loads that are very far beyond one's current capacity, often referred to as "toxic stress" by stress neuroendocrinology researchers, can lead to physical and mental maladaptation through overtraining [14, 16, 31]. A common scenario seen is when gymnasts are exposed to these extraordinarily high training loads, high level skills, and high pressure competition settings at an early age, leading to overuse injuries and nonfunctional overreaching.

In the opposite light, an excessively low level of training may not appropriately prepare athletes for sporting demands [20, 21]. It is important to recognize that a lack of physiological preparation through hybrid strength and conditioning models, a lack of attention to mastery of basic skill technique over multiple months, or not following the cyclical application of training load and recovery to achieve a high chronic training load safely, may lead to elevated injury risk.

The "sweet spot" that appropriately stresses athletes acutely and progressively builds their level of fitness over time may in fact be protective against injury risk [21]. Caution should be taken though, as much of the data has been collected in adult or professional athletes and these patterns may not exist in parallel when considering immature youth athletes like some gymnasts [21, 29, 30].

Very drastic "spikes" in training volume that are not part of a tactical coaching plan have been outlined to be concerning for elevated injury risk, and must be avoided in the rehabilitation process regardless of the presence of pain or the pressure to meet specific timeline goals [29, 32]. This may come in the form of sudden load increases or rapid increases in exercise demand that are not in line with the previously established exercise workloads. To reach this optimal dosage of stress in rehabilitation, both external and internal workloads should be utilized. The culture of gymnastics must change so that it allows for the optimal recovery timeline of injuries based on the biological healing rates of specific tissues, as well as full restoration of mental and physical loading tolerance, instead of returning to sport when pain is no longer present, pressures from coaches or parents, or competitions approach.

11.2.1.3 Tracking External and Internal Workloads

There are a variety of methods to monitor an athlete's training load or workload, most often these include consideration of an "external workload" and "internal workload". The external workload is an objective marker being tracked (number of impacts, pounds of weight lifted, etc.) [20]. In gymnastics, this may be in the form of a certain type of skill (lumbar extension movements for women's gymnastics), impacts (wrist contacts for men's pommel horse, landings for both men's and women's events), or intensity zones for time of a workout spent doing higher intensity activities (warm ups vs. routines or conditioning).

The "internal workload" refers to the global perceived challenge and degree of burden the athlete experiences in response to the external workload. This may be measured on a 1–10 rate of perceived exertion (RPE) scale or through a wellness survey asking health- and mood-related questions. Internal workloads are helpful in factoring in global stress levels that may come from outside sources for athletes like school, competition pressure, family life, or social relationships. Research in the field of stress neuroendocrinology has outlined the importance of factoring in various forms of demand on the young athlete, ranging from physical, to mental, to emotional factors (cumulatively referred to as an "allostatic load") for overall athlete wellness [31, 33]. This is a key concept to understand as the mental and emotional demand placed on athletes in high-pressure sports such as gymnastics is extremely high, as will be discussed in the Sports Psychology section. More advanced and detailed methods for monitoring workload are also available; these include technology to track heart rate variability, zones of heart rate, and accelerometer data. Some methods utilize rate of perceived exertion multiplied by the time of the session, referred to as "session RPE," to create sport-specific workload units. This method offers some lens into the athlete's interpretation of training load for a specific session of training, but not for overall impact of training load offered by internal workload markers.

Although these workload principles have not yet been fully individualized and applied to gymnastics, there are currently models being built that may help with more sensitive and valid measurements of gymnastics workloads. These models blend both internal and external loads by factoring in the time spent on specific apparatus or in physical preparation programs, event-specific RPE numbers, and weighting factors applied to these components based on the relative intensity of training (individual skills vs. half routines vs. full competitions). The multiplication of these variables can yield a "gymnastics training load" that is specific to both the sport and the individual athlete. The hope is that by building a new gymnastics-specific monitoring system on top of the available workload research, a gymnast's fitness and fatigue balance can be more accurately captured.

It cannot be emphasized enough that rehabilitation providers must create and follow objective guidelines for external workloads in rehabilitation. These programs should utilize the most current research in periodization and human adaptation to ensure the steady progression of demand being placed on a gymnast [27, 28, 30]. In similar fashion, constant communication and open discussion between rehabilitation professionals, athletes, parents, sport coaches, and other members of the interdisciplinary team related to workloads must be present for successful return to sport [34]. It is also worth noting that socially supportive training environments and positive coaching styles are essential in the successful rehabilitation of gymnastics injuries, as these factors directly influence acute and chronic workload prescription. Coaches who do not communicate with medical professionals or do not respect healing timelines may push the athlete too fast, too soon, resulting in an elevated risk of re-injury or high mental strain. This is supported by recent observational literature indicating a correlation between dictatorship style leadership, elevated injury risk, and more time missed from practice [35]. Without this supportive environment and social structure, challenges may exist in the successful return to training.

11.2.2 The Five-Stage Rehabilitation Process

Regardless of the specific injury, all instances of pathological tissue damage (overuse, traumatic, or surgical) will be required to move through a natural five-phase progression of injury to reach full recovery. Variations of this model have been successfully implemented in athletes with specific injuries including shoulder injuries in overhead throwing athletes [36], anterior cruciate ligament reconstruction [37], and ulnar collateral ligament reconstruction [38]. Professionals working with gymnasts are encouraged to utilize the same framework as a foundation, while at the same time applying the necessary individualization to the gymnastics athlete during the later stages of rehabilitation.

Depending on many factors (injury severity, concomitant lesions, chronological age, developmental age, pre-training level, training goals, pre-injury fitness, etc.), athletes may progress faster or slower throughout these stages. However, any "skipping" of these stages to achieve an earlier return to training, even if the athlete is pain free, is discouraged as it can be catastrophic for long-term health and career goals.

The reader is advised to educate athletes, coaches, parents, and other support staff on the importance of moving fluidly through all of these stages before attempting to return to full gymnastics training. It is strongly advised that phases are progressed based on both tissue homeostasis timelines as well as subjective and objective measures of athlete readiness, not timelines of competitions, perceived readiness from outside parties, or specific events such as recruiting showcases. The stages, approximate time domains of each, and suggested goals prior to progression proposed are as follows in Table 11.1. Please remember that these stages may vary significantly based on the severity of injuries and many other individual factors. Also, any specific protocol from medical doctors is to be followed specifically if provided to the rehabilitation specialist.

11.2.3 Rationale for the Five-Stage Progression

The principles of periodization, biological tissue healing, human adaptation, and the research in workloads all form the foundation for the five-stage rehabilitation process. In terms of histological adaptations, the appropriate application of increasing mechanical stress as one moves through these phases can promote bioplastic tissue growth within muscle, tendons, cartilage, and bone through the principles of mechanotransduction and Wolff's law. In addition, many other genomic transcription pathways and nongenomic signaling cascades that elicit cellular response to loading stimuli can lead to tissue remodeling and healing through the principles of physiological supercompensation [39–43].

From a neurological perspective, the systematic application of rehabilitation strategies initially assist in reversing inhibitory consequences of injury and helps restore neural pathway activation within the central and peripheral nervous system. In later stages, the intention of rehabilitation is to elicit specific neurological adaptations within local motor units, the peripheral nerves, and central nervous system. These adaptations can range from local neural drive increases, to more global concepts such as motor engram imprinting and new skill acquisition. Appropriate overload principles can rebuild the neurological base for athletic qualities such as coordination, proprioception, and balance. All of the above adaptations are created through functional remodeling of neuroendocrinological circuitry via neuroplasticity and hormonal signaling [28]. Emerging science from the field of human physiology and

Table 11.1 The five-stage rehabilitation criteria

Stage	Goals
Acute (est. weeks 0–4)	Restore local tissue and joint homeostasis Respect biological healing timelines Manage effusion, autogenic inhibition, compensatory adaptations in muscle tone, and protective reductions in lowered motor unit drive Restore basic ROM, tissue flexibility, joint mobility, and ability to perform basic activities of daily living
Subacute (est. weeks 4–8)	Integrate local joint function to kinetic chain function Restore basic strength, dynamic stability, proprioception, and neural drive via motor unit activation through weight-bearing progressions, graded exercise, hands on dynamic stability, and/or proprioceptive drills Return to activities of daily living, as well as school or work demands, as appropriate
Advanced (est. weeks 8–12)	Build local joint function and kinetic chain integrations into foundational movement patterns of squatting, hinging, single leg, pushing, pulling, and holistic core training Teach basic foundational movements that will be used in strength and conditioning for return to sports strength progression Start return to upper extremity weight-bearing progression if applicable through external weight loading and modified loading in quadruped positions, as per MD protocol if necessary
Strength and conditioning (est. weeks 12–20)	Progression from basic foundational movement patterns to exercises training explosive strength, force transference or absorption, power, rate of force development, anaerobic and aerobic capacity, and gymnastics-specific skill progressions Aim to build a general robust athlete first, followed by the second goal of rebuilding gymnastics-specific strength and conditioning, drills, and techniques
Return to sport (est. weeks 20+)	Use best available gymnastics sports science, medical advice, and gymnastics sport coaching advice to create an interdisciplinary program Objective return to sport program highly individualized to age, level, skills, goals, timeline, events, long-term athletic development model Interval program consisting of 2 weeks low impact exposure, then 2 weeks of medium surface exposure, and then 2 weeks of hard surface exposure Typically dosed with 3 days per week, 24–48 hours in between, subjective dosages Tracking external workload as above, but internal workloads with perceived effort and RPE

epigenetics further supports the emerging concept that appropriately dosed stressors may help human tissues adapt and increase their capacity through molecular mechanisms such as DNA methylation, histone modifications, long coding mRNA's, and more [31]. Rehabilitation also aims to restore a normal bandwidth of movement variability in order to accept the large variety of forces seen in sports [44].

Readers are encouraged to view the five-stage progression from a holistic point of view and resist the temptation to be dogmatic or tied to one "system" of rehabilitation. There are an infinite number of tools across many disciplines that can be used to help gymnasts transition throughout the phases of rehabilitation and safely back to sport. Examples include manual therapy, modalities, neuromuscular reeducation, strength and power exercises, advanced plyometrics, bracing or taping, technique improvement, biomechanical analysis, and skill profile modification. The more education and aptitude gained in all of these areas, the greater the chance of success in returning an athlete to training and competition.

11.2.4 Sports Psychology

Before moving on to the specific body regions and injury rehabilitation, an overview of central concepts would not be complete without highlighting the importance of sports psychology in relation to injury rehabilitation in gymnastics. The sport of gymnastics places enormous mental and emotional strain on young developing athletes, and issues related to fear of reinjury, pressure to return to training from coaches, parents, or teammates, and concerns for long-term health all must be considered and addressed. If these issues are not properly approached from a mental health perspective during the rehabilitation process, it can lead to significant negative effects on athlete. As referenced earlier, this cumulative strain is referred to as "toxic stress" or "allostatic overload" in the field of stress neuroendocrinology, and rehabilitation professionals are encouraged to review this work, as well as the chapter on Psychological Aspects of Injury in Gymnastics (Chap. 5) to better understand how fear, anxiety, and social stress play a role in athlete health [31, 33].

Athletes should be encouraged to communicate with the appropriate mental health professionals regarding their concerns for return from injury, and also be taught healthy coping mechanisms to assist in managing these common issues. Rehabilitation providers should serve as a resource and advocate for the athlete in screening for potential mental health concerns.

11.3 Specific Injury Principles and Rehabilitation Concepts: Upper Extremity

11.3.1 Shoulder Injuries

The shoulder joint is a very common source of problems for gymnasts [13, 45, 46]. Male gymnasts are known to have more shoulder injuries, as the nature of men's gymnastics is much more shoulder intensive [13]. This joint often ranks as the number one issue that male gymnasts struggle with throughout their career [3].

Every event in men's gymnastics involves the shoulders, but three more specifically (rings, high bar, and parallel bars) place enormous demands on the shoulder joint and surrounding structures. These forces exist for women's gymnastics, just in different variants and intensities (Fig. 11.2). With this in mind, it is imperative that

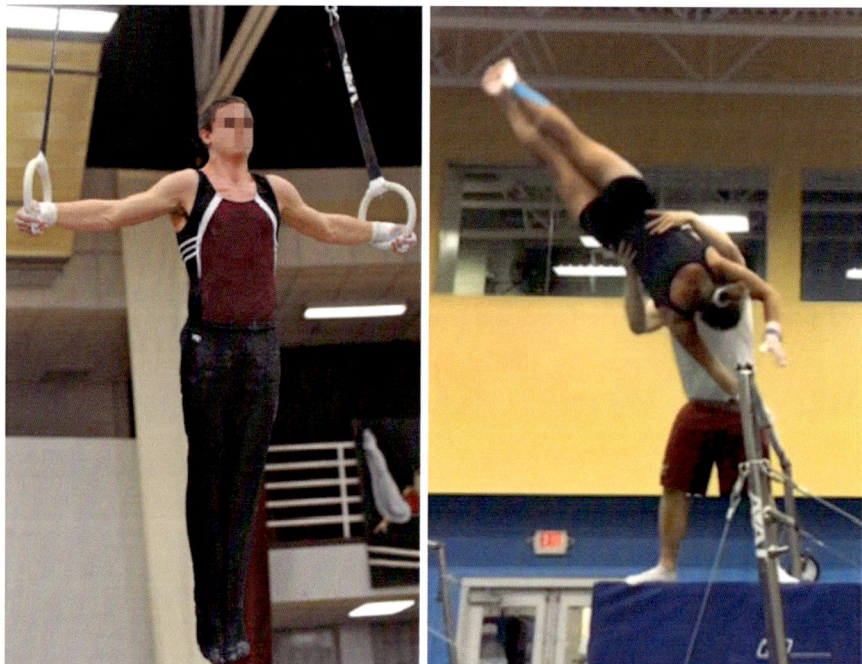

Fig. 11.2 Men's versus women's shoulder demands

rehabilitation professionals understand the unique nature of the shoulder joint as well as the role of the passive and dynamic stabilizers that allow such high degrees of function. Through rehabilitation, professionals should aim to not only restore high levels of strength and dynamic stability to the shoulder, but also increase the joint's tolerance to heavy compression and traction forces that are unique to gymnastics.

There are a variety of shoulder injuries that are seen within gymnastics due to the wide range of forces, ranges of motions, and tissue demands. Examples include mild muscular or rotator cuff strains that can be managed conservatively, to shoulder subluxations, to labral tears, to full musculotendinous ruptures or acute dislocations that may require surgical intervention and extensive rehabilitation [45]. It is beyond the scope of this chapter to fully explore the pathomechanics of each injury or surgical procedure. Readers are encouraged to review the comprehensive texts by Reinold, Wilk, Macrina, and Andrews for more specific pathomechanics, biomechanics, and surgery protocols [47, 48].

Regardless of injury type, the concepts of activity modification with a period of unloading, soft tissue management, rotator cuff and periscapular muscle performance training, rebuilding dynamic stability, progressive single arm overloading programs, and a graded return to sports are typically present within all shoulder rehabilitation programs.

11.3.1.1 Management of Soft Tissue Flexibility

The shoulder joint can be conceptualized as three "layers." The first consists of osseous articulations between the glenoid of the scapula and the humeral head, as well as the acromioclavicular and sternoclavicular attachments [36]. In the second layer lies capsulolabral structures of the various glenohumeral ligaments, the labrum, and neighboring ligamentous structures that provide further passive stability for the large mobility ranges allowed in the shoulder. The main glenohumeral ligaments are thickenings of the capsular tissue broadly categorized as anterior, inferior, and posterior divisions. These static stabilizers help limit excessive glenoid displacement depending on the position of the arm and direction of force being transmitted. In the third layer, various musculotendinous structures make up the more active restraints to the shoulder, working to not only allow dynamic stability against high forces in gymnastics but also to help produce, transfer, and buffer forces [49]. These are appropriately referred to as the "dynamic stabilizers" to the shoulder. Further layers have been outlined by researchers, describing the fourth as the neurovascular layer and the fifth and kinetic chain layer.

Through a process similar to natural selection, gymnastics attracts young athletes who are genetically predisposed to hypermobility, often showing above-average levels of capsular and ligamentous laxity. Although this is not inherently dangerous and allows for extreme ranges of motions to be achieved, it comes with a very important need to not further stress the passive tissues of the capsulolabral and ligamentous layers during rehabilitation, flexibility training, physical preparation programs, or skill training.

It is a misconception that all gymnasts have large ranges of shoulder mobility and do not require management of soft tissue flexibility. As has been noted by other researchers, repetitive overuse for specific sport motions may create adaptive stiffness in muscular soft tissues [50, 51]. This is thought to be from muscular microtrauma that occurs during strenuous exercise from both mechanical overload and acidic environments during exercise. Over time, damage may create changes in muscular stiffness that may negatively impact range of motion. It may also create elevated risk of injuries or increased force being placed upon neighboring joints in the kinetic chain such as the wrist or lower back. Losses of muscle flexibility may also be seen during times of rapid growth, creating further compromised ranges of motion and musculotendinous or osseous growth plate strain [22].

Although no studies exist measuring this specifically in the gymnastics population, it is the authors' experience that athletes develop adaptive stiffness within the latissimus dorsi, teres major, pectoralis major, subscapularis, biceps brachii, and triceps musculature over time. Alongside strength and conditioning and growth as noted above, this adaptation is also theorized to be a result of eccentric stress into overhead motions during bar swings, and from the repetitive shoulder extension needed to create a fundamental "hollow" shape during skills. If not appropriately screened for or managed with manual therapy (Fig. 11.3), appropriate flexibility, and self-soft tissue techniques, these issues may become problematic.

Fig. 11.3 Manual therapy of latissimus dorsi and teres major

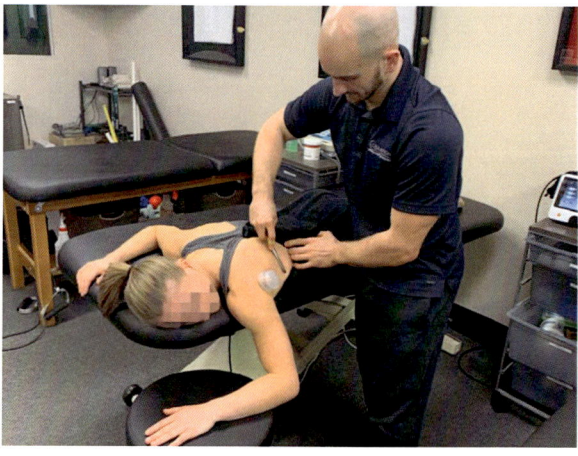

Fig. 11.4 Overhead shoulder mobility screen

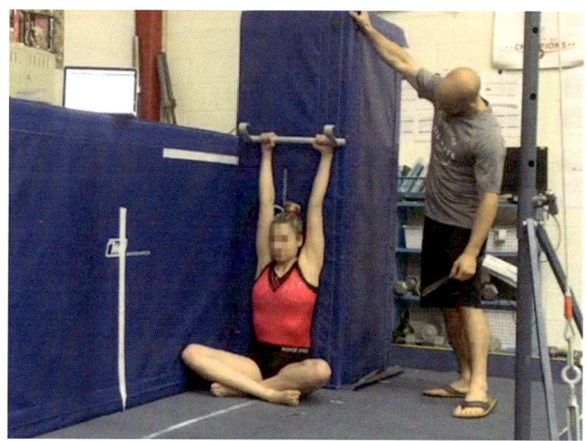

Many different types of shoulder injuries including rotator cuff impingement, labral irritation or SLAP lesions, and acquired microinstability may have a root in this intersection of losses in soft tissue flexibility, underlying capsular laxity, and high forces being repetitively placed on the shoulder at end ranges of motion [36, 48, 49]. These soft tissue changes may lead to altered osteokinematics and localized shoulder pain. Examples include excessive superior humeral head migration leading to subacromial space compression and rotator cuff irritation, or compensatory increased anterior capsular laxity causing anterior labral irritation SLAP tears with or without instability [36, 48, 49].

During the rehabilitation process, professionals are encouraged to use gymnastics specific screening tools to assess for these losses of shoulder motion (Fig. 11.4). In particular, this includes overhead elevation with different degrees of internal rotation, external rotation, and adduction that mimic overhand giant swings, "el-grip" swings, undergrip or "front grip" swings, and skills on balance beam. For male gymnasts, degrees of extreme shoulder extension must also be screened for, as these ranges of motions are seen on parallel bars and pommel horse. Following screening, a variety of manual therapy and soft tissue management techniques can be used to regain ranges of motion that may be lost during repetitive training.

11.3.1.2 Rotator Cuff and Parascapular Muscle Training Programs

The high force demands on the shoulders of gymnasts, combined with a possible lack of passive stability due to ligamentous hyperlaxity, requires special attention be placed on the dynamic stabilizers of the rotator cuff and scapula. Many times, the rehabilitation process does not adequately prepare the shoulder stabilizers of gymnasts prior to return to compression and traction-based skills through high-level exercise programs. Without adequate preparation through the principles of hypertrophy and periodization, gymnasts may be at risk for shoulder reinjury.

Rehabilitation professionals are encouraged to prescribe a core set of rotator cuff and scapular strength exercises that have been outlined by researchers to elicit high levels of EMG activity [52–54]. These include dumbbell side lying external rotation, prone elevation at 120° and 90° of abduction, prone external rotation and upright external rotation at 90° of elevation (Fig. 11.5), and standing front raises in the scapular plane. More traditional exercises for the scapular muscles in the horizontal rowing plane can also be utilized such as single arm dumbbell rows, half kneeling face pulls, and feet-elevated horizontal rows [55]. A variety of manual strengthening drills are also effective to increase strength of these muscle groups. These must be performed in the appropriate sets, repetition, loading, and volume per week to foster adaptations as is outlined in the strength and conditioning or periodization literature.

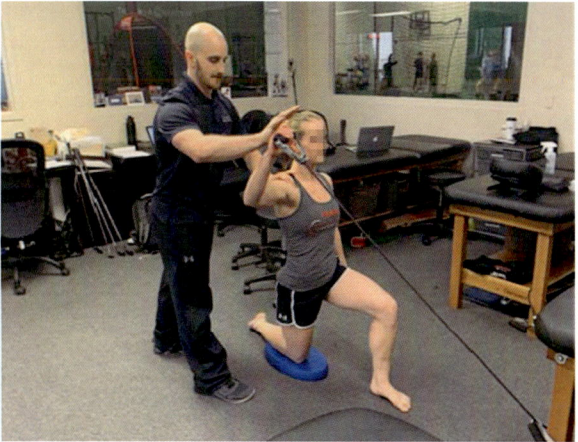

Fig. 11.5 Manual external rotation at 90° of elevation

11.3.1.3 Open and Closed Chain Dynamic Stability Training

Along with developing high levels of rotator cuff and scapular strength, the various muscles of the rotator cuff must also be trained to co-contract to provide further joint stability and centration of the humeral head within the glenoid [36, 49]. This is often referred to as "dynamic stability" of the shoulder joint and is thought to help prevent excessive micro-instability that may cause excessive strain to the structures supporting the glenohumeral joint.

Dynamic stability can be achieved through a combination of hands-on manual proprioception drills and specific exercises. Examples include rhythmic stabilization drills, single arm loaded carry variations, and single arm plyometric neuromuscular drills outlined by Reinold and Wilk [47, 49]. Semi-weight-bearing drills specific to gymnastics can also be used, such as quadruped overhead wall stabilizations (Fig. 11.6). These drills are used in an effort to prepare the upper extremity joints for high traction and compression forces that have been outlined in gymnastics biomechanical research [1, 13].

11.3.1.4 Progressive Single Arm Loading Programs

It must be reemphasized that the joints of the upper extremity are not inherently built for weight bearing. They do not possess the same evolutionary machinery to handle repeated forces as is seen in the lower extremity. These differences include different bony structure, less shock absorbing cartilage, and less robust weight-bearing structures.

During the rehabilitation of any shoulder injury, as well as elbow or wrist injuries, a progressive overload program that utilizes external loading and a progressive return to upper extremity weight bearing is essential. This is in an effort to help close the gap that often exists between the upper extremity's ability to handle repeated force and the high demands that gymnastics requires. Specific exercise

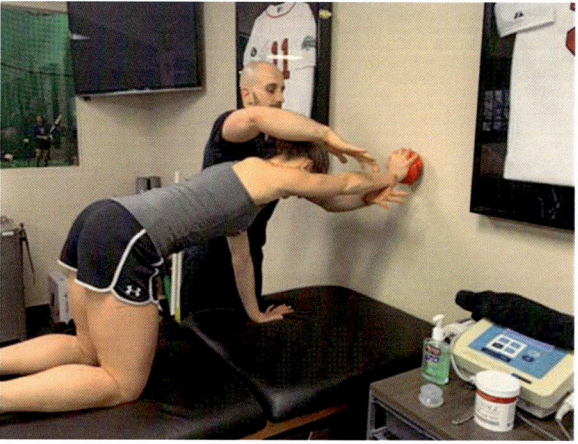

Fig. 11.6 Quadruped single arm wall stabilizations

examples include half kneeling single arm dumbbell landmine or overhead presses, single arm dumbbell floor presses, half kneeling single arm band pull downs, kettlebell or dumbbell Turkish Get Ups, and various single arm loaded carries.

11.3.1.5 Objective Return to Sports Programs for Shoulder-Specific Skills

With all shoulder injuries, one of the most important components in successfully returning to gymnastics is a graded, objective, and progressive return to skill program. This concept has been well outlined in other sports such as returning to throwing in baseball [56, 57], swinging movements in golf and tennis [56], and mileage in running [58], serving as a conceptual foundation for creating gymnastics-specific programs.

Certain skills in gymnastics are inherently more shoulder intensive, while others are not. Through collaboration and interdisciplinary work, gymnasts must be given a specific program that helps reintroduce them to unique shoulder-specific forces. This is typically done by outlining the days per week of training, the skill profile of the gymnast, the events trained per day, and the equipment available. Over the course of 4–6 weeks, the skill demand and total volume is increased, ideally with 24–48 hours between loading sessions to promote optimal adaptation. An example is provided in Table 11.2. Further information on return to gymnastics progressions is included in Chap. 12.

11.3.2 Elbow Injuries and Rehabilitation Considerations

While many of the same principles noted above apply to the elbow joint, there are specific considerations that must be outlined. The most common elbow injuries seen in gymnastics are in the overuse category such as osteochondritis dissecans (OCD),

Table 11.2 Shoulder return to sports progression example

Event	Monday	Tuesday	Wednesday	Thursday	Friday	Saturday		
Vault	No Hyper Ext No Hyper Ext No Hyper Ext PT Home Program	R.Off x 5 Timers x 5 Flip Drills x 5	No Hyper Ext No Hyper Ext No Hyper Ext PT Home Program	R.Off x 5 Timers x 5 Flip Drills x 5	R.Off x 5 Timers x 5 Flip Drills x 5			
Bars	CHS Piro x5 Dismounts x 5 Low Bar Drills	No Hyper Ext No Hyper Ext No Hyper Ext PT Home Program	CHS Piro x5 Dismounts x 5 Low Bar Drills	CHS Piro x5 Pac x 5 Low Bar Drills	CHS Piro x5 Dismounts x 5 Low Bar Drills			
Beam	BHS x 5 Turns x 5 Ariel Drills x 5	SL x 5 B. Tuck x 5 Dismount x 5	BHS x 5 Turns x 5 Ariel Drills x 5	No Hyper Ext No Hyper Ext No Hyper Ext PT Home Program	BHS x 5 Turns x 5 Ariel Drills x 5			
Floor	Back pass x 5 Jumps and leaps Drills	Front Pass x 5 Jumps and leaps Drills	Back Pass x 5 Jumps and leaps Drills	Back Pass x 5 Jumps and leaps Drills	No Hyper Ext No Hyper Ext No Hyper Ext PT Home Program			Week Total
Hyper Ext #	40	45	40	35	25			185
Impact #	35	50	35	35	30			185

Week 4 and 5 - Floor/Hard

triceps apophysitis, and stress fractures. In more rare instances, traumatic falls on an outstretched hand and acute dislocations do occur. OCD specifically refers to an overuse injury that creates cartilage breakdown in the capitellum, often times requiring notable time away from sports and in some cases surgical intervention [59, 60].

Researchers have outlined how the position and mechanisms for OCD in gymnastics (more posterior lesions with compression forces) are different than other sports such as baseball (more anterior lesions with shearing forces) [61]. As a result, the difference in pathomechanics must be considered in the rehabilitation process.

Many gymnastics professionals and rehabilitation specialists have speculated that the drastic increase in OCD injuries are from technical errors, genetic predisposition, or a lack of "mental toughness" from athletes. While these are factors that can be considered, it is the author's opinion that these reasons are not the main contributors for such drastic increases in elbow injury rates seen in the last decade. The more likely reality that many people working in gymnastics fail to admit is that simply too much high force skill volume is being done on hard surfaces (vaulting, tumbling, pommel horse, and balance beam in particular) at an early age when growth plates of the elbow and capitellum cartilage are at high risk of injury. This is often occurring without the prerequisite physical capacity being first developed, or without the necessary patience to resist the temptation of allowing young gymnasts to compete high force skills at a young age.

When this is paired with ongoing cultural resistance to embrace a hybrid model of strength and conditioning that uses external weight lifting, a lack of application of periodization principles or workload ratios, cultural issues of athletes not feeling comfortable to report pain onset early, or the stubbornness of gymnasts choosing to push through injuries, these elbow issues will continue to run rampant.

While specific technical issues such as excessive hand turnout during round-offs have been highlighted as an important risk factor for elbow stress [62], the simple equation of acute elbow loading being more than elbow capacity and cultural issues within training environments appear to be at the epicenter of the problem. Due to the short-term and long-term consequences elbow injuries can present for gymnasts in the forms of pain, lost time from training, and surgical interventions, proactive models of management must become the primary effort.

During the rehabilitation process of gymnastics elbow injuries, a similar program can be utilized during the acute, subacute, and advanced stages as has been outlined by researchers in sports that experience high elbow injury rates [38, 63]. This includes management of acute swelling, pain reduction, reversal of autogenic inhibition, and restoring full elbow range of motion (particularly full extension) early in the rehabilitation sequence. This can be accomplished through various passive and active range of motion techniques, manual therapy, compression garments, modalities, and graded exercise progressions.

Following this, a progressive exercise program utilizing dumbbells should be implemented within the framework of linear loading to regain baseline levels of strength at the elbow and wrist, as well as plyometric drills [63]. If gripping or hand use is not permitted due to protocol guidelines, ankle weights or manual resistance proximal to the elbow joint can be implemented instead of dumbbells. Also, special attention should be given to a progressive flexibility and strength program of the scapulothoracic joint and radiocarpal joint during elbow joint recovery.

11.3.2.1 Return to Weight Bearing and Traction Force Progressions

Of particular importance to elbow injuries, such as OCD, triceps apophysitis, or those requiring surgical management, is a graded return to weight bearing during the advanced stage of rehabilitation. The authors recommend that this is done after a symmetry strength index of 90% is achieved between the involved and uninvolved sides. A symmetry index can be assessed through objective load lifted during single arm exercises or handheld dynamometer. The start of progressive weight bearing is suggested in the form of modified quadruped rocking and crawling drills in multiple directions, ideally with objective feedback from numeric scales or force plates (Fig. 11.7).

For the progression to horizontal pushing strength, the transition from single arm dumbbell floor press exercises can then move to wall push-ups, to table push-ups, to box push-ups of progressively lowered heights, and finally to floor push-ups. This eventually will continue into vertical pressing directions and handstand training, which are essential skills in gymnastics. This can be accomplished by progressing regular push-up positions to piked stacking positions, to 90 degree pike positions with the hips elevated overhead placing the feet on a box, to one-legged elevation stacking in a pike handstand, and finally to wall walk-up progressions and handstand basics. Half kneeling landmine presses and single arm dumbbell presses are also useful during this progression. These exercises must be advanced slowly over multiple weeks, with recovery bouts between sessions to monitor symptoms.

To progress back to hanging traction forces on the upper extremity, athletes are first advised to perform single arm band pull downs in half kneeling, followed by 25–50% weight bearing hanging using a box, to full hanging, and finally to body

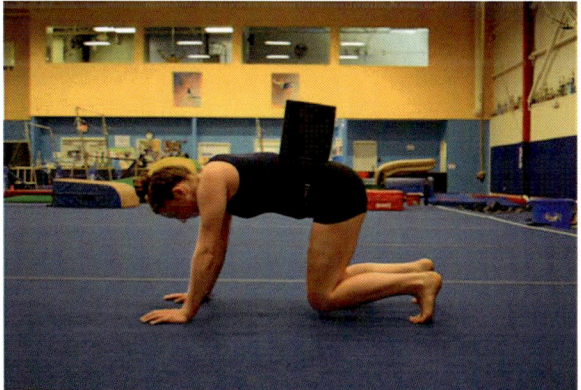

Fig. 11.7 Bear crawl

Fig. 11.8 Wrist loading in men's pommel horse

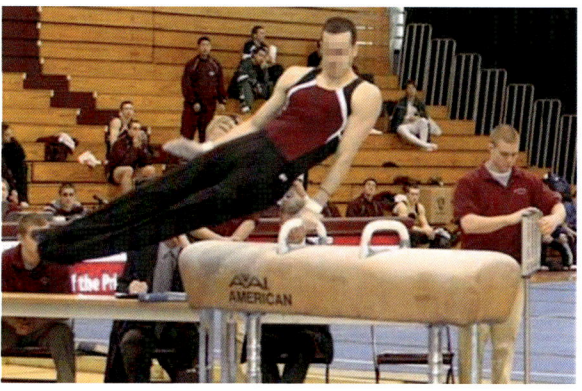

weight and weighted pull-up progressions over a few weeks. This is in conjunction with returning to the horizontal pulling progression outlined above in the shoulder rehabilitation section. Once this is accomplished without pain, the beginning of hanging or swinging gymnastics basics can be implemented through basic gymnastics drills, using spotting to deload body weight percentage, or through modified equipment (e.g., a "strap bar" or "metal bar").

11.3.3 Wrist Injuries and Rehabilitation Considerations

Rehabilitation of the wrist joint uses many of the same concepts as those outlined in the shoulder and elbow section. With this said, there are important differences that must be explored. Due to the fact that the wrist serves as the main interface to ground contact in the upper extremity, much like the ankle joint does to the lower extremity, it is exposed to much higher rates of impact and overuse [64]. Traumatic falls on an outstretched arm can sometimes create acute injuries, but overuse injuries are typically more prominent. Such examples include "gymnast's wrist" that many gymnasts experience from repetitive compression forces during pommel horse (Fig. 11.8), parallel bars, tumbling, and vault [64]. It is worth noting that gymnast's wrist is a large, and often vague, category of diagnosis that the authors discourage medical professionals from using. It is advised that providers discuss further with medical and radiology professionals to narrow in on the exact wrist and hand structures that are involve in the injury to have a better understanding of the mechanisms of injury.

A wide spectrum of wrist issues can exist ranging from growth plate inflammation, to dorsal impact syndrome, to stress fractures, to triangular fibrocartilage complex tears, and more [65, 66]. In particular, the radiocarpal growth plate is a common source of injury when excessively high acute workloads are met with local range of motion limitations (through both osseous and soft tissue changes), a lack of physical preparation to tolerate weight bearing, and impairments being present higher up in the kinetic chain such as limited shoulder range of motion, underdeveloped scapular strength, or suboptimal thoracic spine mobility [64, 65, 67].

11.3.3.1 Screening and Management of Radiocarpal Extension Range of Motion

The wrist joint requires an excessive amount of extension range of motion to stack the athlete's center of mass during handstand skills and also to transfer motion over the wrist during tumbling and vaulting skills. This is similar to the amount of ankle dorsiflexion that is required to show proper force progression of the body's center of mass during gait, running, and squatting movements.

An excessively high volume of gripping, as well as handstand balancing, is required during women's artistic gymnastics uneven bar training, and during men's artistic gymnastics pommel horse, ring, parallel bar, and high bar training. Other disciplines in gymnastics that involve tumbling, hand balancing, and gripping possess similar demands. Over time, these repetitive gripping motions may lead to adaptive stiffness of the flexor pronator muscle groups, which can then, in turn, limit weight bearing wrist extension range of motion. This may create local radiocarpal joint irritation when gymnastics skills that require this flexibility (handstands, tumbling, vaulting) are repeatedly trained. This is similar to the adaptive stiffness of the plantar flexors negatively impacting dorsiflexion range of motion during gait, running, or squatting.

It is important that practitioners screen for this range of motion requirement. For skills that require wrist dorsiflexion with an extended elbow (such a handstands), this can be done with a quadruped rocking screen where athletes are asked to translate their shoulder over their wrists, and the angle of wrist extension is measured (Fig. 11.9). This screen has been created, although not yet validated by normative data, in parallel to those screens for ankle dorsiflexion range of motion. This can also be done manually by a rehabilitation professional with the patient supine, while special attention is taken to fully extend the wrist and thumb joints.

For skills requiring wrist extension with a flexed elbow (dip skills on men's parallel bars and other variants of tumbling drills) wrist range of motion in an extended finger position can be quickly screened in a "prayer" position. Gymnasts are asked

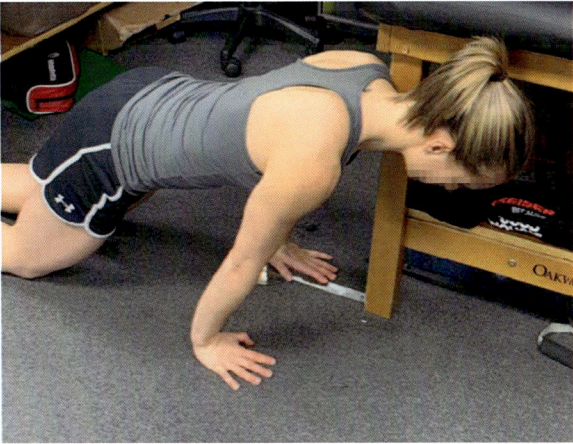

Fig. 11.9 Quadruped weight-bearing wrist extension screen

to place the palms and fingers of both hands together and move their wrists into extension while maintaining the base of the palms in contact. Although normative values do not exist, greater than 90° without pain is recommended.

It is worth noting that due to the nature of demands on the upper body, it has been proposed that limitations in overhead shoulder flexibility may increase the risk of wrist extension overload and possible pain [67]. Overhead shoulder elevation, as well as active use of those ranges of motion during gymnastics skills and proper physical preparation to tolerate weight bearing, must be trained in the rehabilitation progress.

11.3.3.2 Objective Return to Impact Programs for the Upper Extremity

The upper extremity possesses a unique challenge in return to sport criteria in gymnastics, as there are few valid or reliable metrics for upper extremity functional testing. The Closed Chain Kinetic Upper Extremity Stability Test (CKCUEST) has been proposed as a helpful objective measurement of upper extremity sport function, but still lacks markers of normative data and transference to the gymnastics population [68]. Understanding the limited research available in this area, readers are encouraged to use advanced strength and conditioning tests for upper body explosiveness (such as plyometric push-up capacity), upper body force absorption quality, the monitoring of gymnastics-specific physical preparation, and objective return to impact programs as their guide for athlete readiness levels.

Both the elbow and wrist joints require specific and objective return to impact programs, similar to how the shoulder requires a return to traction and compression forces. These programs are similar to return to impact and plyometric programs seen in the lower extremity following knee or ankle injury. However, in the upper body, the program may be more gymnastics specific as most sports do not specifically train for upper body plyometric force absorption and dissipation.

In particular, pommel horse, parallel bars, vault, and floor all require high degrees of wrist and elbow impact for artistic male gymnasts. For female artistic gymnasts, balance beam, vault, and floor possess high volumes of impact on the wrist and elbow. A program that tracks the daily, weekly, and total workload volume of upper body impacts by surface is essential to successful sport return. Following the completion of full strength and conditioning programs, athletes are advised to begin upper extremity loading on trampoline surfaces, and then progress to more firm surfaces such as the floor, and finally back to harder impact surfaces such as pommel horse, balance beam, or vaulting, typically over 6–8 weeks.

11.4 Specific Injury Principles and Rehabilitation Concepts: Lower Extremity

Before delving into the specifics of each joint region, it is pertinent to discuss concepts that will address issues throughout the whole lower extremity. Joint position at time of landing has been linked to a variety of lower extremity pathologies ranging from patellofemoral pain syndrome to anterior cruciate ligament injury [69–71]. Biomechanics literature often refers to "stiff leg" vs. "soft landing" in describing joint kinematics at time of landing in regard to demands put on different tissues of the lower extremity [72–74]. There is some debate in the literature about theoretical transfer of tissue load from internal joint structure to tissues external to the joint (contractile tissues for example) by altering landing form [75, 76].

With this in mind, lab-based research and clinical outcomes literature has advocated to train an athlete to land with more of a "soft landing" that makes the neuromuscular system more responsible for attenuation forces and potentially reduces injury incidence [12, 72, 77–79]. From a practical standpoint, this means greater degrees of knee flexion and hip flexion, the femur being held in a fairly neutral position in regard to rotation, as well as maintenance of a trunk position that is over the pelvis and positions the center of mass within a good base of support. Figures 11.10 and 11.11 provide examples of landing positions that should be discouraged during training, while Figs. 11.12 and 11.13 would be considered more optimal to reduce injury risk and degree of joint impact.

General ballistic training through plyometric drills are a key element for both modifying previously learned landing patterns and producing increased power with better control during final stages of lower extremity rehabilitation. Gymnasts should follow a criteria-based progression of foundational components of recovery prior to beginning ballistic and plyometric programs. This includes muscle-specific strength training and neuromuscular training through balance and proprioceptive challenges. Gymnasts should also have pain-free symmetrical performance on these skills prior

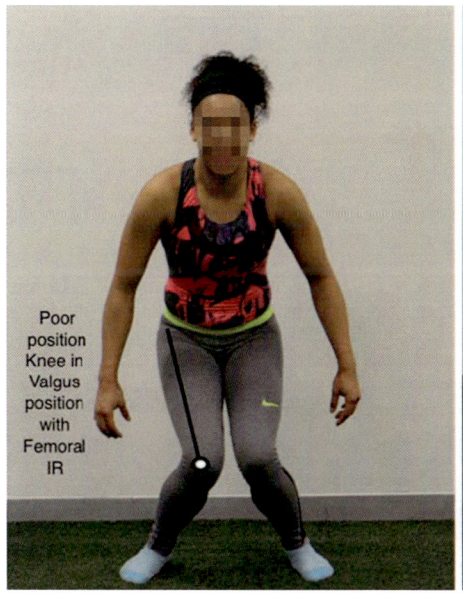 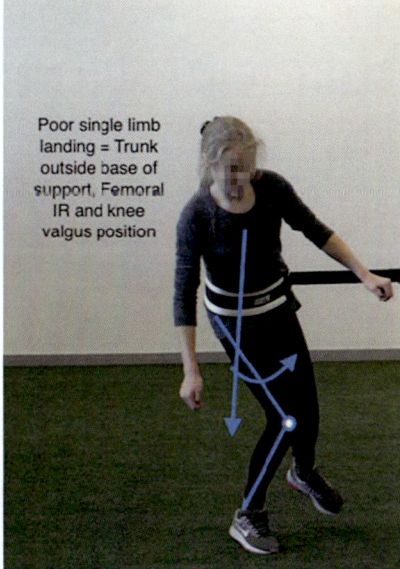

Fig. 11.10 Examples of "poor landing" position

Fig. 11.11 Lateral view of "stiff knee" landing position

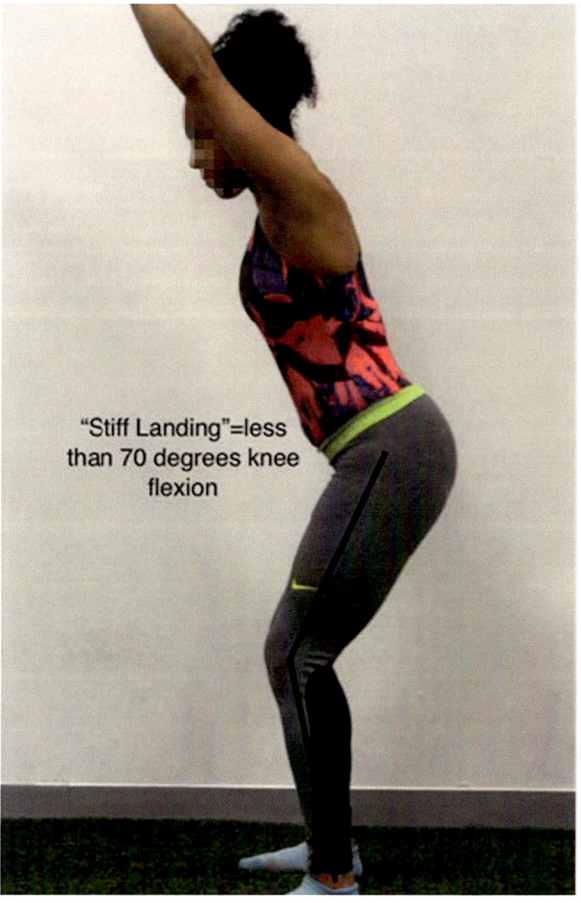

to beginning the foundational ballistics/plyometrics program such as that described in Table 11.3.

During plyometric training, controlled proper form should be established prior to progressive increase in distance, height, and speed of movement for greater power development. Once this foundational level of plyometrics has been completed with satisfactory form, movements specific to the demands of gymnastics should be integrated. It is pertinent to include plyometric training in all directions (forward, back, side to side) as well as rotational movements that involves dropping from a height to mimic skills such as tumbling and dismounts. Table 11.4 describes an example of progression that may be useful for both the hip and knee regions. Figures 11.14 and 11.15 illustrate a few of these exercises.

Although specific lower extremity joints will be addressed below, apophysitis is a common diagnosis that requires specific mention, as it can affect the calcaneus, tibial tuberosity, ischial tuberosity, and other regions of the pelvis and hip

Fig. 11.12 Anterior view of more optimal landing position

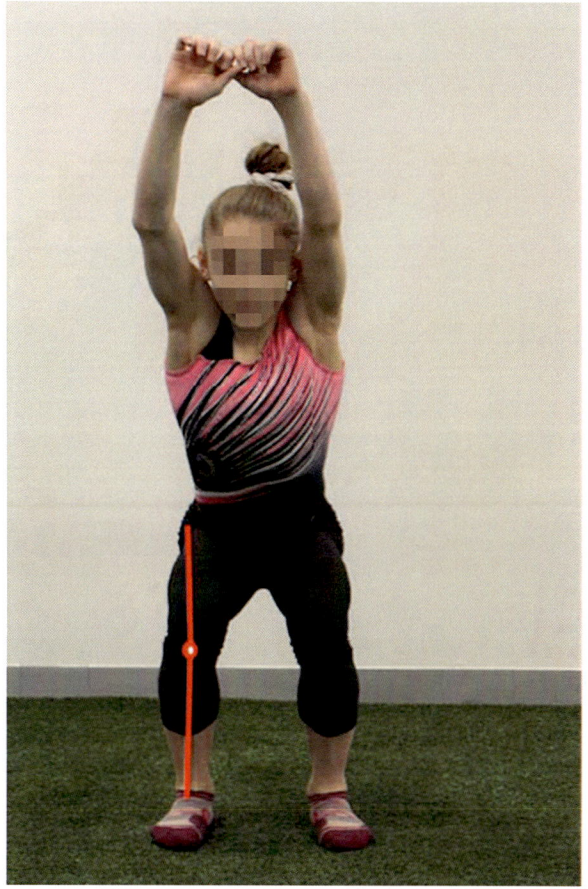

[3, 80–82]. Treatment should focus on reducing the load to the affected tissues through rest and modification of volume of training to prevent continued recurrence at the growth center until the physis at that location has "closed" or ossified. The degree of rest is dictated by severity and irritability of symptoms. In mild cases, this may require only modification of training such as all tumbling being done on Tumbl Trak, avoiding impact loading during strength and conditioning aspects of training, and reducing the number of dismounts performed within a week. On the other hand, more severe cases may require complete rest from training for a period of 3–4 weeks prior to progressive criteria-based return to both strength and conditioning as well as skill-based training [22, 80, 83]. In some cases, it may also be beneficial to implement taping, bracing, or strapping types of interventions for a short period of time until symptoms are reduced. For example, gymnasts may use a cho-pat strap at the knee or a heel cup or strap at the calcaneus. In addition, addressing imbalances in soft tissue flexibility is important, but may require modification of methods or dosage due to typical methods of stretch-

Fig. 11.13 Lateral view of "soft landing"

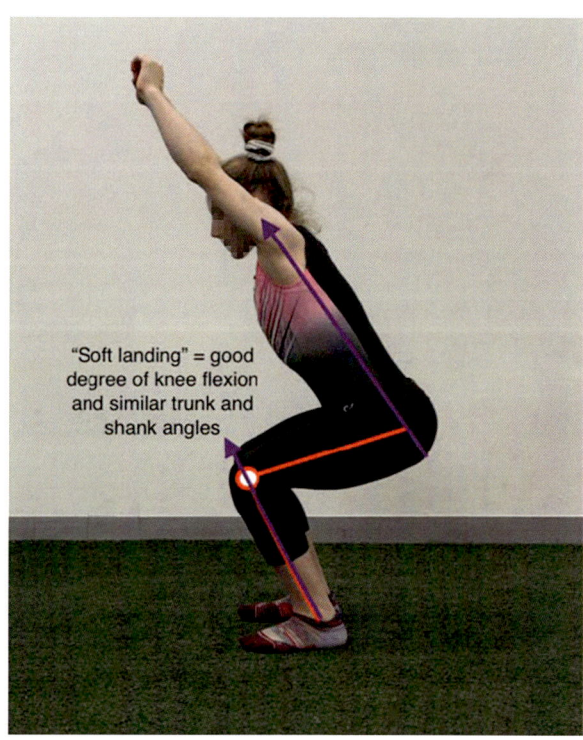

Table 11.3 Lower extremity foundational plyometrics/ballistic training

First phase bilateral	Squat jumps in place
	Broad jumps moving forward
	Box jumps on to box forward (appropriate height progression based on athlete)
	Tuck jumps
	Scissor/lunge jumps in place
Second phase bilateral	180° (1/2 twist) squat jumps
	Broad jumps forward and back in sequence
	Box jumps on and off forward and back
	Box jumps to side on and off
	180° (1/2 twist) tuck jumps
	Lateral movement with scissor jumps
First phase unilateral (following completion of bilateral)	Bilateral squat jump to unilateral landing in place
	Single leg hop forward for progressive distance
	Single leg hop to side for progressive distance
	Single leg cone or hurdle hop
	Single leg forward box jump on only
Second phase unilateral	Single leg triple hop forward
	Single leg triple side/lateral hop
	Single leg forward on/off box jumps
	Single leg side/lateral on/off box jumps
	Single leg 180° (1/2 twist) hop in place progressing to lateral movement

11 Rehabilitation of Gymnasts

Table 11.4 Lower extremity advanced plyometrics/ballistic training

First phase bilateral	Resisted broad jumps Broad jumps with 180° rotation (1/2 twist) Lateral scissor jumps with quick change in direction (side to side) Resisted lateral scissor jumps 180° (1/2 twist) box jump dropping off box of moderate height (18–24 inch initially)
Second phase bilateral to unilateral (controlled landing emphasis)	(Height of box is determined by level of athlete, ability to control the landing, and quality of landing) Box jump drop to single leg landing: forward, backward, and to side Box jump drop to single leg landing with 90° turn (1/4 twist) in the air (all directions of motion) Box jump drop to single leg landing with 180° turn (1/2 twist) in the air Lateral single leg 180° (1/2 twist) hops for distance progressing to distance and speed
Second phase unilateral resisted (power and speed development)	Resisted forward hop progressing from consistent resistance to variable resistance from treating clinician Resisted lateral hops progressing from consistent resistance to variable resistance from treating clinician Resisted change in direction hops (side to side and forward back)

Drop jump with rotation

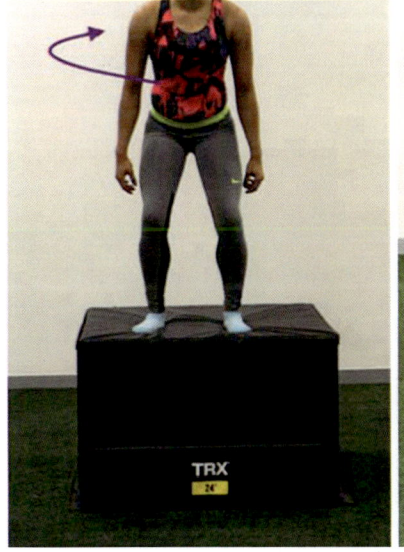
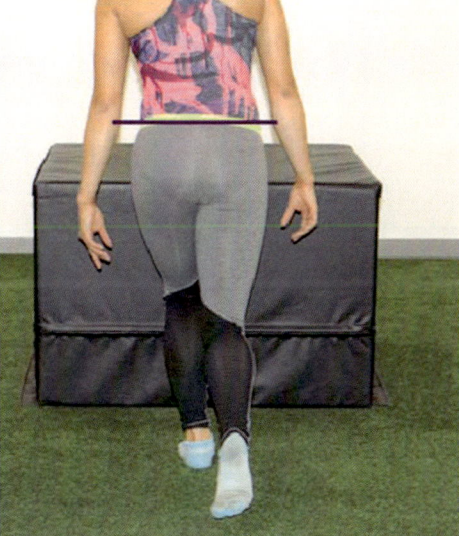

Fig. 11.14 Examples of lower extremity advanced plyometrics

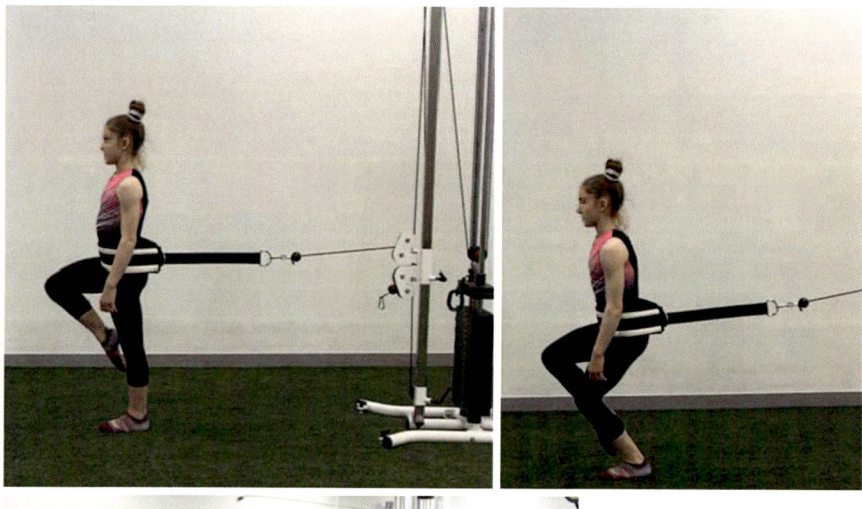
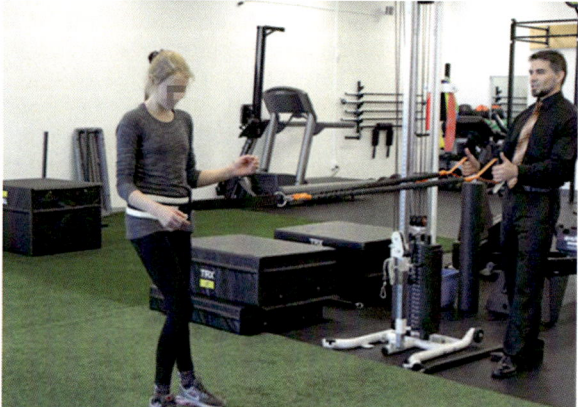
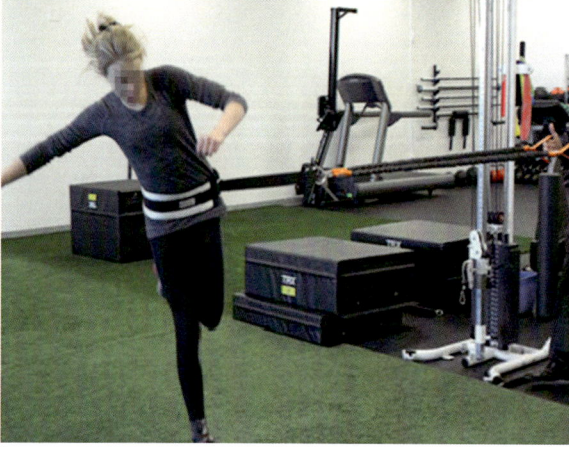

Fig. 11.15 Single leg hop with resistance

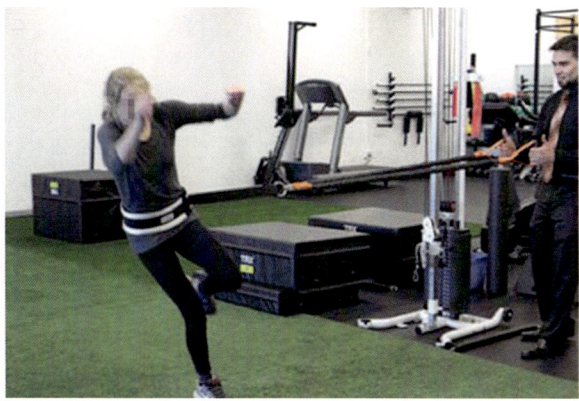

Fig. 11.15 (continued)

ing resulting in a prolonged stress to the growth center. As such, it is advocated to utilize methods of soft tissue mobilization and a modification of stretching parameters including reduced hold times and performing static stretching at a time when the soft tissues are most pliable such as post-activity. Along with addressing impairments in soft tissue mobility, it is important to examine and address any deficits in muscle performance within the whole lower extremity that may be leading to increased forces at the site of pain.

11.4.1 Rehabilitation Considerations for Injuries of the Hip

11.4.1.1 Impingement and Labral Pathology

Gymnastics puts very high demands on the hip region at both the articular level and the surrounding soft tissues. Many of the same "layer concepts" described in the shoulder section can be translated to the hip. The first and deepest layer, the osseous layer that forms the femoracetabular joint, is made up of the acetabular socket within the pelvis and the spherical femoral head [84]. The major difference between the shoulder and the hip is that the acetabular fossa is much deeper, allowing more bony articulation and geometrical support to tolerate weight bearing [85]. The second layer, the capsulolabral layer, is made up of blended thickening of capsular tissue as well as the acetabular labrum. The main static stabilizers of this layer are the iliofemoral ligament, the pubofemoral ligament, the ischiofemoral ligament, and the ligamentum teres [84–86]. The third layer is made up of the dynamic stabilizers. As noted with the shoulder, many practitioners also reference the fourth and fifth layer as the neurovascular and kinetic chain layers, respectively. Within this last layer are many more musculotendinous structures to support weight bearing and locomotion. They are typically broken up into four anatomical groupings (medial, posterior, anterior, and lateral) and compose muscles such as the adductors, hamstrings, quadriceps, glutes, and deep hip rotators [85].

Recent evidence indicates that the most common type of symptoms at the hip region are femoral acetabular impingement (FAI) with associated acetabular labrum pathology [3, 81, 82]. This particular diagnosis and its management is of considerable debate in the literature and at a clinical level [87–91]. While the incidence of acetabular labral pathology on MRI in asymptomatic individuals has been found to be anywhere between 19% and 81% in adults [92–94], the incidence in the pediatric and adolescent age groups has been reported as much lower at 1–2% [95]. The current lack of clarity regarding appropriate management of this particular pathology makes it pertinent to be certain that FAI/labral pathology is the source of pain for the athlete and to exhaust nonoperative management strategies for at least 3–5 months prior to considering surgical intervention [87, 89, 91, 96].

When considering intra-articular pathology of the hip such as FAI or labral pathology, it is important to achieve balance of hip joint range of motion by addressing mobility deficits through manual techniques and quality foundational strength training. This should be guided by those exercises proven to best recruit posterior chain muscles including the gluteus maximus, gluteus medius, gluteus minimus, and the deep hip rotators. Examples include resisted hip ER in various degrees of hip flexion, side bridges, unilateral bridges, resisted lateral walking, retro walking, squats with resistance around the distal femur, Bulgarian split squats, unilateral squat, and many others supported in the literature [87, 97–101].

An individualized impairment-based approach has been described to guide a patient through the early stages of rehabilitation for FAI and labral tears [87, 91]. Additionally, for the subset of patients that require surgical intervention, Heerey et al. have described a basic impairment-based progression [102]. For both the postoperative and nonoperative scenario, a criteria-based progression such as that described by Wahoff et al. is advocated [103].

Upon completing these basic components and entering the finals stages of rehabilitation, the gymnast should be guided through specific plyometric/power training as described at the beginning of the lower extremity section.

In addition to the more commonly considered FAI and anterior labral pathology, it is also important to consider more recently recognized issues at the hip such as microinstability and extra-articular impingements (e.g., ischiofemoral impingement, subspine impingement, and iliopsoas impingement) [84, 104]. Microinstability is a very recently recognized condition that a gymnast may be particularly susceptible to as a result of repeated and high-load movements such as leaps and splits that may result in excessive eccentric load to the anterior structures and migration of the femoral head in an anterior direction [84, 86, 105]. A key element to prevention and treatment of microinstability is implementation of correct position to stretch hip flexor and adductor musculature minimizing femoral head migration. In addition to the above-described interventions for FAI/labrum pathology, microinstability may require very specific low-load muscle recruitment to those muscles most proximal to the joint as described by McNeill and Scoot [106]. A variety of rhythmic stabilization drills and manually resisted exercises specific to the motions in gymnastics can also be used to foster co-contraction of the deep hip stabilizer muscles (Figs. 11.16 and 11.17). Management of most extra-articular impingement syndromes will involve similar treatment strategies to those described in the following section.

11.4.1.2 Soft Tissue and Repetitive Tissue Stress Injuries

Soft tissue and overuse injuries, such as hip flexor tendonitis, hamstring muscle strains, and iliopectineal or trochanteric bursitis, should be managed with particular attention to progressive tissue loading from both a tissue mobility/flexibility perspective and muscle performance perspective. As has been discussed throughout this chapter, progressive loading based both on time and criteria will be the optimal

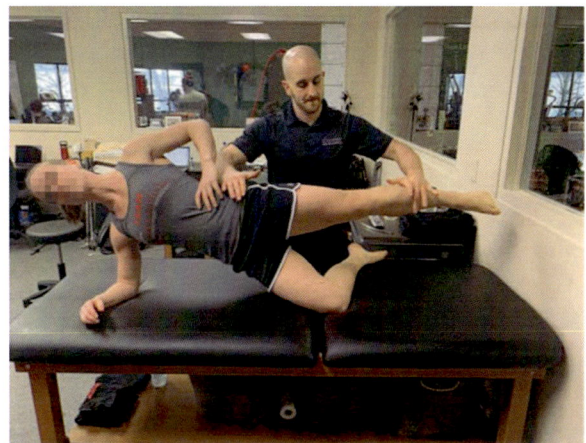

Fig. 11.16 Manual hip abduction in side plank

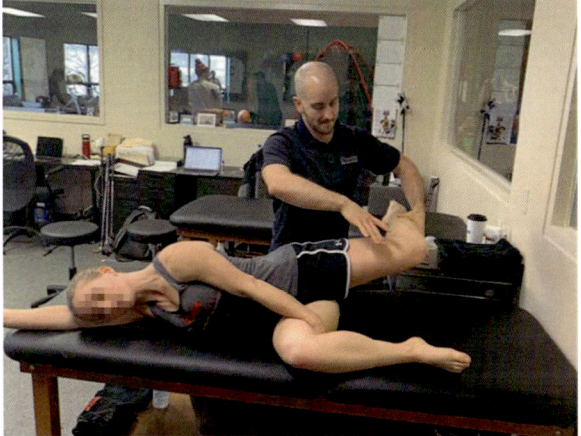

Fig. 11.17 Side-lying split pelvis rhythmic stabilizations

management strategy. At the hip, it is important to fully assess soft tissue flexibility deficits that may exist not only in the symptomatic tissues but also in those soft tissues that are in opposition to the symptomatic area. Should a deficit in soft tissue mobility be identified, manual techniques and stretching techniques should be implemented, and an assessment of the athlete's typical flexibility routine should be performed. For example, in many cases, the typical hip flexor stretching position and technique may result in motion at the lumbar spine or anterior femoral-acetabular joint instead of at the hip flexor muscle (Fig. 11.18). It is also important to address any muscle performance deficits and imbalances, since in many cases the basic gluteal muscles mentioned above will be a staple of the rehabilitation process.

Once the athlete has completed the typical foundational components of rehabilitation and balanced the force production and soft tissue mobility around the hip, he or

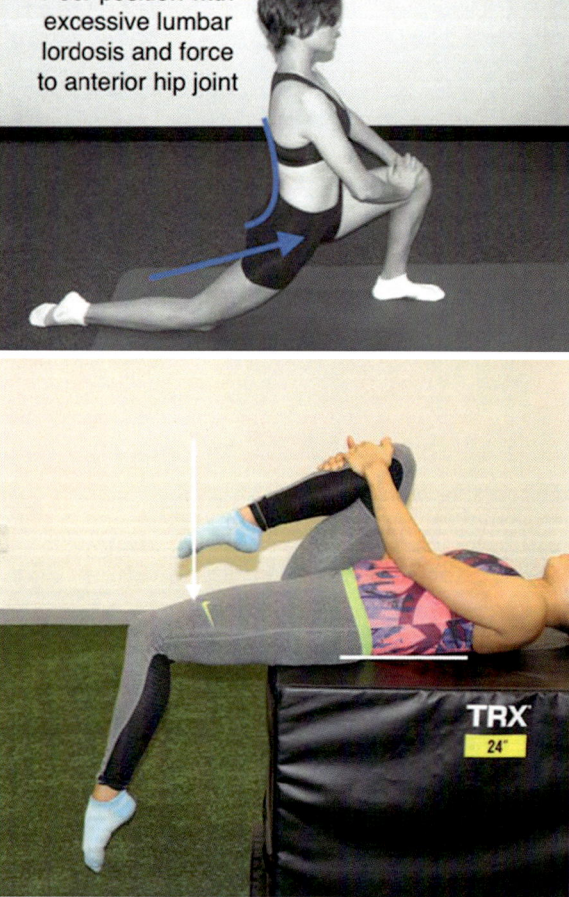

Fig. 11.18 Improper hip flexor stretching with increased lumbar lordosis versus proper position with lumbar spine neutral position

she will be ready to enter the last two phases of rehabilitation. At the hip, there are two key elements to address specific to preparing to return to gymnastics. The first is to provide specific exercises to address muscle performance at the very terminal degrees of motion, especially in hip extension and flexion positions (Fig. 11.19). Performance should be trained in both concentric and eccentric manners to provide necessary joint control and support in the positions required for many skills of the sport. The second element is to train hip muscles in conjunction with the lower trunk for both force production and power components of performance. Progressing from resistance applied at the pelvis to resistance applied at the arms facilitates progressive loading of segments to improve coordination and power of movement for the full body skills required by the sport of gymnastics. Figure 11.20 provides just a few examples of these concepts. These exercises should initially begin with muscle performance in mind, then move toward production of power through plyometric movements.

Fig. 11.19 Examples of hip muscle terminal motion training

Resisted hip abduction-extension in single limb stance

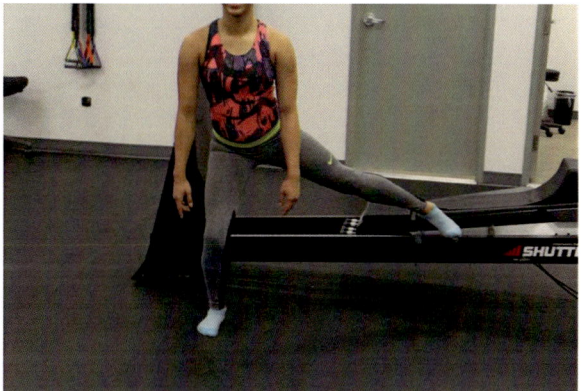

Hip extension in single limb stance

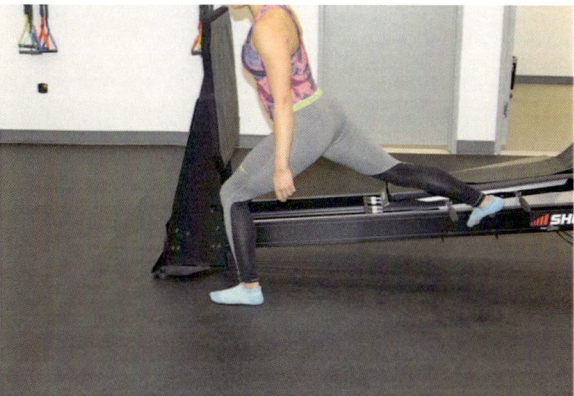

Fig. 11.19 (continued)

Hip flexor and abductor training through abduction motion

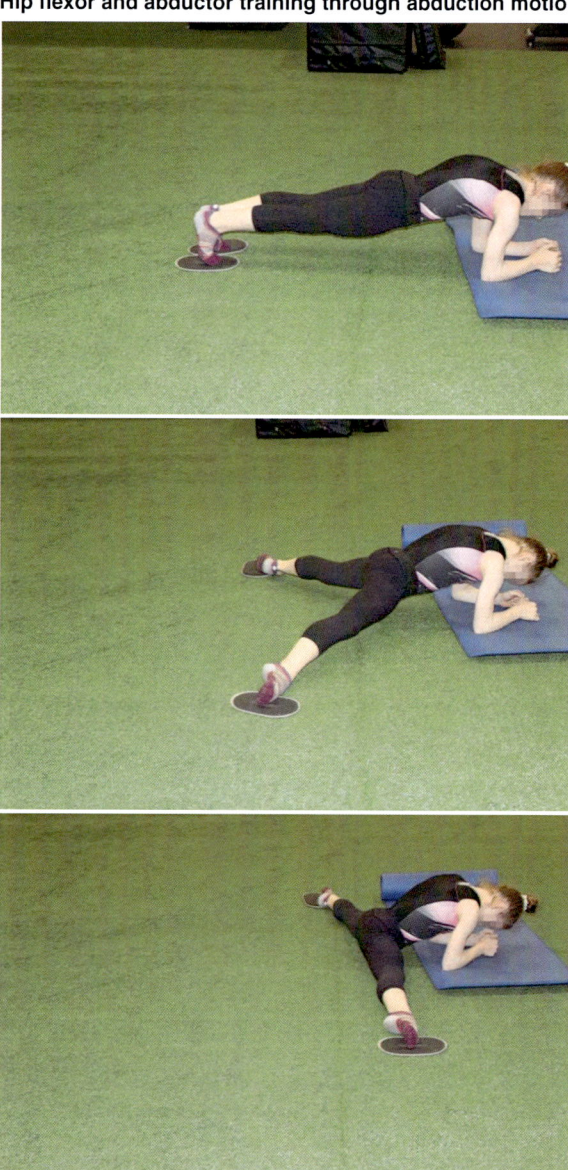

Fig. 11.19 (continued)

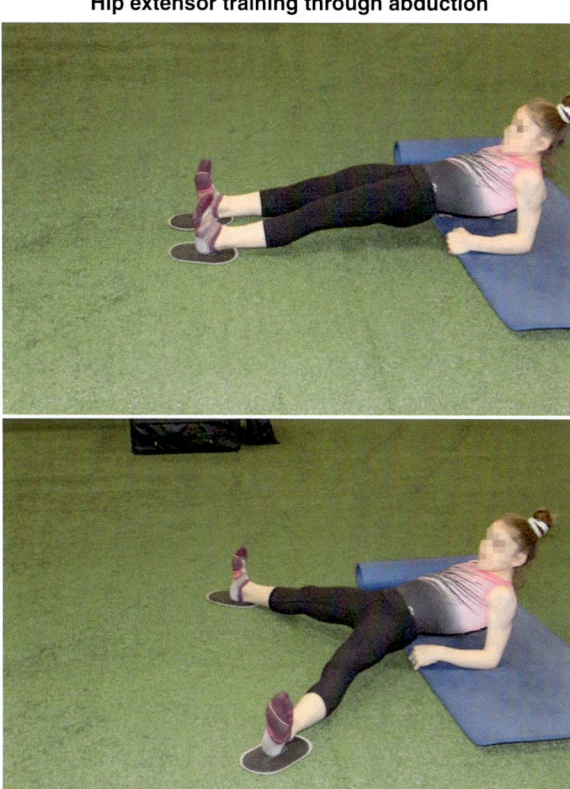

Hip extensor training through abduction

11.4.2 Rehabilitation Considerations for Injuries of the Knee

The knee is one of the most frequently injured joint regions in the body in gymnastics [3, 82]. Similar to other body parts discussed in this chapter, the approach to rehabilitation at the knee will be broken into categories. The first category will include ligamentous type injuries, including the anterior cruciate, posterior cruciate, medial collateral, and lateral collateral ligaments, as well as patellar instability injuries. The second category will focus on repetitive stress injuries including patellofemoral pain syndrome, patellar tendinopathy and iliotibial band compression syndrome. As previously noted, in the lower body, peak ground reaction forces have been recorded between 8.8 and 14.2 times body weight [8] and 15 times body weight in laboratory settings [9]. The knee is responsible for distributing a great

Fig. 11.20 Examples of lower extremity strengthening with associated trunk muscle activation

Single leg squat with rotational resistance

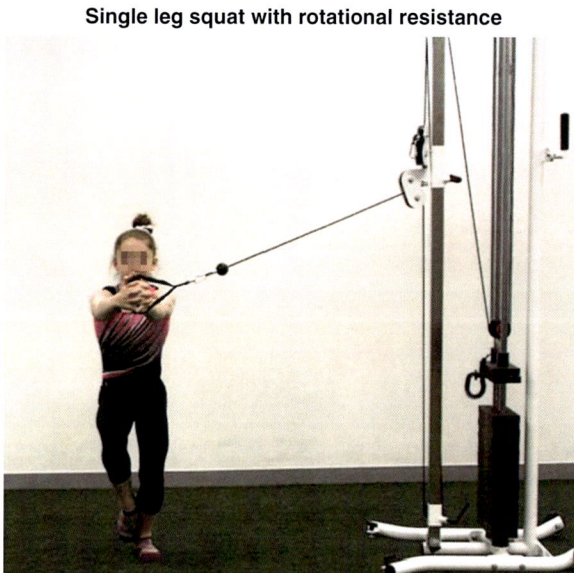

Single leg squat with lateral resistance

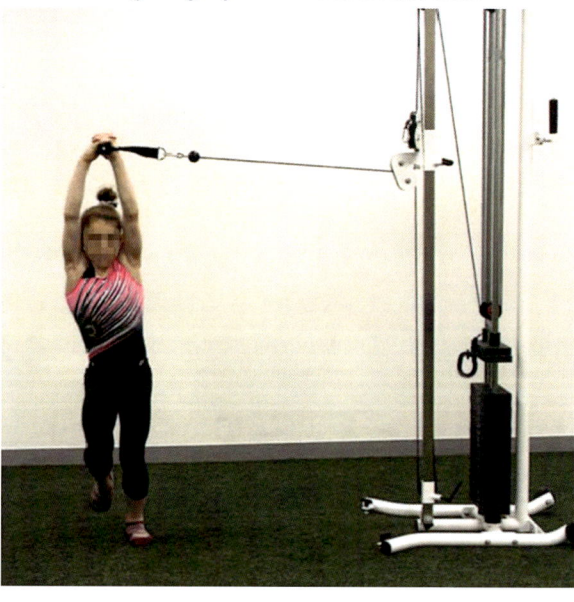

deal of this force. For both categories, the position of the knee during landing and in unilateral stance tasks is of utmost importance. Therefore, training the athlete to land with proper "soft landing" technique is a mainstay of treating all issues around the knee.

11.4.2.1 Ligamentous and Instability Injuries

Both anterior cruciate ligament (ACL) injury and patellar dislocation have been correlated to knee position at landing or planting the foot during pivoting movement [69–71, 77, 79, 107]. Specifically, a more "stiff knee" (less than 70° of knee flexion) and/or increased position of femoral internal rotation and adduction at peak loading has been linked to higher incidence of injury. As such, for all gymnasts that undergo rehabilitation for a ligamentous injury or patellar dislocation, whether surgical reconstruction/intervention was required or not, an emphasis on correct knee and trunk positions during landing and agility-based movements is absolutely essential. In addition, even up to 2 years after ACL reconstruction, individuals continue to exhibit motor control deficits and neuromuscular deficits which reinforces the need for continued training in this area [108, 109].

While it has not been specifically studied, similar deficits are likely to exist with other ligament injuries making it prudent to adopt strategies to train motor control and neuroplasticity during the course of rehabilitation [37, 110, 111]. A combination of neuromuscular training, balance task progression, and appropriate progression of foundational strengthening exercises that include proper trunk and hip positioning (e.g., squats, Bulgarian split squats, lunges in multiple planes, step up and retro step down, single leg squats) should be the basis for the intermediate portion of rehabilitation. A criteria-based progression as described in several sources is advocated [37, 112, 113].

In addition to these basic progressions, variation in visual input and perturbations to the trunk and lower limb should be integrated once the individual is proficient at the basic movements. Once the individual has gained 90% symmetry on functional assessments such as star excursion balance test (SEBT), single leg squat repetitions for time, and unilateral leg press 10 repetition max, ballistic and agility-based interventions can be initiated [114–117]. Once the proper landing mechanics and symmetry of movement have been attained in plyometric movements, another assessment should be completed.

Valid and reliable functional movement assessments such as the landing error scoring system (LESS), tuck jump assessment, and drop jump vertical assessment are advocated [11, 70, 116, 118–121]. These assessments could also be utilized in screening athletes that would benefit from interventions to improve landing mechanics in hopes to reduce injury risk potential. Once acceptable movement patterns are re-established for symmetry and proper landing position and limb position with agility maneuvers, training specific to gymnastics can be initiated. This would include variations of height, distance, and speed, and should include bilateral training in both narrow and medium base of support/foot placement position. In addition, unilateral power training should be included with an emphasis on control of joint position and trunk relative to the joint in order to attenuate forces during landing. Similar to the hip region, key components specific to gymnastics would include progressive training of unilateral rotational movements, dropping from height, and "blind" landing training in a controlled environment. A basic example would be having an athlete drop from an 18–24 inch height (plyo box or mats) with a 180° twist in the air. The gymnast should be able to control the landing, initially with landing on 2 feet followed by unilateral landing. As the athlete becomes more competent in attenuating forces in the lower extremity and controlling the trunk during these tasks, he/she can begin the return to sport progression as outlined in the following chapter.

11.4.2.2 Repetitive Tissue Stress Injuries at the Knee

When considering repetitive tissue stress injuries such as patellofemoral pain syndrome (PFPS), iliotibial band compression syndrome, patella tendon pathology, and pes anserine bursitis, reduction of tissue stress through modification of training parameters for both skill development and strength and conditioning is critical. In addition, research indicates that deficits in hip muscle performance, specifically femoral external rotators (ER), abductors and extensors, are associated with PFPS and other overuse injuries [67, 71, 122–124]. Both as a means to prevent onset of symptoms and in rehabilitation process, a series of exercises directed at improving force production and control of these muscle groups at the hip are fundamental. Some of the key exercises include unilateral bridge, side plank, resisted ER in side lying, resisted lateral walking, single leg dead lift/functional reach in multiple planes, single limb squat, crossover step up, squats with resistance against femoral external rotation, and "hip thrusters." These exercises have the highest muscle recruitment and are effective in reducing symptoms at the knee [97–101, 125]. In some cases, basic training of landing mechanics, as previously described, may be warranted; however, the volume of plyometric training should be monitored closely with repetitive tissue loading injuries. As with other injuries of this nature, progressive return to gymnastics training volume over the course of time will be central to successful return without recurrence of symptoms.

11.4.3 Rehabilitation Considerations for Lower Leg, Ankle, and Foot Injuries

The lower leg, ankle, and foot are very common areas of injury for the gymnast [3, 82, 126]. This is likely due to the extraordinarily high degree of forces put through this region of the body [7]. The management strategies previously described in regard to repetitive tissue stress injuries as well as the importance of proper landing mechanics also hold true for this region. In addition, biomechanical research indicates that stiffness, friction, and density of mats utilized in training can influence the amount of force experienced by this region. Therefore, patient education regarding use of mats to modify impact to the joints or surrounding muscles is important [127, 128].

11.4.3.1 Ligamentous Injury Considerations

Lateral ankle ligamentous injury, or lateral ankle instability, is common in many sports, including gymnastics [3, 46, 81, 82, 126, 129]. Research has revealed that lateral ankle injury and chronic instability are associated with proprioceptive deficits, postural stability deficits, and neuromuscular deficits [130, 131]. As such, specific foundational exercises to address each of these impairments are advocated in the early to intermediate stages of recovery [130, 132–134]. This is true for both nonoperative and postoperative rehabilitation, once joint motion is at least 80% with minimal effusion. Progression of static and dynamic balance tasks on stable and compliant surfaces with varied perturbation, compromised visual input, and dual-task activity are essential for all gymnasts with ankle instability [135, 136]. As the athlete transitions to the strength and conditioning stage of recovery, ankle-specific power and plyometric training would be essential. A suggested progression can be found in Table 11.5.

Before transitioning to gymnastics-specific training and the return to sport stage of rehabilitation, some functional assessment such as SEBT, 30 cm hop test, figure of

Table 11.5 Example of ankle-specific plyometric progression

	Plantarflexed position should be emphasized for all movements to use calf muscles for ballistic movement
Bilateral phase 1	Bilateral side to side 45° diagonal forward hops across a line Bilateral forward/backward 45° diagonal to the side hops across a line Hurdle or cone side to side hops Hurdle or cone forward back hops 90° progressing to 180° twist/turn with quick movement
Bilateral phase 2 (compliant surfaces)	Bilateral on/off of foam block/pad side to side and forward/backward Bilateral on/off foam block/pad with 90° or 180° twist in the air Bilateral over hurdle to landing on compliant surface side to side and forward back
Unilateral phase 1	Single leg side to side hops over line Single leg forward/backward hops over line Single leg triple hop to stick landing forward Single leg triple hop to stick landing lateral and medial 30 cm square drills with determined pattern
Unilateral phase 2 (compliant surfaces and cued direction change)	30 cm square drills with verbal cue to change direction (side to side, forward/backward, diagonal relative to square outlined on floor) Side to side on/off foam pad Forward/backward on/off foam pad On/off foam pad with 90° or 180° twist in air Progress to combining the above drills with one another, i.e., single leg hop over hurdle with twist in air to land on foam pad then hop forward with twist to the ground
Unilateral phase 2 – resistance/emphasis on power and speed	Same progression as per general lower extremity described in Table 11.3 just with ankle strategy emphasis

8 hop test, and single leg triple hop crossover for distance test should be performed. The athlete should be able to perform these tests within 90% of the contralateral limb [130, 133, 134, 137]. Once this has been achieved, high-level agility and plyometric tasks that mimic some of the demands of gymnastics should be incorporated including hops in all planes on and off varied surfaces with and without rotation as well as reactionary training. It is important to note that both maintenance proprioceptive/balance exercise and ankle bracing have proven to reduce the risk of lateral ankle sprain in many other sports [135, 136, 138]. Therefore, maintenance exercises and bracing may be recommended once the gymnast has returned to gymnastics. Although there is less research-based evidence regarding rehabilitation of other ligamentous injuries at the ankle, a similar method of rehabilitation is recommended.

11.4.3.2 Repetitive Tissue Stress Injuries

A variety of foot and ankle injuries have been associated with a lack of dorsiflexion range of motion secondary to gastrocnemius and soleus muscle tightness/shortness. Prevention and management of these injuries should include gastrocnemius- and soleus-specific flexibility testing and stretching as well as weight bearing assessment with goniometry or utilizing a weight bearing lunge measurement [133, 139]. When possible, reducing risk of injuries such as anterior talocrural impingement, posterior impingement, and Achilles tendinopathy through preventative screening and stretching is advocated. In addition to flexibility measures, full lower body strengthening programs with an emphasis on hip muscle performance can help to further attenuate forces away from the foot and ankle. Repetitive stress injuries such as OCDs, metatarsal stress fractures, and tibial stress fractures should be managed through modification of tissue loading, controlled progressive exposure of tissues to the necessary demands of the sport, and specific movement training for proper landing mechanics to better distribute forces throughout the body.

11.5 Rehabilitation Considerations for Lumbar Spine Injuries in Gymnastics

Next to the lower extremity, the spine is one of the most commonly injured sites in gymnastics [3]. This is largely due to extremely high forces being placed on the spine of a gymnast who is not yet fully matured. It is also due to the large range of forces gymnastics subjects the athlete's spine to, and the high workload of repetitions required to master and compete skills. Despite injuries occurring to the thoracic and cervical spine, the focus of this section will remain on the lumbar spine due to its high prevalence as a site of pain and pathology in gymnasts.

The average compressive forces at the thoracolumbar junction during landings have been recorded at 11.6 times body weight, while peak forces have reached 20 times body weight [1]. Forces during the takeoff phase of tumbling to the same area have been estimated at 6.5–8.5 times body weight (Fig. 11.21). Shearing forces at the L5/S1 disc have been recorded at 3.5 times body weight, while shearing load to the L5/S1 disc and pars interarticularis have been recorded at 2000 N [13]. Compression forces to the spine during horizontal bar giants have been measured at just below 4.5 times body weight and shearing forces of near 3.0 times body weight [1, 7].

It is worth noting that while these studies are extremely valuable to understanding the forces in gymnastics, there is no data on many of the highest force skills seen in gymnastics (e.g., floor skills with multiple flips or twists and the highest difficulty release skills on bars) The available studies also do not account for imperfect landing positions or falls that occur many times during the training week. Although more data is needed, it is likely that the most intense aspects of gymnastics would reveal even higher compressive and shearing forces to the spine of a gymnast. In addition, these forces are being placed on a gymnast's spine hundreds of times per month during training, depending on the competition level.

It is also critical to consider that in many cases a gymnast may not report their back pain due to the fear of being held out of training or competition, as well as the inherent culture of the sport that sometimes encourages expectation of working through early signs of injury. This creates an under representation of the severity of this issue within the sport [3]. When looking at surveys of former gymnasts, it is clear that many gymnasts suffer from back pain during and after their careers, with some studies reporting greater than 90% of elite-level gymnasts having had back pain [1, 3].

Fig. 11.21 Compression loading during tumbling takeoff

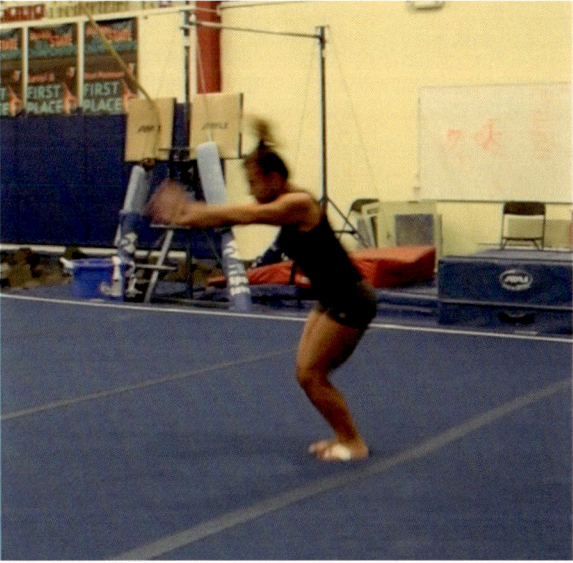

11.5.1 Skill Profiles for Accurate Diagnosis and Treatment Programs

As mentioned, the artistic gymnast's spine is subject to a large variety of movements and forces that are specific to the skills trained. While there is some variability in skill forces, it is not as much the case with other disciplines as trampoline and rhythmic gymnastics. This is referred to as a "skill profile" and it is essential to understand for successful diagnosis, treatment, and rehabilitation of spine injuries in this population. For example, gymnasts who are proficient at back bending (spine extension) type skills when younger may adopt more of an "extension"- based skill profile as they move to the higher levels of gymnastics. This may include back handspring-type movements on vault (Yurchenko entry), bars (Pac or Shaposhnikova release), beam (back handspring series or layout step-outs), and floor (back handspring entry to perform more advanced skills). Similarly, male gymnasts who demonstrate a natural propensity to extension skills may perform back handspring-type movements on floor (back handspring entry), rings (giant swings), vault (Yurchenko entry), parallel bars (Moy, Tipelt, or Bhavsar), and high bar ("Chinese" style dismount tap, Tkachev release). While at younger ages and lower levels this skill profile is much more consistent as the skills competed are part of set routines. This is a crucial piece to working with gymnasts who compete in optional levels that have much wider skill diversity.

The very nature of this skill profile will expose gymnasts to a significantly higher extension-based workload volume during training, which has been shown to be a main mechanism of common injuries in gymnastics [140, 141]. This repetitive extension may place excessive forces on the posterior elements of the spine including the facets, neural arch, and pars interarticularis [140, 142]. Repetitive movement under high load and volume predisposes this subset of athletes to extension-based spine pathology such as facet syndrome, spinous process impingement, and bone pathology such as stress reactions or spondylolisthesis [140, 141, 143]. When combined with twisting skills that also expose the spine to extension and rotation forces, pain and overuse injuries may quickly surface. Specific movement testing to bias these structures, such as the seated extension/compression test, prone extension and rotation overpressure test, and posterior to anterior (PA) shearing at individual levels in suspicion of pathology are warranted to confirm this diagnosis in conjunction with diagnostic imaging (Fig. 11.22).

This is in contrast to a young gymnast who does not possess a natural propensity to this extension-based movement, due to mobility, motor control, and/or strength-related factors. These gymnasts often gravitate to learning more flexion or impact-based skills on each event, creating a skill profile that exposes the spine to high compressive forces.

Building off the example above, female gymnasts who are naturally good at creating rotation in skills may learn higher compression force skills on vault (Tsukahara or front handspring entry), bars (toe-on or stalder skills), beam (salto-based series), and floor (double flipping skills). Male gymnasts may follow this trend learning

Fig. 11.22 Seated extension/compression, prone extension rotation, and PA shearing tests

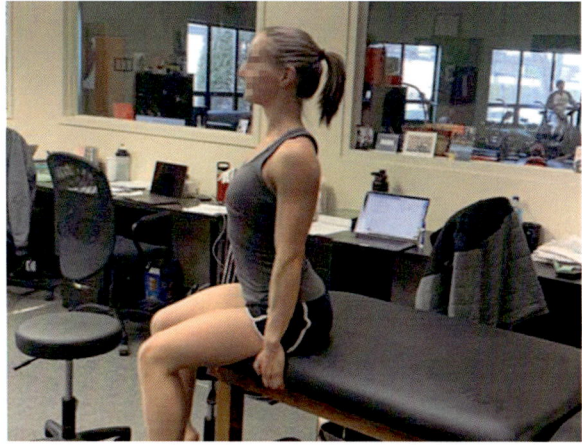
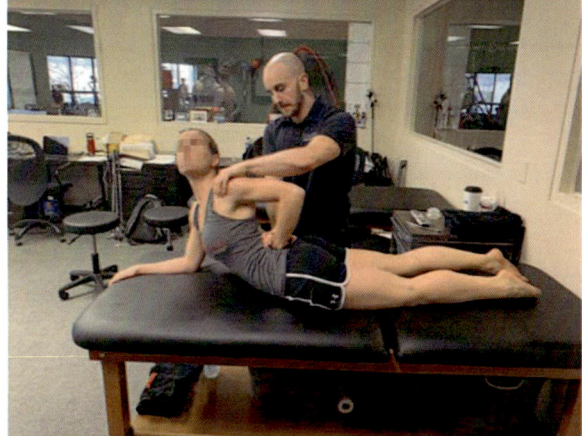
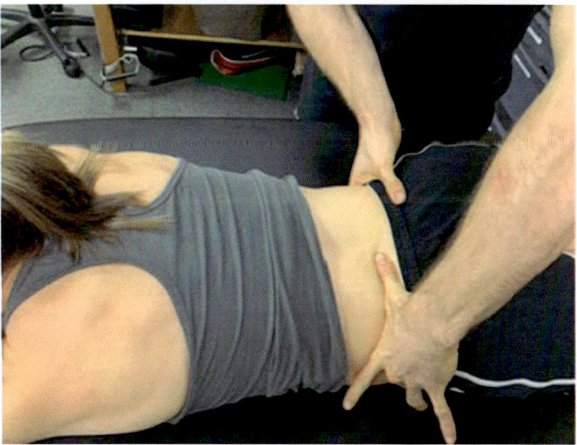

higher flexion or compression skills on floor (multiple flipping and twisting skills), rings (Yamawakis), vault (Tsukahara and Front handspring entry), parallel bars (peach basket-based skills), and high bar (in-bar stalders and "jam" based skills). These athletes are exposed to a high degree of flexion and compression movements. This may create a propensity to discogenic pathology, end-plate fractures, or spinal segmental nerve irritation, as repetitive flexion cycles or end-range flexion forces have been shown to stress these structures significantly [140, 142]. Clinicians should utilize a thorough history and quality physical examination for these injuries including seated compression/flexion tests, neural tension tests including passive straight leg raise (SLR), and contralateral straight leg raise test. Appropriate diagnostic imaging combined with clinical reasoning should be used to determine the category of movement that is most provocative and also is in line with pathological findings or skills that first created pain (Table 11.6).

11.5.2 General Spine Rehabilitation Based on Five-Stage Progression

During the acute and subacute phase of rehabilitation, the structures of the lumbar spine are typically extremely hypersensitized and possess a low tolerance to loading. Research indicates that the spine has considerable acute neurophysiological,

Table 11.6 Spine loading, pathology, and movement categories

Provoking movement	Provoking skills	Suspected structure involved	Suspected pathology	Screens/test
Flexion (Pike)	Tuck/pike flipping In bars	Muscular Discogenic Nerves	Strain/sprain Disc injury Adv. neural tension	MSF Rock back SLR + slump
Extension (Back bend)	BHS/FHS based skill Yurchenko	Facet Pars interarticularis Spinous process	Stress Rxn/Frx Spinous process Impingement	MSE Stork Press up PA shearing
Rotation (Turning)	Twisting	Muscle/ligament Facet	Strain/sprain Stress Rxn/Frx	MSR Prone stork PA shearing
Compression (Landing)	Dismounts Tumbling/VT impact	Muscle/ligament End plate (Above in combo)	End plate irritation Facet or disc (Above in combo)	Heel drop test Seated compression
Traction (Swinging)	Swinging Giants/release	Muscle/ligament (Above in combo)	Strain/sprain (Above in combo)	Prone traction

MSF multisegmental flexion, *SLR* straight leg raise, *Stress Rxn/Frx* stress reaction/fracture, *MSE* multisegmental extension, *PA* posterior-anterior, *MSR* multisegmental rotation biomechanical, and movement-based adaptive changes in response to nociception [144–146]. In an effort to reduce pain levels, reduce hypersensitivity, and restore normal amounts of movement variability in the beginning stages of spinal rehabilitation, clinicians are encouraged to use multiple tools based on what the literature suggests, what the patient expresses comfort with, and what will progress towards their goals. These could include pain science education, pathoanatomical education, loading modification, graded exercises, manual therapy, breathing exercises, biomechanical-based movement correction, and modalities.

Orthoric spinal bracing is sometimes recommended for extension-based injures, although conflict exists in the research on the best protocol for this intervention or whether there is any benefit to it [143]. The use, timeline, and type of brace are typically dictated by the medical doctor overseeing the patients case, and rehabilitation professionals are encouraged to defer to their individual guidelines. Regardless of the decision to use bracing or not, during the rehabilitation process, lower trunk muscle control and core training exercises typically begin in the "neutral" position. Gymnasts must be educated on proper neutral position muscle activation strategies that use diaphragmatic breathing as extensive research into spinal biomechanics has demonstrated dynamic stability is required to support the inherent passive stability of the spine [142, 147, 148].

Proper spine position is typically taught through exercise progressions specific to the gymnast such as hook-lying breathing progressions, quadruped reaching, supine alternating arm drops, modified side or front planking, and half kneeling band press outs. Following the clearance of restricted movement outside of neutral, gymnasts must be progressively exposed to higher degrees of muscle control and strength exercises (Table 11.7). The next progression remains in relative neutral spine with increasing demand of exercise through the use of crawling, adding manual rhythmic stabilizations to exercises noted above, and increasing the resistance through elastic, pulley or dumbbell loading.

As the gymnast begins to wean out of movement restrictions, it is imperative that the demand on the lower trunk and hip muscles to maintain dynamic bracing and spinal control in the presence of high forces is a main focus of exercise progressions. The integration of exercises that have high EMG activation of the gluteal muscles are combined with higher threshold trunk exercises that integrate movement of the extremities around the stable spine. Examples include side plank with clamshells using external resistance bands, side plank with leg abduction using external resistance bands, various single or double leg hip lift progressions, various single or double leg deadlift progressions, loaded squatting and lunging, loaded farmer or suitcase carries, sled pushing and pulling variations, chops and lifts, and basic medicine ball slam/throw drills (Fig. 11.23) [28, 101, 125, 145, 148, 149]. In addition, the introduction of resistance to trunk on pelvis motion with emphasis on spinal control during motions such as rotation, flexion/extension, and side bending, required by a variety of gymnastics skills, can be incorporated.

Table 11.7 Exercise progression example for spine extension pathology

Phase	Exercises
1	Hook lying breathing Quadruped reaching Supine alternating arm and leg drops Modified side and front planks Half kneeling band press outs
2	Bear crawling Supine wall press with leg lowers Side plank and front planks Split stance band press outs
3	Plank up downs Multidirectional bear crawl Side plank with clamshells and leg lifts Weighted step ups and single leg RDLs
4	Sled push, pull, and lateral drag Medball throws/slams Plank drag through Suitcase and farmer carries Lunging, squatting, step ups Kettlebell deadlifting
5	Broad and vertical jumps Sprinting drills Explosive medball work Gymnastics-specific drills

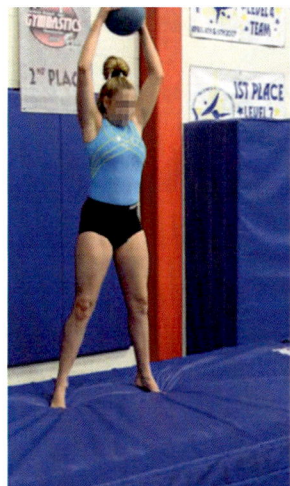 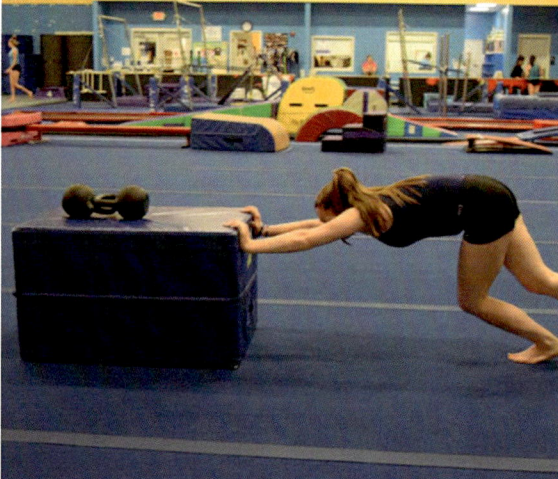

Fig. 11.23 Medicine ball slams and weighted sled push

These exercises progress naturally through the advanced and strength phases of spinal rehabilitation to restore the spine's tolerance to loading and capacity to produce, transfer, and absorb force. Examples include various high-threshold plank variations, more advanced medicine ball throws and slams, sled pushing or pulling variations, loaded carries, kettlebell swing progressions, rebounding and plyometric drills, and sprinting drills.

Regardless of the pathology or main movement pattern that generated pain, gymnasts must progress back through gymnastics-specific drills and skills. During this program, the gymnast can be taught to have global extension, flexion, and squatting patterns that reduce load on the spine during high force movements.

Typically, gymnastics-specific core training and skill basics start the return to sport progression, followed by the reintroduction of technical drills specific to gymnastics skills they train. This can be built into an objective workload program that prescribes specific numbers of spinal loading skills (impacts, compression, or extension skills) throughout the week, similar to throwing programs for baseball or running programs for field athletes. The surface of impacts, starting with foam pits or trampolines and progressing to hard floor, as well as the quantity can be manipulated over 4–6 weeks. It must be emphasized that a collaborative, interdisciplinary approach must be taken to this progression to ensure full and safe return to training.

11.5.3 Specific Spine Rehabilitation Based on Movement Category and Pathology

11.5.3.1 Extension and/or Rotation Pathologies

For injuries to the spine that are provoked during extension or rotations skills, it is important that the quantity and quality of motion at the shoulder, hip, and thoracic spine are evaluated. Gymnastics skills require an excessive amount of multisegmental extension throughout the body. If range of motion is not available at the shoulder, thoracic, and hip joints, it is common to see gymnasts make up for this motion with excessive lumbar extension motion. During the acute phase of rehabilitation when gymnasts have a low tolerance to exercise or loading, in-depth evaluations of overhead shoulder mobility, thoracic spine extension/rotation, and hip extension/rotation should be evaluated. This is best done through regular soft tissue care, specific stretching, and eccentric exercises, all of which have support in the literature for increasing range of motion [150–152].

As noted above, losses in motion often occur due to rapid growth spurts and through adaptive stiffness of musculature through repetitive training. Evaluating the gymnast's entire body and educating the athlete on the need to reduce load on the lumbar spine by using the entire kinetic chain will improve end-range rehab and return to sport progressions. This is best done through regular soft tissue care, specific stretching, and eccentric exercises, all of which have support in the literature for increasing range of motion [150–152]. If mobility in these areas is not found to be an issue, strength and motor control deficits should be addressed. This too can be addressed with specific strength and conditioning or home exercise programs.

It is also important that gymnasts are taught proper global extension patterns prior to the reintroduction of gymnastic-specific skill basics. This is best done through the use of tall kneeling multi-extension drills that emphasize the use of hip extension, thoracic extension, and overhead shoulder elevation as the main sites for movement while preventing excessive use of lumbar spine extension (Figs. 11.24 and 11.25). If it is found that excessive lumbar hyperextension is used during skill movements, most commonly seen at the thoracolumbar joint or lumbosacral joint, it is imperative this movement pattern be corrected and retaught prior to gymnastics skill exposure.

Basic motor control drills can be built into more dynamic exercises that focus on tolerating multisegmental eccentric spinal overload like standing medball slams, seated overhead medball throws, sprinting drills, and gymnastics-specific extension drills. It is also important that gymnasts learn jumping and landing mechanics using proper hip declaration, and do not use excessive lumbar extension during impact, as these have been sources of ongoing pain generation for gymnasts returning back to training.

Resisted trunk on pelvis flexion with rotation

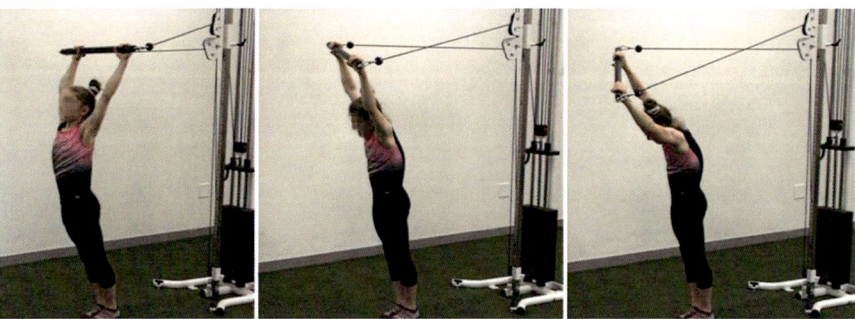

Trunk on pelvis side bend

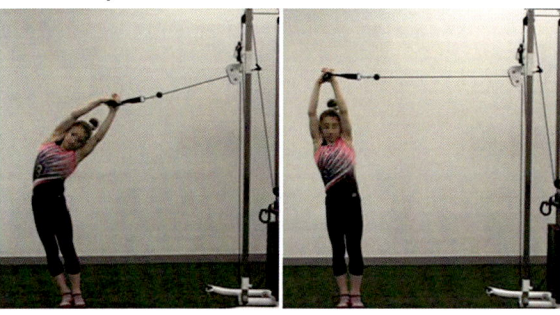

Fig. 11.24 Examples of trunk on pelvis motion for controlled spine motion

Fig. 11.25 Tall kneeling banded multisegmental extension drill

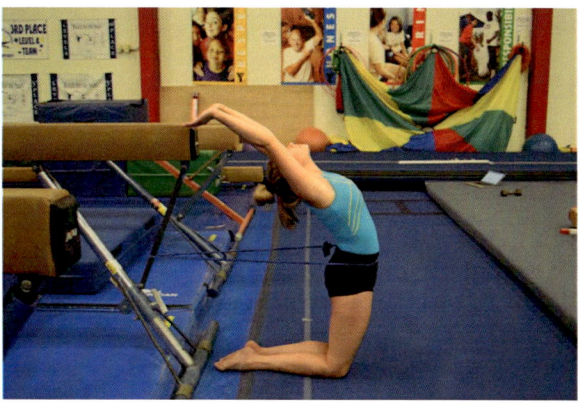

11.5.3.2 Flexion and/or Rotation Pathologies

With regard to flexion-based injuries, it is important to evaluate the mobility of the posterior chain as well as the upper body. Limitations in multisegmental flexion, either through protective guarding of the hamstring soft tissue or true bioplastic tissue stiffness, must be addressed to prevent lower back flexion reinjury. This is best done through daily self-soft tissue work (i.e., foam rolling), manual therapy, hamstring stretching that incorporates core control, eccentric exercises, and correction of excessive anterior pelvic tilt which may predispose neural tension in the posterior neural structures. Again, these methods are best supported in literature for increasing joint range of motion [151].

It is the authors' experience that adverse neural tension is another common complaint of gymnasts who must endure supraphysiologic ranges of motion during compression-based skills, stretching, or advanced jumps and leaps (Fig. 11.26). Athletes often report transient neurological symptoms within various dermatome patterns, which is thought to be a result of rapid eccentric stretching of posterior neural structures. The first line of defense of this is gymnast and coach education on the difference between moderate stretching discomfort and adverse responses of neurological symptoms such as paresthesias. Second, pending the athlete being cleared of all "sinister pathology" by a medical doctor, it is the authors' experience that soft tissue mobilizations and neural mobilizations in the forms of nerve glides can be beneficial for these challenging cases. Butler and Ellis describe specific exercise prescriptions related to this topic [114, 153].

11.5.3.3 Compression and Traction Pathologies

For compression-based mechanisms of pain provocation, gymnasts should be encouraged to land with proper deceleration-based landing mechanics [9, 10] and also given specific exercises that help build tolerance to compression forces on the spine. Examples may include loaded farmer or suitcase carries (Fig. 11.27), specific

Fig. 11.26 Switch leap

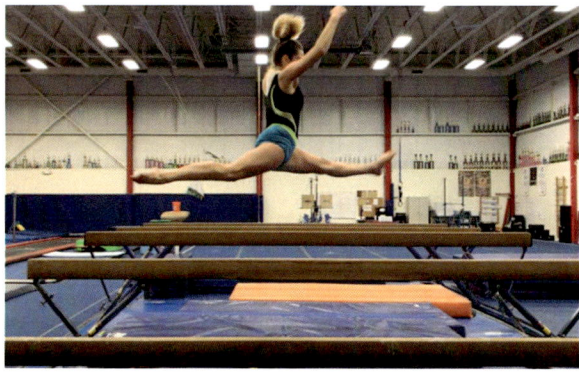

Fig. 11.27 Farmer carries

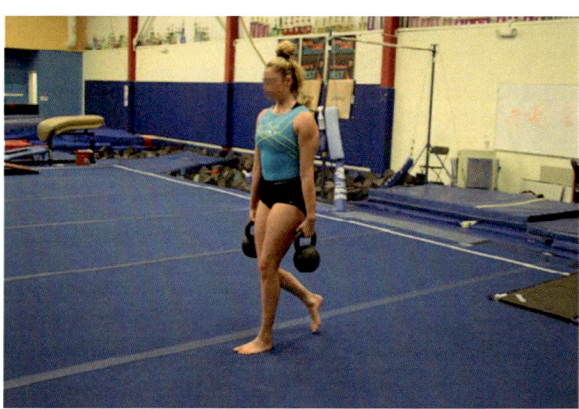

deadlifting or squatting variations that are appropriate for the athlete, and various sled pushing/pulling drills [148, 149]. During the reintroduction of compression based skills, specific exposure to impact from trampoline surfaces first, and with the use of padded landing cushions, is recommended.

Similar progressions may be done for traction intolerance through the use of hanging progressions, weighted pull-ups, and basic tap swing drills within the gymnastics arena. For both of these scenarios, gymnasts must specifically be taught to recruit their trunk muscles for global bracing with proper breathing mechanics during provocative skills.

Typically for traction forces, giant swings on high bar and rings are common generators of pain. For compression forces, dismount landings and bounding tumbling on floor are common generators of pain. Within the rehabilitation context, and also through communication to gymnastics coaches, the gymnast must be taught how to maintain dynamic stability of the trunk musculature through muscle activation and control to protect themselves from "buckling" during these skills.

As has already been outlined in other sections, the spine also must be exposed to a graded return of objective skill volume. The authors suggest that gymnasts are exposed to the least provocative movement categories first while continuing to regain gymnastics-specific strength, basic movements, drills, and impact tolerance. This is best done through modified impact surfaces such as softer mats or Tumbl Trak, by exposing the athlete to skill workload 3× per week with 24 hours in between sessions to monitor symptom responses, and also by working specific pieces of skill technique typically referred to as "drills" in the gymnastics training culture. Over the course of 4–8 weeks, the amount of force per skill, total skill workload, days per week of loading, impact surface, and difficulty of skills can be increased. This is continued until the most provocative skills (i.e., those that initially caused the injury) and highest training load is restored.

References

1. Caine DJ, Russell K, Lim L. Handbook of sports medicine and science: gymnastics. Oxford: Wiley-Blackwell; 2014.
2. Sweeney EA, Howell DR, James DA, Potter MN, Provance AJ. Returning to sport after gymnastics injuries. Curr Sports Med Rep. 2018;17(11):376–90.
3. Thomas RE, Thomas BC. A systematic review of injuries in gymnastics. Phys Sports Med. 2019;47(1):96–121.
4. Hart E, Meehan WP 3rd, Bae DS, d'Hemecourt P, Stracciolini A. The young injured gymnast: a literature review and discussion. Curr Sports Med Rep. 2018;17(11):366–75.
5. Penitente G, Sands WA. Exploratory investigation of impact loads during the forward handspring vault. J Hum Kinet. 2015;46:59–68.
6. Koh TJ, Grabiner MD, Weiker GG. Technique and ground reaction forces in the back handspring. Am J Sports Med. 1992;20(1):61–6.
7. Bruggemann GP. Mechanical load in artistic gymnastics and its relation to apparatus and performance. In: Leglise M, editor. Symposium medico-technique. Lyss: International Gymnastics Federation; 1999. p. 17–27.
8. Panzer V, Bates BT, Wood GA, Mason B. Lower extremity loads in landings of elite gymnasts International Society of Biomechanics. Amsterdam: Free University Press; 1988. p. 727–35.
9. McNitt-Gray JL, Yokoi T, Millward C. Landing strategy adjustments made by female gymnasts in response to drop height and mat composition. J Appl Biomech. 1993;9(3):173–90.
10. Ardern CL, Ekås GR, Grindem H, Moksnes H, Anderson AF, Chotel F, et al. 2018 International Olympic Committee consensus statement on prevention, diagnosis and management of paediatric anterior cruciate ligament (ACL) injuries. Br J Sports Med. 2018;52:422.
11. Hewett TE, Ford KR, Hoogenboom BJ, Myer GD. Understanding and preventing ACL injuries: current biomechanical and epidemiologic considerations—update 2010. N Am J Sports Phys Ther. 2010;5(4):234–51.
12. Nessler T, Denney L, Sampley J. ACL injury prevention: what does research tell us? Curr Rev Musculoskelet Med. 2017;10(3):281–8.
13. Jemni M. The science of gymnastics: advanced concepts, vol. 2018. 2nd ed. New York: Routledge; 2018. 380 p.
14. DiFiori JP, Benjamin HJ, Brenner J, Gregory A, Jayanthi N, Landry GL, et al. Overuse injuries and burnout in youth sports: a position statement from the American Medical Society for Sports Medicine. Clin J Sport Med. 2014;24(1):3–20.

15. Feeley BT, Agel J, LaPrade RF. When is it too early for single sport specialization? Am J Sports Med. 2016;44(1):234–41.
16. Kellmann M. Preventing overtraining in athletes in high-intensity sports and stress/recovery monitoring. Scand J Med Sci Sports. 2010;20 Suppl 2:95–102.
17. Soligard T, Schwellnus M, Alonso JM, Bahr R, Clarsen B, Dijkstra HP, et al. How much is too much? (part 1) International Olympic Committee consensus statement on load in sport and risk of injury. Br J Sports Med. 2016;50(17):1030–41.
18. Faigenbaum AD, Kraemer WJ, Blimkie CJ, Jeffreys I, Micheli LJ, Nitka M, et al. Youth resistance training: updated position statement paper from the national strength and conditioning association. J Strength Cond Res. 2009;23(5 Suppl):S60–79.
19. Lloyd RS, Faigenbaum AD, Stone MH, Oliver JL, Jeffreys I, Moody JA, et al. Position statement on youth resistance training: the 2014 international consensus. Br J Sports Med. 2014;48(7):498–505.
20. Bourdon PC, Cardinale M, Murray A, Gastin P, Kellmann M, Varley MC, et al. Monitoring athlete training loads: consensus statement. Int J Sports Physiol Perform. 2017;12(Suppl 2):S2161–s70.
21. Gabbett TJ. The training—injury prevention paradox: should athletes be training smarter and harder? Br J Sports Med. 2016;50(5):273–80.
22. Arnold A, Thigpen CA, Beattie PF, Kissenberth MJ, Shanley E. Overuse physeal injuries in youth athletes. Sports Health. 2017;9(2):139–47.
23. Gabbett TJ. Reductions in pre-season training loads reduce training injury rates in rugby league players. Br J Sports Med. 2004;38(6):743.
24. Malone S, Owen A, Newton M, Mendes B, Collins KD, Gabbett TJ. The acute:chonic workload ratio in relation to injury risk in professional soccer. J Sci Med Sport. 2017;20(6):561–5.
25. Timoteo TF, Debien PB, Miloski B, Werneck FZ, Gabbett T, Bara Filho MG. Influence of workload and recovery on injuries in elite male volleyball players. J Strength Cond Res. 2018; https://doi.org/10.1519/JSC.0000000000002754.
26. Murray NB, Gabbett TJ, Townshend AD, Blanch P. Calculating acute:chronic workload ratios using exponentially weighted moving averages provides a more sensitive indicator of injury likelihood than rolling averages. Br J Sports Med. 2017;51(9):749–54.
27. Bompa TO, Haff GG. Periodization: theory and methodology of training. Champaign: Human Kinetics; 1999.
28. Lorenz D, Morrison S. Current concepts in periodization of strength and conditioning for the sports physical therapist. Int J Sports Phys Ther. 2015;10(6):734–47.
29. Gabbett T. Workload monitoring and athlete management. In: Turner A, Comfort P, editors. Advanced strength and conditioning: an evidence based approach. New York: Routledge; 2018. p. 137–50.
30. Blanch P, Gabbett TJ. Has the athlete trained enough to return to play safely? The acute:chronic workload ratio permits clinicians to quantify a player's risk of subsequent injury. Br J Sports Med. 2016;50(8):471–5.
31. McEwen BS. In pursuit of resilience: stress, epigenetics, and brain plasticity. Ann N Y Acad Sci. 2016;1373(1):56–64.
32. Hulin B, Gabbett T, Blanch P, Chapman P, Bailey D, Orchard JW. Spikes in acute workload are associated with increased injury risk in elite cricket fast bowlers. Br J Sports Med. 2014;48:675–6.
33. Condon EM. Chronic stress in children and adolescents: a review of biomarkers for use in pediatric research. Biol Res Nurs. 2018;20(5):473–96.
34. Dijkstra HP, Pollock N, Chakraverty R, Alonso JM. Managing the health of the elite athlete: a new integrated performance health management and coaching model. Br J Sports Med. 2014;48(7):523.
35. Ekstrand J, Lundqvist D, Lagerbäck L, Vouillamoz M, Papadimitiou N, Karlsson J. Is there a correlation between coaches' leadership styles and injuries in elite football teams? A study of 36 elite teams in 17 countries. Br J Sports Med. 2018;52(8):527.

36. Reinold MM, Curtis AS. Microinstability of the shoulder in the overhead athlete. Int J Sports Phys Ther. 2013;8(5):601–16.
37. Wilk KE, Macrina LC, Cain EL, Dugas JR, Andrews JR. Recent advances in the rehabilitation of anterior cruciate ligament injuries. J Orthop Sports Phys Ther. 2012;42(3):153–71.
38. Ellenbecker TS, Wilk KE, Altchek DW, Andrews JR. Current concepts in rehabilitation following ulnar collateral ligament reconstruction. Sports Health. 2009;1(4):301–13.
39. Humphrey JD, Dufresne ER, Schwartz MA. Mechanotransduction and extracellular matrix homeostasis. Nat Rev Mol Cell Biol. 2014;15(12):802–12.
40. Khan KM, Scott A. Mechanotherapy: how physical therapists' prescription of exercise promotes tissue repair. Br J Sports Med. 2009;43(4):247.
41. Wang N. Review of cellular mechanotransduction. J Phys D Appl Phys. 2017;50(23):233002.
42. Warden SJ, Thompson WR. Become one with the force: optimising mechanotherapy through an understanding of mechanobiology. Br J Sports Med. 2017;51(13):989.
43. Wippert P-M, Rector M, Kuhn G, Wuertz-Kozak K. Stress and alterations in bones: an interdisciplinary perspective. Front Endocrinol. 2017;8:96.
44. Latash ML. Movements that are both variable and optimal. J Hum Kinet. 2012;34:5–13.
45. Hinds N, Angioi M, Birn-Jeffery A, Twycross-Lewis R. A systematic review of shoulder injury prevalence, proportion, rate, type, onset, severity, mechanism and risk factors in female artistic gymnasts. Phys Ther Sport. 2018;35:106–15.
46. Saluan P, Styron J, Ackley JF, Prinzbach A, Billow D. Injury types and incidence rates in precollegiate female gymnasts. Orthop J Sports Med. 2015;3(4):2325967115577596.
47. Reinold MM, Gill TJ, Wilk KE, Andrews JR. Current concepts in the evaluation and treatment of the shoulder in overhead throwing athletes, part 2: injury prevention and treatment. Sports Health. 2010;2(2):101–15.
48. Wilk KE, Reinold MM, Andrews JR. The athlete's shoulder. 2nd ed. Philadelphia: Churchill Livingstone; 2009. 876 p.
49. Wilk KE, Macrina LC. Nonoperative and postoperative rehabilitation for glenohumeral instability. Clin Sports Med. 2013;32(4):865–914.
50. Gadomski SJ, Ratamess NA, Cutrufello PT. Range of motion adaptations in powerlifters. J Strength Cond Res. 2018;32:3020.
51. Reinold MM, Wilk KE, Macrina LC, Sheheane C, Dun S, Fleisig GS, et al. Changes in shoulder and elbow passive range of motion after pitching in professional baseball players. Am J Sports Med. 2008;36(3):523–7.
52. Paine R, Voight ML. The role of the scapula. Int J Sports Phys Ther. 2013;8(5):617–29.
53. Reinold MM, Escamilla RF, Wilk KE. Current concepts in the scientific and clinical rationale behind exercises for glenohumeral and scapulothoracic musculature. J Orthop Sports Phys Ther. 2009;39(2):105–17.
54. Reinold MM, Macrina LC, Wilk KE, Fleisig GS, Dun S, Barrentine SW, et al. Electromyographic analysis of the supraspinatus and deltoid muscles during 3 common rehabilitation exercises. J Athl Train. 2007;42(4):464–9.
55. Andersen CH, Zebis MK, Saervoll C, Sundstrup E, Jakobsen MD, Sjogaard G, et al. Scapular muscle activity from selected strengthening exercises performed at low and high intensities. J Strength Cond Res. 2012;26(9):2408–16.
56. Reinold MM, Wilk KE, Reed J, Crenshaw K, Andrews JR. Interval sport programs: guidelines for baseball, tennis, and golf. J Orthop Sports Phys Ther. 2002;32(6):293–8.
57. Sgroi TA, Zajac JM. Return to throwing after shoulder or elbow injury. Curr Rev Musculoskelet Med. 2018;11(1):12–8.
58. Nielsen RO, Parner ET, Nohr EA, Sorensen H, Lind M, Rasmussen S. Excessive progression in weekly running distance and risk of running-related injuries: an association which varies according to type of injury. J Orthop Sports Phys Ther. 2014;44(10):739–47.
59. Churchill RW, Munoz J, Ahmad CS. Osteochondritis dissecans of the elbow. Curr Rev Musculoskelet Med. 2016;9(2):232–9.
60. Wu M, Eisenberg K, Williams K, Bae DS. Radial head changes in osteochondritis dissecans of the humeral capitellum. Orthop J Sports Med. 2018;6(4):2325967118769059.

61. Kajiyama S, Muroi S, Sugaya H, Takahashi N, Matsuki K, Kawai N, et al. Osteochondritis dissecans of the humeral capitellum in young athletes: comparison between baseball players and gymnasts. Orthop J Sports Med. 2017;5(3):2325967117692513.
62. Farana R, Jandacka D, Irwin G. Influence of different hand positions on impact forces and elbow loading during the round off in gymnastics: a case study. Sci Gymnast J. 2013;5(2):5–14.
63. Wilk KE, Macrina LC, Cain EL, Dugas JR, Andrews JR. Rehabilitation of the overhead athlete's elbow. Sports Health. 2012;4(5):404–14.
64. DiFiori JP, Caine DJ, Malina RM. Wrist pain, distal radial physeal injury, and ulnar variance in the young gymnast. Am J Sports Med. 2006;34(5):840–9.
65. Benjamin HJ, Engel SC, Chudzik D. Wrist pain in gymnasts: a review of common overuse wrist pathology in the gymnastics athlete. Curr Sports Med Rep. 2017;16(5):322–9.
66. Webb BG, Rettig LA. Gymnastic wrist injuries. Curr Sports Med Rep. 2008;7(5):289–95.
67. McLaren K, Byrd E, Herzog M, Polikandriotis JA, Willimon SC. Impact shoulder angles correlate with impact wrist angles in standing back handsprings in preadolescent and adolescent female gymnasts. Int J Sports Phys Ther. 2015;10(3):341–6.
68. de Oliveira VMA, Pitangui ACR, Nascimento VYS, da Silva HA, Dos Passos MHP, de Araújo RC. Test-retest reliability of the Closed Kinetic Chain Upper Extremity Stability Test (CKCUEST) in adolescents: reliability of CKCUEST in adolescents. Int J Sports Phys Ther. 2017;12(1):125–32.
69. Paterno MV, Schmitt LC, Ford KR, Rauh MJ, Myer GD, Huang B, et al. Biomechanical measures during landing and postural stability predict second anterior cruciate ligament injury after anterior cruciate ligament reconstruction and return to sport. Am J Sports Med. 2010;38(10):1968–78.
70. Paterno MV, Rauh MJ, Schmitt LC, Ford KR, Hewett TE. Incidence of second ACL injuries 2 years after primary ACL reconstruction and return to sport. Am J Sports Med. 2014;42(7):1567–73.
71. Boling MC, Padua DA, Marshall SW, Guskiewicz K, Pyne S, Beutler A. A prospective investigation of biomechanical risk factors for patellofemoral pain syndrome: the Joint Undertaking to Monitor and Prevent ACL Injury (JUMP-ACL) cohort. Am J Sports Med. 2009;37(11):2108–16.
72. Bradshaw EJ, Hume PA. Biomechanical approaches to identify and quantify injury mechanisms and risk factors in women's artistic gymnastics. Sports Biomech. 2012;11(3):324–41.
73. d'Hemecourt PA, Luke A. Sport-specific biomechanics of spinal injuries in aesthetic athletes (dancers, gymnasts, and figure skaters). Clin Sports Med. 2012;31(3):397–408.
74. Gittoes MJR, Irwin G. Biomechanical approaches to understanding the potentially injurious demands of gymnastic-style impact landings. Sports Med Arthrosc Rehabil Ther Technol. 2012;4(1):4.
75. Mills C, Pain MT, Yeadon MR. Reducing ground reaction forces in gymnastics' landings may increase internal loading. J Biomech. 2009;42(6):671–8.
76. Slater A, Campbell A, Smith A, Straker L. Greater lower limb flexion in gymnastic landings is associated with reduced landing force: a repeated measures study. Sports Biomech. 2015;14(1):45–56.
77. Padua DA, Distefano LJ. Sagittal plane knee biomechanics and vertical ground reaction forces are modified following ACL injury prevention programs: a systematic review. Sports Health. 2009;1(2):165–73.
78. Alentorn-Geli E, Myer GD, Silvers HJ, Samitier G, Romero D, Lazaro-Haro C, et al. Prevention of non-contact anterior cruciate ligament injuries in soccer players. Part 1: mechanisms of injury and underlying risk factors. Knee Surg Sports Traumatol Arthrosc. 2009;17(7):705–29.
79. Silvers HJ, Mandelbaum BR. Prevention of anterior cruciate ligament injury in the female athlete. Br J Sports Med. 2007;41(Suppl 1):i52–9.
80. Longo UG, Ciuffreda M, Locher J, Maffulli N, Denaro V. Apophyseal injuries in children's and youth sports. Br Med Bull. 2016;120(1):139–59.

81. Tirabassi J, Brou L, Khodaee M, Lefort R, Fields SK, Comstock RD. Epidemiology of high school sports-related injuries resulting in medical disqualification: 2005–2006 through 2013–2014 academic years. Am J Sports Med. 2016;44(11):2925–32.
82. Westermann RW, Giblin M, Vaske A, Grosso K, Wolf BR. Evaluation of men's and women's gymnastics injuries: a 10-year observational study. Sports Health. 2015;7(2):161–5.
83. Schiller J, DeFroda S, Blood T. Lower extremity avulsion fractures in the pediatric and adolescent athlete. J Am Acad Orthop Surg. 2017;25(4):251–9.
84. Safran MR. Microinstability of the hip-gaining acceptance. J Am Acad Orthop Surg. 2019;27(1):12–22.
85. Nho SJ, Lunig M, Larson CM, Bedi A, Kellly BT. Hip arthroscopy and hip joint preservation surgery, vol. 1. New York: Springer; 2015.
86. Kalisvaart MM, Safran MR. Microinstability of the hip-it does exist: etiology, diagnosis and treatment. J Hip Preserv Surg. 2015;2(2):123–35.
87. Cianci A, Sugimoto D, Stracciolini A, Yen YM, Kocher MS, d'Hemecourt PA. Nonoperative management of labral tears of the hip in adolescent athletes: description of sports participation, interventions, comorbidity, and outcomes. Clin J Sport Med. 2019;29(1):24–8.
88. Weber AE, Bedi A, Tibor LM, Zaltz I, Larson CM. The hyperflexible hip: managing hip pain in the dancer and gymnast. Sports Health. 2015;7(4):346–58.
89. Amanatullah DF, Antkowiak T, Pillay K, Patel J, Refaat M, Toupadakis CA, et al. Femoroacetabular impingement: current concepts in diagnosis and treatment. Orthopedics. 2015;38(3):185–99.
90. Bolia I, Utsunomiya H, Locks R, Briggs K, Philippon MJ. Twenty-year systematic review of the hip pathology, risk factors, treatment, and clinical outcomes in artistic athletes-dancers, figure skaters, and gymnasts. Clin J Sport Med. 2018;28(1):82–90.
91. Wall PD, Dickenson EJ, Robinson D, Hughes I, Realpe A, Hobson R, et al. Personalised hip therapy: development of a non-operative protocol to treat femoroacetabular impingement syndrome in the FASHIoN randomised controlled trial. Br J Sports Med. 2016;50(19):1217–23.
92. Lee AJ, Armour P, Thind D, Coates MH, Kang AC. The prevalence of acetabular labral tears and associated pathology in a young asymptomatic population. Bone Joint J. 2015;97–B(5):623–7.
93. Schmitz MR, Campbell SE, Fajardo RS, Kadrmas WR. Identification of acetabular labral pathological changes in asymptomatic volunteers using optimized, noncontrast 1.5-T magnetic resonance imaging. Am J Sports Med. 2012;40(6):1337–41.
94. Tresch F, Dietrich TJ, Pfirrmann CWA, Sutter R. Hip MRI: prevalence of articular cartilage defects and labral tears in asymptomatic volunteers. A comparison with a matched population of patients with femoroacetabular impingement. J Magn Reson Imaging. 2017;46(2):440–51.
95. Georgiadis AG, Seeley MA, Chauvin NA, Sankar WN. Prevalence of acetabular labral tears in asymptomatic children. J Child Orthop. 2016;10(2):149–54.
96. Herickhoff PK, Safran MR. Surgical decision making for acetabular labral tears: an international perspective. Orthop J Sports Med. 2018;6(9):2325967118797324.
97. Distefano LJ, Blackburn JT, Marshall SW, Padua DA. Gluteal muscle activation during common therapeutic exercises. J Orthop Sports Phys Ther. 2009;39(7):532–40.
98. Dolak KL, Silkman C, Medina McKeon J, Hosey RG, Lattermann C, Uhl TL. Hip strengthening prior to functional exercises reduces pain sooner than quadriceps strengthening in females with patellofemoral pain syndrome: a randomized clinical trial. J Orthop Sports Phys Ther. 2011;41(8):560–70.
99. Philippon MJ, Decker MJ, Giphart JE, Torry MR, Wahoff MS, LaPrade RF. Rehabilitation exercise progression for the gluteus medius muscle with consideration for iliopsoas tendinitis: an in vivo electromyography study. Am J Sports Med. 2011;39(8):1777–85.
100. Reiman MP, Bolgla LA, Loudon JK. A literature review of studies evaluating gluteus maximus and gluteus medius activation during rehabilitation exercises. Physiother Theory Pract. 2012;28(4):257–68.
101. Selkowitz DM, Beneck GJ, Powers CM. Which exercises target the gluteal muscles while minimizing activation of the tensor fascia lata? Electromyographic assessment using fine-wire electrodes. J Orthop Sports Phys Ther. 2013;43(2):54–64.

102. Heerey J, Risberg MA, Magnus J, Moksnes H, Odegaard T, Crossley K, et al. Impairment-based rehabilitation following HIP arthroscopy: postoperative protocol for the HIP arthroscopy international randomized controlled trial. J Orthop Sports Phys Ther. 2018;48(4):336–42.
103. Wahoff M, Dischiavi S, Hodge J, Pharez JD. Rehabilitation after labral repair and femoroacetabular decompression: criteria-based progression through the return to sport phase. Int J Sports Phys Ther. 2014;9(6):813–26.
104. Nakano N, Yip G, Khanduja V. Current concepts in the diagnosis and management of extra-articular hip impingement syndromes. Int Orthop. 2017;41(7):1321–8.
105. Dangin A, Tardy N, Wettstein M, May O, Bonin N. Microinstability of the hip: a review. Orthop Traumatol Surg Res. 2016;102(8S):S301–S9.
106. McNeill W, Scott S. Treatment of hip microinstability and gluteal tendinopathies involves movement control and exercise. J Bodyw Mov Ther. 2016;20(3):588–94.
107. Lewallen LW, McIntosh AL, Dahm DL. Predictors of recurrent instability after acute patellofemoral dislocation in pediatric and adolescent patients. Am J Sports Med. 2013;41(3):575–81.
108. Johnston PT, McClelland JA, Webster KE. Lower limb biomechanics during single-leg landings following anterior cruciate ligament reconstruction: a systematic review and meta-analysis. Sports Med. 2018;48(9):2103–26.
109. Mueske NM, Patel AR, Pace JL, Zaslow TL, VandenBerg CD, Katzel MJ, Edison BR, Wren TAL. Improvements in landing biomechanics following anterior cruciate ligament reconstruction in adolescent athletes. Sports Biomechanics. 2018; https://doi.org/10.1080/14763141.2018.1510539.
110. Gokeler A, Benjaminse A, Hewett TE, Paterno MV, Ford KR, Otten E, et al. Feedback techniques to target functional deficits following anterior cruciate ligament reconstruction: implications for motor control and reduction of second injury risk. Sports Med. 2013;43(11):1065–74.
111. Grooms D, Appelbaum G, Onate J. Neuroplasticity following anterior cruciate ligament injury: a framework for visual-motor training approaches in rehabilitation. J Orthop Sports Phys Ther. 2015;45(5):381–93.
112. Adams D, Logerstedt DS, Hunter-Giordano A, Axe MJ, Snyder-Mackler L. Current concepts for anterior cruciate ligament reconstruction: a criterion-based rehabilitation progression. J Orthop Sports Phys Ther. 2012;42(7):601–14.
113. Myer GD, Paterno MV, Ford KR, Quatman CE, Hewett TE. Rehabilitation after anterior cruciate ligament reconstruction: criteria-based progression through the return-to-sport phase. J Orthop Sports Phys Ther. 2006;36(6):385–402.
114. Ellis RF, Hing WA. Neural mobilization: a systematic review of randomized controlled trials with an analysis of therapeutic efficacy. J Man Manip Ther. 2008;16(1):8–22.
115. Barber-Westin SD, Noyes FR. Factors used to determine return to unrestricted sports activities after anterior cruciate ligament reconstruction. Arthroscopy. 2011;27(12):1697–705.
116. Kong DH, Yang SJ, Ha JK, Jang SH, Seo JG, Kim JG. Validation of functional performance tests after anterior cruciate ligament reconstruction. Knee Surg Relat Res. 2012;24(1):40–5.
117. Munro AG, Herrington LC. Between-session reliability of the star excursion balance test. Phys Ther Sport. 2010;11(4):128–32.
118. Narducci E, Waltz A, Gorski K, Leppla L, Donaldson M. The clinical utility of functional performance tests within one-year post-acl reconstruction: a systematic review. Int J Sports Phys Ther. 2011;6(4):333–42.
119. Fox AS, Bonacci J, McLean SG, Spittle M, Saunders N. A systematic evaluation of field-based screening methods for the assessment of anterior cruciate ligament (ACL) injury risk. Sports Med. 2016;46(5):715–35.
120. Kyritsis P, Bahr R, Landreau P, Miladi R, Witvrouw E. Likelihood of ACL graft rupture: not meeting six clinical discharge criteria before return to sport is associated with a four times greater risk of rupture. Br J Sports Med. 2016;50(15):946–51.
121. Padua DA, Marshall SW, Boling MC, Thigpen CA, Garrett WE Jr, Beutler AI. The Landing Error Scoring System (LESS) is a valid and reliable clinical assessment tool of jump-landing biomechanics: the JUMP-ACL study. Am J Sports Med. 2009;37(10):1996–2002.

122. Tyler TF, Nicholas SJ, Mullaney MJ, McHugh MP. The role of hip muscle function in the treatment of patellofemoral pain syndrome. Am J Sports Med. 2006;34(4):630–6.
123. Post WR, Dye SF. Patellofemoral pain: an enigma explained by homeostasis and common sense. Am J Orthop (Belle Mead NJ). 2017;46(2):92–100.
124. Collado H, Fredericson M. Patellofemoral pain syndrome. Clin Sports Med. 2010;29(3):379–98.
125. Andersen V, Fimland MS, Mo D-A, Iversen VM, Vederhus T, Rockland Hellebø LR, et al. Electromyographic comparison of barbell deadlift, hex bar deadlift, and hip thrust exercises: a cross-over study. J Strength Cond Res. 2018;32(3):587–93.
126. Chilvers M, Donahue M, Nassar L, Manoli A 2nd. Foot and ankle injuries in elite female gymnasts. Foot Ankle Int. 2007;28(2):214–8.
127. Mills C, Yeadon MR, Pain MT. Modifying landing mat material properties may decrease peak contact forces but increase forefoot forces in gymnastics landings. Sports Biomech. 2010;9(3):153–64.
128. Xiao X, Hao W, Li X, Wan B, Shan G. The influence of landing mat composition on ankle injury risk during a gymnastic landing: a biomechanical quantification. Acta Bioeng Biomech. 2017;19(1):105–13.
129. Kay MC, Register-Mihalik JK, Gray AD, Djoko A, Dompier TP, Kerr ZY. The epidemiology of severe injuries sustained by National Collegiate Athletic Association Student-Athletes, 2009–2010 through 2014–2015. J Athl Train. 2017;52(2):117–28.
130. McCriskin BJ, Cameron KL, Orr JD, Waterman BR. Management and prevention of acute and chronic lateral ankle instability in athletic patient populations. World J Orthop. 2015;6(2):161–71.
131. Simpson JD, Stewart EM, Macias DM, Chander H, Knight AC. Individuals with chronic ankle instability exhibit dynamic postural stability deficits and altered unilateral landing biomechanics: a systematic review. Phys Ther Sport. 2019;37:210–9.
132. Burcal CJ, Sandrey MA, Hubbard-Turner T, McKeon PO, Wikstrom EA. Predicting dynamic balance improvements following 4-weeks of balance training in chronic ankle instability patients. J Sci Med Sport. 2019;22(5):538–43.
133. Clanton TO, Matheny LM, Jarvis HC, Jeronimus AB. Return to play in athletes following ankle injuries. Sports Health. 2012;4(6):471–4.
134. Shawen SB, Dworak T, Anderson RB. Return to play following ankle sprain and lateral ligament reconstruction. Clin Sports Med. 2016;35(4):697–709.
135. Anguish B, Sandrey MA. Two 4-week balance-training programs for chronic ankle instability. J Athl Train. 2018;53(7):662–71.
136. Wortmann MA, Docherty CL. Effect of balance training on postural stability in subjects with chronic ankle instability. J Sport Rehabil. 2013;22(2):143–9.
137. Caffrey E, Docherty CL, Schrader J, Klossner J. The ability of 4 single-limb hopping tests to detect functional performance deficits in individuals with functional ankle instability. J Orthop Sports Phys Ther. 2009;39(11):799–806.
138. Barelds I, van den Broek AG, Huisstede BMA. Ankle bracing is effective for primary and secondary prevention of acute ankle injuries in athletes: a systematic review and meta-analyses. Sports Med. 2018;48(12):2775–84.
139. Bennell KL, Talbot RC, Wajswelner H, Techovanich W, Kelly DH, Hall AJ. Intra-rater and inter-rater reliability of a weight-bearing lunge measure of ankle dorsiflexion. Aust J Physiother. 1998;44(3):175–80.
140. Kruse D, Lemmen B. Spine injuries in the sport of gymnastics. Curr Sports Med Rep. 2009;8(1):20–8.
141. Petering RC, Webb C. Treatment options for low back pain in athletes. Sports Health. 2011;3(6):550–5.
142. McGill S. Low back disorders: evidence based prevention and rehabilitation. Champaign: Human Kinetics; 2007.
143. Garet M, Reiman MP, Mathers J, Sylvain J. Nonoperative treatment in lumbar spondylolysis and spondylolisthesis: a systematic review. Sports Health. 2013;5(3):225–32.

144. Hainline B, Turner JA, Caneiro JP, Stewart M, Lorimer Moseley G. Pain in elite athletes-neurophysiological, biomechanical and psychosocial considerations: a narrative review. Br J Sports Med. 2017;51(17):1259–64.
145. Hodges PW, Cholwicki J, van Dieen JH. Spinal control: the rehabilitation of back pain: state of the art and science. London: Churchill Livingstone; 2013. 338 p.
146. Moseley GL, Hodges PW. Reduced variability of postural strategy prevents normalization of motor changes induced by back pain: a risk factor for chronic trouble? Behav Neurosci. 2006;120(2):474–6.
147. Chaitow L, Bradley D, Gilbert C. Recognizing and treating breathing disorders: a multidisciplinary approach. 2nd ed. Edinburgh: Churchill Livingstone; 2013. 320 p.
148. McGill S. Ultimate back fitness and performance. 5th ed. Waterloo: Wabuno Publishers; 2014. 319 p.
149. McGill SM, McDermott A, Fenwick CM. Comparison of different strongman events: trunk muscle activation and lumbar spine motion, load, and stiffness. J Strength Cond Res. 2009;23(4):1148–61.
150. Beardsley C, Skarabot J. Effects of self-myofascial release: a systematic review. J Bodyw Mov Ther. 2015;19(4):747–58.
151. O'Sullivan K, McAuliffe S, Deburca N. The effects of eccentric training on lower limb flexibility: a systematic review. Br J Sports Med. 2012;46(12):838–45.
152. Thomas E, Bianco A, Paoli A, Palma A. The relation between stretching typology and stretching duration: the effects on range of motion. Int J Sports Med. 2018;39(4):243–54.
153. Butler D. The sensitive nervous system. Adelaide City West: Noigroup Publications; 2000. 431 p.

Chapter 12
Return to Play in Gymnastics

Marla Ranieri, Morgan Potter, Melissa Mascaro, and Marsha Grant-Ford

12.1 Introduction

Injuries in gymnastics present many clinical challenges due to the development and maintenance of unique motor skills required in the various events, training protocols that increase as skill levels escalate with no traditional offseason, and the age at which training commences [1]. However, in the current body of literature, there are limited evidence-based return to play (RTP) protocols specific to the unique demands of gymnastics [1]. As such, the purpose of this chapter is to first review the unique demands of gymnastics that must be understood when designing a RTP protocol. Second, we will review general principles of RTP protocols, and how these principles relate to gymnastics. Third, we will go through general guidelines for progressive protocols for injuries to the head/neck (concussion), upper extremity (UE), lumbar spine, and lower extremity (LE) in gymnasts.

12.1.1 Unique Demands of Gymnastics

There are a number of factors that must be taken into consideration when developing a RTP protocol for gymnasts following injury, including the athlete's age, developmental abilities, and the biomechanical demands. In order for gymnasts to reach their peak performance by late adolescence or early adulthood, gymnasts spend many hours training from a young age. Lower levels may train up to 9 hours a week and elite gymnasts train upward of 40 hours per week [2]. These rigorous training hours can cause injuries to their developing bodies. Another factor that should be considered when designing a RTP progression are the forces placed on the body in gymnastics. This includes distractive, compressive, and rotational forces. While learning new skills or practicing mastered skills, gymnasts must perform many repetitions and can experience forces up to 13 times their body weight during dismounts [3]. Likewise, gymnasts are required to utilize their wrists, arms, elbows, and shoulders as weight-bearing joints in a similar fashion as their lower extremities. Allowing specific injured body regions to rest while still training others presents many obstacles for clinicians and gymnasts as they attempt to balance the modified training without causing a new injury [1, 4]. Through better understanding of the sport and proper modifications, a safe RTP protocol can be developed.

12.1.2 RTP Principles and Gymnastics

Before beginning the RTP process, the medical team, coaching staff, and the athlete must define their idea of a successful RTP by discussing their expectations and goals. The following influential factors must be taken into consideration when creating the plan: age of the athlete, biomechanical and physical requirements of each apparatus, level of competition, upcoming events (such as important competitions), and the injury type (chronic vs acute injury) [5, 6]. This discussion and effective communication among everyone involved is vital to a successful RTP protocol. The authors recommend that the athlete carry a journal to record these goals. In addition, the journal should be taken to all medical appointments and practices in order to record medical instructions, progress in the gym, and any questions that may arise. A gymnast may begin their RTP protocol once the following are met: resolution of pain, restoration of normal joint function, completion of a progressive rehabilitation program, execution of proper technique for skills, and approval from the medical team [6].

In order to minimize the risk for reinjury or new injury, RTP protocols must be a progressive stepwise process focused on enhancing range of motion, strength, and symmetry to ensure the athlete is ready for the various muscular, cardiovascular, and technical demands of their sport [6]. For gymnasts, both hours spent training and the skills must be progressive. As such, when a gymnast begins their RTP protocol, the number of training hours must progressively increase, rather than resuming the same hours of training before the injury. In addition, zealous adherence to any one linear formula should be undertaken with caution. Simply adding repetitions and increasing skill difficulty weekly does not ensure the athlete is properly rehabilitating their injury. The "ten percent rule" is often cited anecdotally as a rule of thumb to gauge the rate of rehabilitative progress. The suggestion is that rehabilitation activity should increase no more than 10% per week in intensity, duration of sessions, repetitions, and weight/resistance. Despite controversies about its effectiveness, the suggestion of gradual increases in workload is not a bad one and certainly provides guidelines for coaches who lack optimal rehabilitative guidance.

The progressive nature of the RTP protocol can be implemented by executing sequential steps in the protocol. Successful completion of each step can be measured by meeting predetermined criteria, such as contralateral symmetry in strength, or specific functional test scores [5–7]. However, multiple steps of the protocol should not be done in 1 day [7, 8]. Once a gymnast has successfully completed one step, he or she may begin the next step the following day. The amount of time on each step is not always equal or linear in fashion. A gymnast may need to spend multiple days, weeks, or months on one step before meeting the requirements to advance to the next step.

The RTP process can be filled with many emotions. We recommend that gymnasts keep the following three items in mind when they start their RTP protocol in order to achieve a successful progression back to gymnastics.

1. *Mental vs. physical readiness:* The medical team supervising the RTP, as well as the athlete, must be aware of the psychosocial factors that can affect RTP. Specifically, it is not uncommon for an athlete to be physically ready to begin the RTP protocol before he or she is psychologically ready [9, 10].
2. *RTP takes time*: The athlete should understand that he or she will not start on skills he or she was training before the injury. Likewise, even with the same injury, full progression back to sport may take longer for some athletes.
3. *Stay positive and practice "active rest":* The medical team and coach should remind the athlete to focus on what he or she can do, rather than what he or she cannot. It is always encouraged to give the athlete an athletic goal (e.g., improve flexibility, improve bars if it is a lower extremity injury, etc.).
4. *Continue to attend practice:* Being in the gym allows the athlete to maintain camaraderie with teammates, work on prior existing deficits not related to the injury, continue skill learning by observation, and listen to corrections and feedback from the coaches.

12.2 Return to Play After Concussion

Conventional management for concussion previously recommended complete rest and then progressive return to activity. Recent evidence challenges this notion and suggests that active approaches may be effective for many patients [11, 12].

Gymnasts, however, must be able to complete the basic stepwise progression completely symptom-free before advancing to the next stage in recovery.

There have been few high-quality prospective studies conducted regarding the effectiveness of rest and concussion recovery in gymnasts. A concussed gymnast is under incredible stress to get back to the gym and, due to the injury, may already feel isolated and emotional. These athletes may exhibit a number of concussion-related symptoms. Many of these symptoms resolve with the injury, but it is imperative to not add undue stress to the burden of recovery. By allowing the athlete to return to academics first, the pressure of the initial stages of concussion rehabilitation is reduced.

12.2.1 Return to Learn

Most kids and teens will only need help through informal, academic modifications as they recover from a concussion. However, for kids and teens with ongoing symptoms or postconcussive syndrome (PCS), a variety of formal support services may be available to help them during their recovery. These support services may vary widely among states and school districts. The type of support will differ based on the academic needs of each student. Some of these support services may include a Response to Intervention Protocol, a 504 Plan, or even an Individualized Education Plan (IEP) [13].

Concussed athletes should begin a "return to learn protocol" provided by their physician as soon as possible. First, a student-athlete should be able to tolerate 10–15 minutes of concentration which may include listening to audio books, reading class notes in large font, or reading textbooks. The use of computers, smart boards, and other screens may be used as long as they are tolerated by the gymnast. As the symptoms decrease, the amount of time spent in direct schoolwork should increase. It is important to include rest breaks to avoid worsening of symptoms.

Early on in recovery, a half-day of school or limited time in the classroom may be advised given the increase in stimulation. Physicians may give other accommodations to help with a return to full classwork in both the home instruction and the traditionally schooled athletes. This may include dismissal from class a few minutes early to avoid noisy hallways and transitioning of classes, occasional breaks in a quiet place, and providing extra time on assignments and exams. If symptoms reoccur or worsen, it may be that the student-athlete tried to do too much cognitive activity too quickly. Finally, standardized testing should be avoided until clearance is provided by a physician.

12.2.2 Return to Gymnastics

Most concussions resolve within 2–4 weeks, but some do not [14]. Once an athlete is symptom-free and has completed a "return to learn" program, a return to gymnastics (RTG) assessment and plan should be initiated. The standard RTP programs do not provide good structure for returning a gymnast [8]; however, a six-stage return to gymnastics protocol has been published and is described below [15]. Each stage correlates to a day of practice, and practice should only occur once a day. Activity should stop immediately if symptoms return at any stage of a progression. In this situation, it may be in the gymnast's best interest to be sent home for the day. If that is not possible, the athlete may need to go into a private room or office to rest until a parent can come to pick them up. If symptoms develop, the athlete should rest the following day and return to the stage in which symptoms did not occur. During this recovery phase, the athlete should be checking in with his/her physician, and it is important to encourage honesty at these visits.

12.2.2.1 Stage 1

Typically, a gymnast will come into the gym and perform 15–20 minutes of light cardio. This may include light jogging or biking. There should be no inverted stretching or skills at the gym. Keep in mind while this seems minimal, the athlete is also incorporating and adjusting to the lighting, the noise, the stimulation of driving/being in a car, and being in a gym setting. If a gymnast is unable to do light cardio, he or she should be sent home to rest [14]. This stage may last a day or can last weeks depending on how the athlete feels the following day. With concussion symptoms often taking 24 hours to appear, it may be helpful for the athlete to keep track of their symptoms at home on a SCAT 5 or similar tool.

12.2.2.2 Stage 2

If there are no symptoms present 24 hours after completing stage 1, the athlete may increase the activity level to 20–30 minutes of moderate aerobic activity and body weight strength training and then incorporate some balance skills such as walking on a balance beam with eyes open [16]. No inversion skills or flipping allowed. High kicks and landing drills may be incorporated with limited numbers (e.g., up to five).

12.2.2.3 Stage 3

This stage can include the introduction of vertical (handstand) work as well as jumps, leaps, turns, and walkovers. The increase in skills may bring on symptoms, so it is important for the coach and athlete to continue to monitor for symptoms. Floor work is advised first before progression to a balance beam; low beam should be utilized before attempting skills on a high beam. Tap swings, casts on bars, and run through on vault may be appropriate based on the athlete's skill level.

12.2.2.4 Stage 4

The next stage progresses the inversion skills to add in handsprings and saltos. Basic skills on bars such as clear hips, stalders, and giants on bars may be introduced, based on the athlete's level. Handsprings and Tsuk or Yurchenko timers may also be performed as long as these skills had been mastered prior to injury. Keep in mind, single rotations should be done before double rotations, and single twists should be done before multiple. Much of this stage involves rebuilding the confidence in the athlete, particularly with advanced skills and release moves on bars; numbers should be reduced, and symptoms checked regularly.

12.2.2.5 Stage 5

After medical clearance, the gymnast may progress to stage 5. All skills may be incorporated into practice, but the athlete should be monitored periodically throughout practice for any symptoms. If symptom-free, the gymnast may progress to partial and then full routines.

12.2.2.6 Stage 6

The final stage is full return to competition and may occur after successful completion of stage 5.

12.2.3 Clearance and Final Follow-Up

It is recommended that gymnasts with concussions be treated by a physician with gymnastics and concussion knowledge. Individualized RTG progressions may need to be altered based on the level of the gymnast and should be made based on state guidelines. Some gymnasts may take longer to return to sport than others. Factors that may prolong recovery include young age, previous concussions, coexisting learning disorders (i.e., ADHD, ADD, dyslexia), migraines, seizures, and other coexisting conditions such as anxiety and depression [17].

The treating physician, through the interpretation of all testing and the gymnast's ability to tolerate the RTG protocol, determines the rate of progression and final clearance. Some athletes may require additional rehabilitation, which may include visual and/or ocular rehabilitation before final clearance. Persistent dizziness or imbalance may indicate a need for these referrals [18]. For a gymnast, dizziness or imbalance may inadvertently cause catastrophic injury if not addressed early, particularly in the higher-level athletes.

While progressing through the RTG program, continual education should be done with athletes, coaches, and parents regarding:

1. The importance of reporting symptoms [19]
2. The risk of recurrent concussion
3. The risk for delayed recovery with subsequent injury
4. Proper supervision and the utility of standardized baseline and post injury testing once the injury has recovered completely [20]

It is the responsibility of the coaches, parents, teachers, and entire medical staff to help the gymnast transition back into class and athletics without causing unnecessary pressure or stress on an already stressed athlete. The time out of the gym may cause social isolation, so it is important to remember to include the athlete in as many team meetings or other team events as possible without overwhelming him/her. The pressure felt to return quickly may mean an athlete may downplay symptoms hoping for a faster return. The medical team and coaches should make sure to protect the gymnasts in order to allow for a safe recovery [21, 22].

12.3 RTP After Upper Extremity Injuries

Because gymnasts use their wrists, elbows, and shoulders as weight-bearing joints, the RTP process for upper extremity (UE) injuries is similar to that for the lower extremity [23, 24]. The following areas must be considered when designing the athlete's RTP program: proper UE weight-bearing progression, UE mobility, grip strength, elbow stability, core and scapular stability, muscular endurance, plyometric power, and the mechanics of skills.

12.3.1 Upper Extremity Weight-Bearing Progression

It is important to learn how to walk before you run and how to run before you leap. The same concepts pertain to the weight-bearing athlete after a UE injury. A gymnast cannot transition from a non-weight-bearing status during the healing phase to an immediate return to impact skills such as tumbling on floor or vault. This is a common mistake that leads to setbacks or reinjury. There must be a functional progression [25] in place with each successive progression being pain-free.

A functional weight-bearing progression seen in Fig. 12.1 involves moving from quadruped position (a), to push-up position (b), to piked handstand position (c), to supported handstand position (d), and finally to nonsupported handstand position (e).

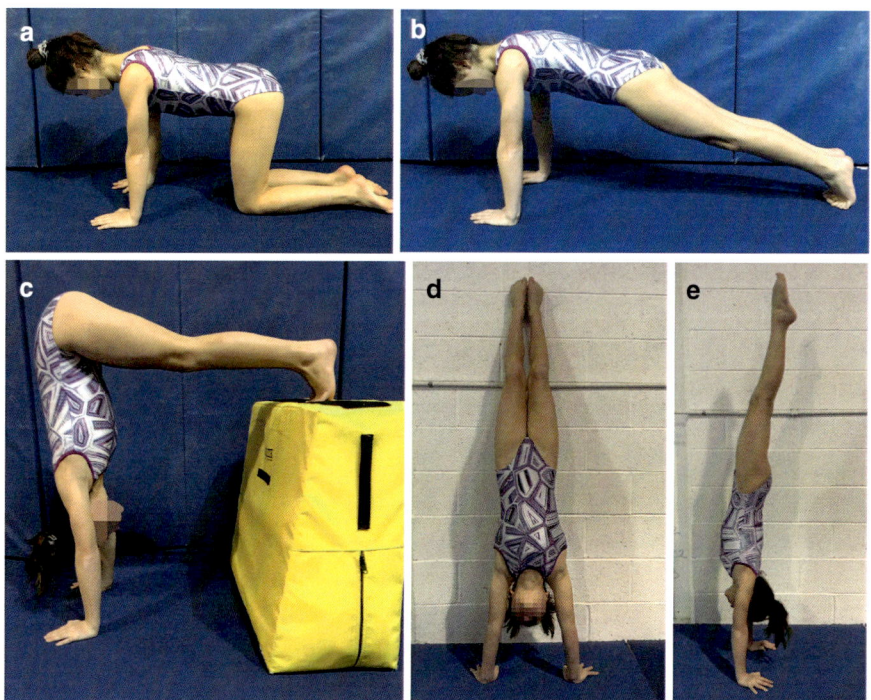

Fig. 12.1 Upper Extremity progression from quadruped position (**a**) to push up position (**b**), to piked handstand position (**c**), to supported handstand position (**d**), and finally to non-supported handstand position (**e**)

Throughout these progressive positions, the athlete must be challenged in the following ways:

1. Using a stable surface and then a nonstable surface
2. Being in a static position and then a dynamic position
3. Progressing from bilateral UE weight-bearing to single UE weight-bearing
4. Increasing endurance and time of weight-bearing
5. Increasing speed, power, and plyometrics in each position

Examples of plyometric weight-bearing progressions (Fig. 12.2) are kneeling push-up claps (a), push-up claps (b), piked handstand push-up jumps (c), supported handstand pops (d), and nonsupported handstand pops (e).

Sweeney et al. have developed a detailed progression for UE injuries for female (Table 12.1) and male gymnasts (Table 12.2) that correlates well with the above functional weight-bearing progression [1]. Each UE injury is different, and there is no guideline or time component related to how quickly or slowly to move through these functional weight-bearing progressions and functional skill progressions. Quality is more important than quantity, and therefore, control, stability, and lack of pain are the guides to progressing the gymnast.

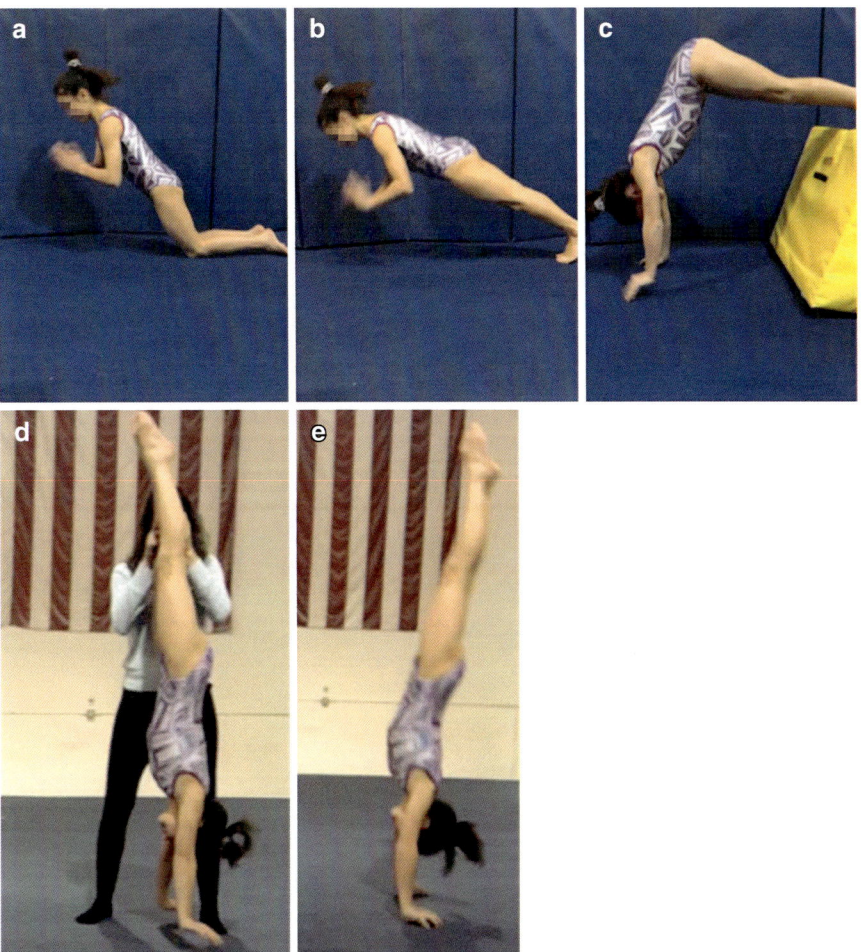

Fig. 12.2 Kneeling push up claps (**a**), push up claps (**b**), piked handstand push up jumps (**c**), supported handstand pops (**d**), and non-supported handstand pops (**e**)

12.3.2 Upper Extremity Mobility

Whether the athlete endures a wrist, an elbow, or a shoulder injury, the entire UE complex has to be taken into consideration [26]. Further, all joints throughout the kinetic chain must be returned to full active range of motion (AROM) and passive range of motion (PROM) in open-chain and closed-chain movements. It has been shown that lack of wrist or shoulder mobility in a weight-bearing athlete can lead to wrist [27], elbow, and shoulder injuries [27–31]. Therefore, not regaining the proper range of motion can lead to reinjury during the RTP progression or can lead to a new injury somewhere else along the kinetic chain.

Table 12.1 Return to gymnastics skill progression for UE injuries for female artistic gymnasts [1]

Step	Vault	Uneven bars	Balance beam	Floor	Tumble track
Women: Wrist					
1		Hang on bar 10–60 s		Push-up with shoulder shrug (protraction) × 10–15 Push-up position: rock forward and back × 10–15	
2		Tap swings on bars (~3 sets of 5)		Handstand hold against the wall × 10–60 s (facing the wall will be easier on wrist than facing away from wall in the handstand position)	
3				Free-standing handstands Cartwheels[a]	Roundoffs × 10
4		Glide and long-hang kips[b]		Press to handstand (up to 10) Front and/or back walkovers (up to 10)	Roundoff, back handspring (may add single saltos[c])
5		Cast handstand[d] and back giants[e]	Cartwheels and handstands	Roundoffs[a] Pirouetting skills	Front handsprings (may add single saltos[c])
6		Clear hips and stalders[f]	Front and back walkovers (progressing from low to high beam)	Roundoff, back handspring (add single saltos[c])	Standing back handsprings
7	Handstand hops and blocking drills on floor (use softer mats initially if gymnast had impact-type injury)	Front giants[e] Pirouetting skills[g]	Standing back handspring on a line	Standing back handspring Front handsprings	
8	Handspring and Tsuk[a,h] timers Roundoff entry only for Yurchenko[i]	Release skills Eagle giants[j]	Roundoffs and back handsprings (progressing from low to high beam)		

Table 12.1 (continued)

Step	Vault	Uneven bars	Balance beam	Floor	Tumble track
9	Yurchenko[i] timers Flipping handsprings and Tsuk[h] vaults		One arm skills[a] (e.g., one arm back handspring)		
10	Flipping Yurchenko[i] vaults				
Women: Elbow					
1		Hang on bar 10–60 s (may need to delay step 2 or 3 for elbow stability issues)		Shoulder shrug (protraction in push-up position × 10–15) Handstand at wall 10–60 s Front and back walkovers (up to 10)	
2				Push-up with shrug (protraction) × 10–15 Cartwheels[a] (up to 15)	Roundoff[a] × 10
3		Tap swings (10–20) (may need to delay until step 4 for elbow stability issues)		Press to handstand	Roundoff, back handspring Front handsprings (may add single saltos[c])
4			Walkovers and cartwheels on low then high beam	Roundoff, back handspring and front handspring (may add saltos[c])	Standing back handsprings
5		Glide and long-hang kips[b] Cast[d] to handstand	Roundoff and back handsprings on line on floor	Pirouetting skills[g]	
6	Handstand hops/blocking drills	Back giants[e] and circling elements Dismounts	Roundoff and back handsprings		
7	Handsprings Roundoff entry for Yurchenko[i]	Pirouetting skills[g]			
8	Yurchenko[i] and Tsuk[h] vaults	Front[e] and eagle[f] giants Release elements			

(continued)

Table 12.1 (continued)

Step	Vault	Uneven bars	Balance beam	Floor	Tumble track
Women: Shoulder					
1		Hang on bar × 10–60 s	Leaps and jumps	Shoulder shrug (protraction in push-up position × 10–15) Handstand at wall 10–60 s Front and back walkovers (up to 10)	
2		Cast[d] to horizontal	Cartwheels Handstands	Push-up with shrug (protraction) × 10–15 Cartwheels[a] (up to 15)	Roundoff[a] × 10
3		Tap swings (~10–20) Kips[b] and casts[d] to handstand	Roundoffs[a]	Press to handstand	Roundoff, back handspring Front handsprings (may add single saltos[c])
4		Clear hips and stalders[f]	Walkovers (start on low beam)	Roundoff, back handspring and front handspring (may add saltos[c])	Standing back handsprings Twisting saltos[c]
5	Handstand hops and blocking drills	Back giants[e]	Roundoff to dismount saltos[c]	Pirouetting skills[g]	Add double saltos[c]
6	Handspring and Tsuk[a,h] timers Roundoff entry for Yurchenko[i]	Front giants[e] Pirouetting skills[g]	Back handsprings		
7	Yurchenko[i] timers	Release moves		Twisting and double saltos[c]	
8	Flip all vaults	Eagle giants[j]			

[a]If the leading arm is the gymnast's injured arm, this may be more difficult
[b]Kip: Gymnast swings from under the bar and then, pushing down on the bar, ends in a front support with the bar at her hips and next to her thighs
[c]Salto: A front or back flip without hands in a tuck, pike, or straight position
[d]Cast: Gymnast starts in front support and swings legs backward into a handstand position
[e]Giants: Circling backward or forward around the bar with the body extended straight in a handstand position
[f]Stalders: Backward or circling element in which gymnast is in a straddle-pike position without touching her feet to the bar
[g]Pirouetting skills: If pivoting base arm is the injured arm, this may be more difficult
[h]Tsuk: (Tsukahara) A vault in which the gymnast hits the springboard, then does a half-turn (roundoff) onto the vault, and then flips backward off the vault
[i]Yurchenko: A vault in which the gymnast does a roundoff onto the board, then jumps backward onto her hands on the vault, and then flips backward off the vault
[j]Eagle giants: Gymnast circles forward around the bar but forearms are fully pronated with shoulders internally rotated so that palms are facing upward (thumbs away from the body)

Table 12.2 Return to gymnastics skill progression for UE injuries for male gymnasts [1]

Step	Floor	Pommel horse	Rings	Vault	Parallel bars	High bar	Tumble track
Men: Wrist							
1	Push-up with shoulder shrug (protraction) × 10–15 Push-up position: rock forward and back × 10–15		Hang on rings 10–60 s			Hang on 10–60 s	
2	Handstand hold against the wall × 10–60 s (facing the wall will be easier on wrist than facing away from wall in the handstand position)					Tap swings on bars (~3 sets of 5)	
3	Free-standing handstands Cartwheels[a]				Under bar hangs		Roundoffs[a]
4	Press to handstand		Swings		Support swings Above bar basics	Long-hang kips[b]	Roundoff, back handsprings (may add single saltos[c])
5	Roundoffs[a]	Basic circles on mushroom[d] Scissors	Front support holds		Above bar sequences[a]	Kips[b] and casts[e] to handstand	Front handsprings (may add single saltos[c])
6	Roundoff back handsprings (may add saltos[c])	Double pommel basic skills	Handstand and basic swinging skills			Clear hips and stalders[f] Back giants[g]	Standing back handsprings
7	Standing back handsprings Front handsprings	Single pommel basics[a] Leather basics	More difficult swinging skills	Handstand hops and blocking drills on floor (use softer mats initially if gymnast had impact-type injury)	Under bar drills	Front giants[g] and pirouetting[a] skills	

(continued)

Table 12.2 (continued)

Step	Floor	Pommel horse	Rings	Vault	Parallel bars	High bar	Tumble track
8	Flare/circle[h] and hold skills	More difficult skills and single pommel work	Strength and planche[i] holds	Handspring and Tsuk[j] timers	Under bar skills	Release moves Eagle[k] and invert[l] skills	
9		Connect multiple skills		Yurchenko[a,m] timers Flipping handspring and Tsuk[a,j] vaults	Release skills		
10				Flip Yurchenko[a,m] vaults			

Men: Elbow

Step	Floor	Pommel horse	Rings	Vault	Parallel bars	High bar	Tumble track
1	Shoulder shrug (protraction in push-up position × 10–15) Handstand at wall 10–60 s		Hang on rings 10–60 s (may need to delay to step 2 or 3 for elbow stability issues)			Hang on high bar 10–60 s (may need to delay to step 2 or 3 for elbow stability issues)	
2	Push-up with shrug (protraction) × 10–15 Cartwheels[a] (up to 15)						Roundoff[a] × 10
3	Press to handstand Roundoffs[a]				Under bar hangs (may need to delay for elbow stability issue)	Tap swings on high bar (may need to delay to step 4 for elbow stability issues)	Roundoff back handsprings Front handsprings (may add saltos[c])
4	Roundoff back handsprings (may add saltos[c]) Front handsprings		Below ring swings		Support swings Above bar basics		Standing back handsprings

#	Floor	Pommel	Rings	Vault	Vault (handspring)	Parallel/Above bar	High bar	Uneven
5	Standing back handsprings							Kips[b] and casts[e]
6	Flare/circle[h] skills	Scissor skills, Circles on mushroom[d]						Back giants[g], Stalders[f], Dismounts
7	All tumbling	Basic skills on 2 pommels and the leather	Handstand and basic swinging skills	Tsuk[a-j] and Yurchenko[a-m] timers	Handspring timers	Pirouette skills[a], Under bar basics		Pirouette skills[a]
8		Single pommel work[a]	More difficult swinging skills	Handspring vaults		Under bar skills		Front giants[g], Release skills
9		Connect multiple skills	Strength and planche[i] holds	Tsuk[a-j] and Yurchenko[a-m] vaults		Release skills		Eagles[g] and invert[l] giants

Men: Shoulder

#	Floor	Pommel	Rings	Vault	Vault (handspring)	Parallel/Above bar	High bar	Uneven
1	Shoulder shrug (protraction in push-up position × 10–15), Handstand hold against wall × 10–60 s, Cartwheels[a] (10–15)		Hang on rings 10–60 s				Hang on high bar 10–60 s	
2	Push-up with shrug (protraction)							
3	Roundoffs[a]						Cast[e] to horizontal	Roundoffs[a]
4	Roundoff back handsprings (may add saltos[c]), Front handsprings	Scissor swings, Mushroom[d] circles	Front support holds, Below ring swings			Support swings, Under bar hangs	Below bar tap swings	Roundoff back handsprings (may add saltos[c]), Front handsprings
5	Standing back handsprings		Handstands	Handstand hops and blocking drills		Above bar skills	Clear hips, Stalders[f]	Standing back handsprings, Add twisting saltos[c]
								Add double saltos[c]

(continued)

Table 12.2 (continued)

Step	Floor	Pommel horse	Rings	Vault	Parallel bars	High bar	Tumble track
6	Add twisting and double saltos[c]		Bail drills	Handspring and Tsuk[a,j] timers	Advance above bar sequences and under bar skills, no Tippelt	Back giants[g] Dismounts	
7	Flare/circle[h] skills	Basic skills on 2 pommels and on the leather	Basic strength skills	Yurchenko timers[a,m]	Pirouette skills[a] Advance under bar skills	Pirouette skills Front giants[g]	
8		Single pommel work[a]	Moderate strength skills Full-swing skills and sequences	Flipping vaults	Release moves including Tippelt	Release elements	
9		Connect multiple skills	All strength holds			Eagle[k] and invert[l] giants	

[a]If the injured arm is the lead arm for roundoffs or vaulting and the base arm for pirouettes, above bar swinging skills, or single pommel work, then the progression may be more difficult and may be delayed

[b]Kip: Gymnast swings from under the bar and then, pushing down on the bar, ends in a front support with the bar at his hips and next to his thighs

[c]Salto: A front or back flip without hands in a tuck, pike, or straight position

[d]Mushroom: A short cylinder with a rounded top that is a training tool for learning skills on pommel horse

[e]Cast: Gymnast starts in front support and swings legs backward into a handstand position

[f]Stalders: Backward or circling element in which gymnast is in a straddle-pike position without touching his feet to the bar

[g]Giants: Circling backward or forward around the bar with the body extended straight in a handstand position

[h]Flare/circle: Gymnast circles legs around torso/shoulders while weight-bearing only on the hands

[i]Planche: Gymnast uses his arm strength to hold his body in a horizontal position

[j]Tsuk: (Tsukahara) A vault in which the gymnast hits the springboard, then does a half-turn (roundoff) onto the vault, and then flips backward off the vault

[k]Eagle giants: Gymnast circles forward around the bar, but forearms are fully pronated with shoulders internally rotated so that palms are facing upward (thumbs away from the body)

[l]Invert: Skills with the shoulders fully extended backward and internally rotated

[m]Yurchenko: A vault in which the gymnast does a roundoff onto the board, then jumps backward onto his hands on the vault, and then flips backward off the vault

Table 12.3 Normative values specific to male and female gymnasts for the UE joints [27, 32–35]

Motion	ROM (open chain)		ROM (closed chain)	
	Female	Male	Female	Male
Wrist extension	85	85	95	95
Elbow pronation	90	90	90	90
Elbow supination	80	80	90+	90+
Elbow flexion	140+	140+	NA	NA
Elbow extension	0	0	0	0
Shoulder flexion	190+	190	220+	220
Shoulder extension	45+	45+	75–90	75–90
Shoulder external rotation (at 90° abduction)	90+	120	90+	120
Shoulder internal rotation (at 90° abduction)	80+	90	80+	90
Shoulder horizontal abduction	45	100	NA	110+
Shoulder abduction	180	180	180	180

It is imperative to restore normal motion for the UE joints after injury. However, gymnasts have different requirements for UE range of motion [27] than standardized normative values [32] for a generic population due to the demands of their sport. Table 12.3 presents normative values specific to male and female gymnasts for the UE joints. This table has been created with expert opinion by prominent physical therapists in the field. When these range of motion values are obtained, the gymnast will typically have the appropriate range of motion to move their UE through the air in non-weight-bearing positions. For some UE injuries, gymnasts may be able to start some of these non-weight-bearing movements prior to having full motion (e.g., a gymnast may perform full leaps if she is in a short arm cast for a stable fracture of the distal radius). However, this will need to be determined by the medical team on an individual basis.

12.3.3 Grip Strength

Grip strength has been shown to correlate with strength of the UE, measures of the shoulder stabilizing muscles, and as an objective measure of UE function [36–39].

Therefore, lack of grip strength can indicate wrist, elbow, or shoulder injuries. A dynamometer can be used to test grip strength in gymnasts after UE injuries in order to clear them for the RTP progression [36, 40]. Grip strength should be tested for strength and power (one-time quick squeeze of the dynamometer) and for endurance (hanging on a bar for 30 seconds and then immediately testing grip strength after the hang using a dynamometer). Hand dominance should be considered when measuring grip strength. The dominant hand can be 10% stronger than the non-dominant hand during dynamometer measurements [41]. A gymnast should pass grip strength testing before he/she returns to events that require gripping such as the uneven bars, pommel horse, rings, parallel bar, and high bar.

12.3.4 Elbow Stability

Elbow stability should be a point of focus for gymnasts during the RTP process. It is common for many gymnasts to have elbow hypermobility [42], which is excessive laxity and range of motion in the elbow joint. This is seen when a gymnast has greater than 0 degrees of extension (i.e., hyperextension) that increases with weight-bearing activities (Fig. 12.3). A change or alteration anywhere in the body can lead to injury or dysfunction above or below that joint due to the kinetic chain theory [43–45]. Elbow hypermobility has been shown to alter the kinetic chain during overhead weight-bearing and can, therefore, lead to an increased risk of wrist, elbow, and shoulder injuries [28]. Therefore, constant education and cueing regarding elbow hypermobility needs to be considered throughout the rehabilitation and RTP phases.

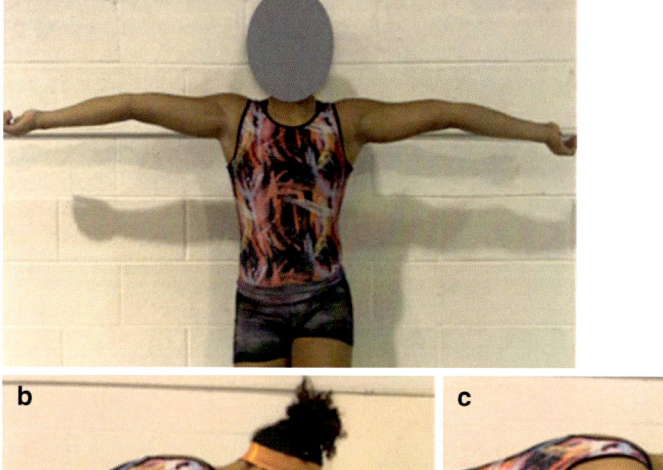

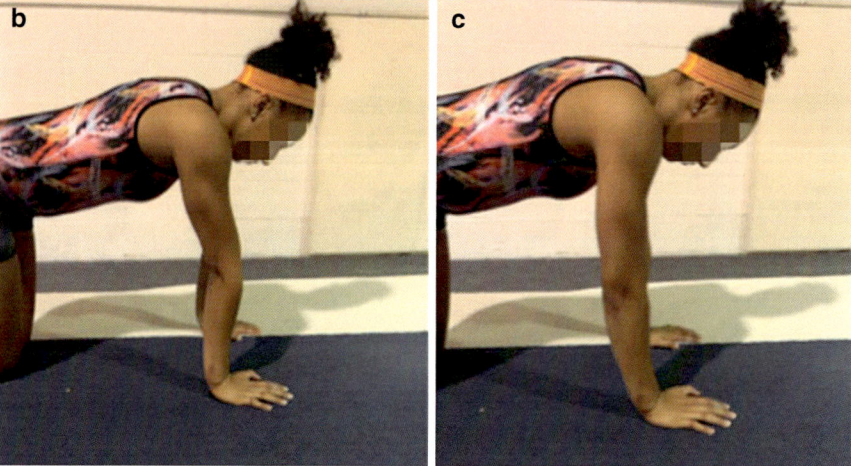

Fig. 12.3 Hyperextended elbows in non-weight-bearing (**a**) and weight-bearing (**b**) with corrected "soft elbows" (**c**)

Gymnasts with excessive elbow mobility need to be taught how to maintain a "soft elbow" (Fig. 12.3) with neutral elbow pronation/supination during open-chain movements and during closed-chain movements of the UE. Many gymnasts with hyperextended elbows tend to lock the elbows out in end range elbow extension with elbow supination. Maintaining proper elbow stability requires constant education and verbal cues during the rehabilitation phase and during the RTP phase. Elbow stability in addition to core stability and scapula stability should be a continued point of focus throughout the UE weight-bearing progression.

Functional tests appropriate for assessing elbow stability are the Closed Kinetic Chain Upper Extremity Stability Test (CKCUEST) [46] and Upper Quarter Y Balance Test (UQYBT) [47]. Gymnasts should be reminded to maintain soft elbows throughout these tests. Gymnasts should pass these tests before returning to non-plyometric UE weight-bearing skills such as handstands, cartwheels, back walkovers, cyclical swinging on bars, etc.

12.3.5 Scapula and Core Stability

Core stability is essential in daily living and athletic activities as it is the primary component of functional movement [48]. Core stability has been defined as "the ability to control trunk position and motion for the purpose of optimal production, transfer, and control of forces to and from the arms and legs during functional activities" [49]. Core stability is commonly overlooked in gymnastics because gymnasts have visually well-defined "six packs" which give them the appearance of being strong. However, the "six pack" (rectus abdominis) muscle is only one of many muscles that make up the core, and in reality, gymnasts tend to be lacking in their deeper local (transversus abdominis) core muscles. Therefore, gymnasts may appear to look strong, but functionally are lacking significant core control and stability.

Research studies have shown that deficits in core stability may lead to shoulder [50–53] and/or elbow [28, 49, 54] injuries. Since the scapula is the sole connection between the core and the UE complex, it is also very important to include the scapula muscles as part of core stability for gymnasts. The scapula muscles (serratus anterior, rhomboids, trapezius, levator scapulae) provide a stable base [26, 27, 51–53, 55] for shoulder mobility to occur. When weakness or dyskinesis [56] of the scapula is present, poor neuromuscular control of the shoulder, elbow, and, wrist can also occur, ultimately leading to a greater chance of injury and reinjury [53, 57, 58].

Core and scapular stability are important for distal mobility, which means a gymnast requires a strong stable base (core and scapula) in order to perform full, controlled UE movements [27, 59]. If there is a lack of core and scapular stability, there will be greater forces exerted on the shoulder, elbow, and wrist joints during weight-bearing activities [27, 53, 59].

The core and scapula stability muscles should be a point of focus in the UE RTP process. The scapula should be flush against the body during open-chain arm move-

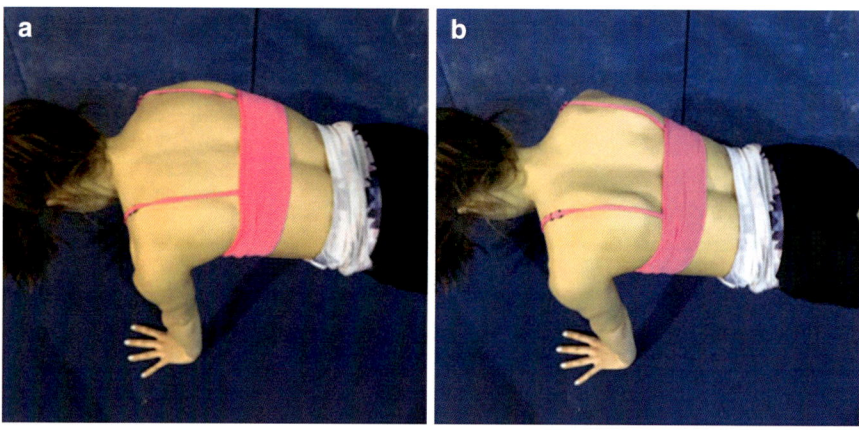

Fig. 12.4 Scapula stability during high plank (**a**) and scapula instability during high plank (**b**)

ments and closed-chain weight-bearing activities [56]. Scapular instability or dyskinesis [56] can be seen when the medial border of the scapula protrudes away from the body or the inferior border tilts forward or the superior border tilts backward. The athlete in Fig. 12.4 demonstrates scapula stability (a) and scapula instability during a high plank (b) [28].

The same functional tests to evaluate elbow stability can also be used to test scapular stability: these are the Closed Kinetic Chain Upper Extremity Stability Test (CKCUEST) [46] and the Upper Quarter Y Balance Test (UQYBT) [47], but there should be a focus on the scapula position throughout the tests. Functional tests appropriate to use for core stability are the double-leg-lowering test (DLL) [60], Sorensen test [61], side bridge test [62], and plank test [63]. Gymnasts should pass these tests before returning to higher-level weight-bearing skills, such as presses, pommel horse skills, pirouetting on bars, and light UE plyometric activities, such as standing roundoffs, standing back handsprings, and front handsprings.

12.3.6 *Muscular Endurance*

In addition to having full ROM, gymnasts should score a 5/5 on manual muscle testing [64] for all UE strength tests before beginning the RTP progression. Manual muscle testing is a basic way to test that the gymnast has recovered strength sufficient for daily life activities such as opening and closing doors, lifting a heavy bag, etc. It is also a good test to indicate that a gymnast is ready to start performing progressive weight-bearing strengthening exercises. However, this test does not indicate that a gymnast is ready to perform full gymnastics skills as it lacks the functional weight-bearing component and endurance component of strength, which is imperative to gymnastics. A bar routine, pommel horse routine, and ring routine may last up to a minute, and this will require not only strength but also endurance

12 Return to Play in Gymnastics

Table 12.4 Mean functional test scores for levels 4 through 10 female [65] and male [66] gymnasts

	Rope climb test (secs)	Over grip pull up test (reps)	Push-up test (reps)	Handstand test (secs)	Handstand push-up test (reps)	Ring hold test (cm from axilla/cm arm length)
Mean score (sd) in females	12.40 (6.9)	–	24.52 (9.2)	23.48 (29.5)	–	–
Mean score (sd) in males	–	–	9.2 (5.5)	–	6.8 (7.2)	0.39 (0.13)

Adapted from Sleeper et al. [65, 66] and used with permission of the International Journal of Sports Physical Therapy

of the UE muscles. For this reason, the RTP protocol for UE must progressively build muscle endurance in non-weight-bearing and weight-bearing positions.

Sleeper et al. developed a way to measure fitness in female [65] and male [66] gymnasts called the Functional Measurement Tool. In this test, the authors used the rope climb test, the over grip pull up test, the push-up test, the handstand test, the handstand push-up test, and the rings hold test as ways to measure UE fitness in gymnasts. These tests can be used as benchmark values for the RTP protocol of gymnastics as they help give normative values for strength and endurance during functional gymnastics movements (Table 12.4). When a gymnast is able to pass these fitness tests, it shows they are ready to start increasing the number of repetitions of skills performed in practice and may start putting skills together in combinations.

12.3.7 Plyometric Power

Gymnasts jump, land, and rebound with forces distributed throughout the entire UE chain [67, 68]. Therefore, plyometric power tests and plyometric power exercises should be incorporated in the UE RTP protocol. Functional tests appropriate for assessing plyometric power and speed are the plyometric push-up test [69], one arm hop test [70], seated medicine ball throw [71], and single-arm seated shot put test [72]. When gymnasts are able to complete these tests with quality, control, and no complaints of pain, then they are able to continue the progression toward UE plyometric gymnastics activities such as tumbling, release skills, and vaulting.

12.3.8 Mechanics of Skill

While progressing through the RTP protocol and slowly integrating gymnastics skills back into the athlete's daily tasks, it is crucial to make sure the form and mechanics of the skill are executed correctly [73]. For example, gymnasts may obtain full strength and ROM and progress through the UE weight-bearing progression with ease; however, when they return to a back handspring on floor, they may continue to exhibit a decreased shoulder angle during the handstand phase of the back handspring (Fig. 12.5) [27]. This will put the athlete back at risk for a wrist, elbow, shoulder, or back injury even though full healing of the initial injury has occurred. This may be due to the repetitive increased loads and abnormal forces on the UE.

If the root problem of improper skill acquisition has not been addressed during the RTP protocol, then the repetitive motion of that skill will lead to future injury or reinjury. The athlete and coach should consider the time in rehabilitation as a time to relearn UE movement patterns and skill acquisitions with special attention on the

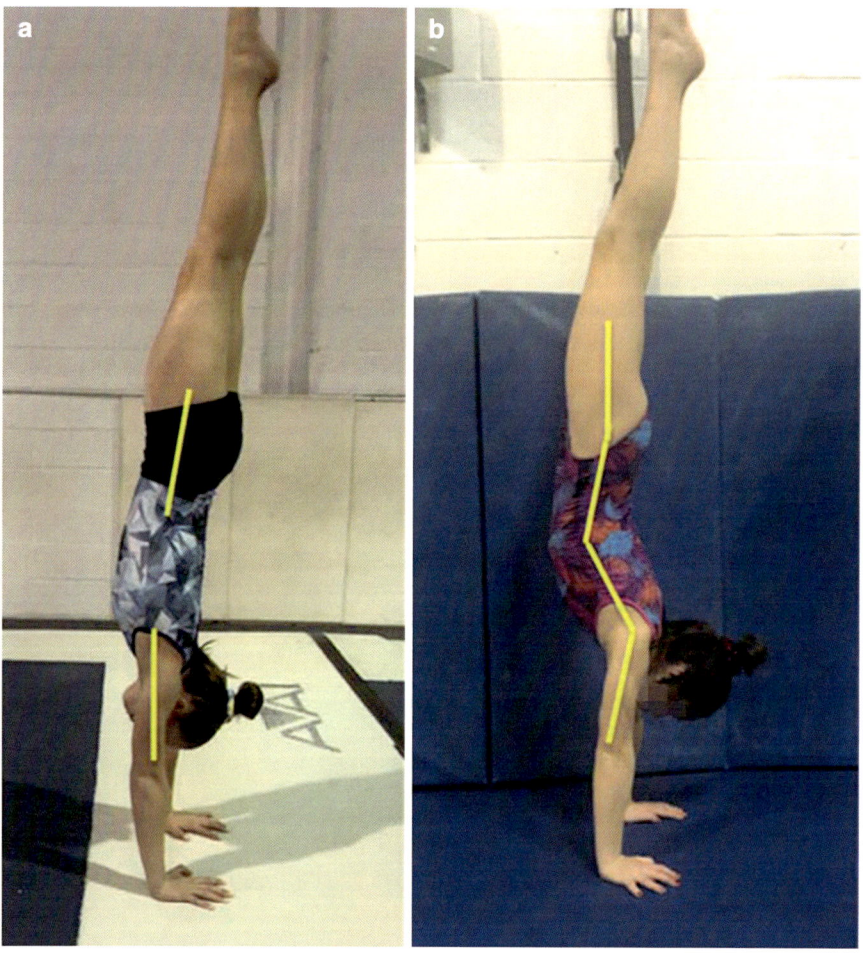

Fig. 12.5 Handstand position with proper (**a**) and improper (**b**) shoulder flexion, thoracic extension, pelvic mobility, and hip extension range of motion

handstand. When gymnasts are able to display appropriate mechanics of skills, then they are ready to start progressing toward combining skills in a routine and performing those skills in competitions.

In conclusion, there are many factors to consider during the RTP progression after an UE injury. Gymnasts should be working on their scapula strength, core strength, and grip strength throughout their rehabilitation phase and should continue to work on these areas during the RTP phase. When creating the RTP program, make sure to consider a proper UE weight-bearing progression, proper elbow stability, appropriate muscular endurance, plyometric power, and mechanics of skill. As these areas start to improve, the gymnast's skill level and repetitions of skills can start to progress as well.

12.4 RTP After Lumbar Spine Injuries

Gymnastics is a unique sport when considering RTP guidelines after lumbar spine injuries, as a gymnast is required to perform skills that involve high repetitions of spinal hyperextension, flexion, and rotation combined with reaction forces to the spine of up to 11–18 times their body weight [3, 4, 74–78]. The RTP guidelines presented in this section will focus specifically on the lumbar spine given the higher incidence of lumbar injuries in gymnastics compared to cervical or thoracic injuries [74, 79]. Lumbar spine injuries will be discussed as flexion-based spine injuries (FBSI) or extension-based spine injuries (EBSI). FBSI (tucking or bending forward) are related to the repetitive exposure to high-impact landings, especially those experienced during dismounts [3, 80, 81]. EBSI (arching or extending) are related to the repetitive exposure of lumbar hyperextension motions (e.g., back walkovers, back handsprings, Yurchenkos) and lumbar rotation motions (e.g., fulls, double fulls, front fulls) seen in training and competition [82, 83]. Examples of FBSI and EBSI are shown in Table 12.5.

Recommendations regarding RTP after spine injuries are specific to each athlete and will vary depending on anatomic location of the spine injury, mechanics and type of injury, how long the athlete has been dealing with the injury, competition level of gymnast, and whether there was surgical involvement or not. Sweeney et al. have developed a general progression for spine injuries for female (Table 12.6) and male gymnasts (Table 12.7) [1]. After the medical team has determined the athlete's lumbar spine pathology is healed and the athlete has been cleared to start the RTP progression, the following areas must be considered when designing the athlete's RTP program: total functional range of

Table 12.5 Examples of common flexion-based spine injuries (FBSI) and extension-based spine injuries (EBSI) in gymnasts

FBSI	EBSI
Herniated disc/disc disease	Spondylolysis
Ring apophysis fracture	Spondylolisthesis
Compression fracture	Facet syndrome

Table 12.6 Return to gymnastics skill progression for back injuries for female gymnasts [1]

Step	Vault	Uneven bars	Balance beam	Floor	Tumble track
Women: Back					
1		Hang on bar 10–60 s	Turns Kicks forward and sideways	Handstand against wall × 10–60 s Cartwheels Straight jumps with good landing technique	Roundoffs
2		Glide and long-hang kips[a]	Cartwheels Handstands	Tuck, straddle, and pike jumps with good landings	
3		Tap swings (10–20) Kip[a] to cast[c] handstand (lower-level gymnasts may need to delay this step if not proficient) Clear hips and stalders[e]	Basic jumps	Leaps and split jumps (without arch)	Roundoff back handsprings Front handsprings
4		Back and front giants[d] Dismount timers onto soft mat	Roundoffs Leaps and split jumps (without arch)	Roundoff back handsprings Front handsprings	Standing back handsprings Non-twisting saltos[b] (no double layouts); land on soft mat
5	Handspring and Tsuk[f] timers onto soft mat	Limited release moves (no Tkatchev, Pak, or Hechts which requiring arching)	Back/front handsprings on line on floor Dismount timers onto soft mat	Single saltos[b] without twisting (standing and tumbling) Leaps and jumps with arch	Twisting saltos[b]
6		All release skills Dismounts onto regular mats	Back handsprings Leaps and jumps with arch	Twisting skills Walkovers (if required)	Double layouts
7	Yurchenko[g] timers onto soft mat	All skills	Layout step outs Saltos[b] on the beam	Double layouts Walkover on line (if required)	

Table 12.6 (continued)

Step	Vault	Uneven bars	Balance beam	Floor	Tumble track
8	Start flipping vaults onto soft mat		Walkovers (if required)		

^aKip: Gymnast swings from under the bar and then, pushing down on the bar, ends in a front support with the bar at her hips and next to her thighs
^bSalto: A front or back flip without hands in a tuck, pike, or straight position
^cCast: Gymnast starts in front support and swings legs backward into a handstand position
^dGiants: Circling backward or forward around the bar with the body extended straight in a handstand position
^eStalders: Backward or circling element in which gymnast is in a straddle-pike position without touching her feet to the bar
^fTsuk: (Tsukahara) A vault in which the gymnast hits the springboard, then does a half-turn (roundoff) onto the vault, and then flips backward off the vault
^gYurchenko: A vault in which the gymnast does a roundoff onto the board, then jumps backward onto her hands on the vault, and then flips backward off the vault

motion, posture, core stability, gluteal activation, lumbopelvic dissociation, muscular endurance, plyometric power, and mechanics of skill.

12.4.1 Total Functional Range of Motion

In order to start the RTP progression, it is imperative that the athlete has full, pain-free lumbar AROM with good quality of movement. This means the athlete should be able to bend forward and touch his/her toes (especially for a FBSI), should be able to arch backward displaying 35 degrees of lumbar extension (especially for EBSI), should be able to side bend equally with fingers surpassing crease of knee, and should be able to perform lumbar rotation equally to at least 18 degrees (Table 12.8) [84].

In addition to obtaining proper lumbar AROM, it is also important that the athlete obtains Total Functional Motion (TFM) (Table 12.9). TFM is the result of multiple levels of the spine (lumbar and thoracic) in addition to the joints above and below the spine (pelvis, hips, and shoulders) working together to accomplish a TFM goal that requires more motion than one level can accomplish on its own [34]. TFM can be observed in a handstand and a back bridge (especially for EBSI) (Fig. 12.6). If the athlete is unable to obtain proper shoulder flexion, thoracic extension, hip extension, and posterior pelvic tilt mobility, then an increase in lumbar extension or "hinging" at a specific segment of the spine will occur with additional loads placed on that lumbar spine segment [34, 85]. TFM can also be observed in an overhead

Table 12.7 Return to gymnastics skill progression for back injuries for male gymnasts [1]

Step	Floor	Pommel horse	Rings	Vault	Parallel bars	High bar	Tumble track
Men: Back							
1	Handstand holds against wall (10–60 s) Cartwheels Straight jumps with good technique						Roundoffs
2	Roundoffs	Scissor swings	Basic swings Front support holds		Above bar support swing basics	Kips[a] Tap swings	Roundoffs back handsprings Front handsprings
3	Roundoffs back handsprings Front handsprings Flare/circle[f] skills	Basics on pommels and leather, no dismounts	Handstand and basic strength skills Bail drills	Handspring and Tsuk[g] timers	Above bar support swing skills Under bar drills	Cast[c] to handstand (lower-level gymnasts may need to delay this step if not proficient) Clear hips Stalders[d]	Standing back handsprings Non-twisting saltos[c] (no double layout)
4	Add single saltos[b] without twisting Standing back handsprings	All skills and sequences	Back giants[e]	Handspring and Tsuk[g] vaults	Under bar skills, no Tippelt	Back and front giant[e] Dismounts into pit	Add double layout
5	Add double Salto[b] skills	Add dismounts	Front giants[e]	Yurchenko[h] timers	Full dismounts	All release moves	
6	Add twisting skills		Add dismounts	Full vaults	Full under bar skills and Tippelt		

[a]Kip: Gymnast swings from under the bar and then, pushing down on the bar, ends in a front support with the bar at his hips and next to his thighs
[b]Salto: A front or back flip without hands in a tuck, pike, or straight position
[c]Cast: Gymnast starts in front support and swings legs backward into a handstand position
[d]Stalders: Backward or circling element in which gymnast is in a straddle-pike position without touching his feet to the bar
[e]Giants: Circling backward or forward around the bar with the body extended straight in a handstand position
[f]Flare/circle: Gymnast circles legs around torso/shoulders while weight-bearing only on the hands
[g]Tsuk: (Tsukahara) A vault in which the gymnast hits the springboard, then does a half-turn (roundoff) onto the vault, and then flips backward off the vault
[h]Yurchenko: A vault in which the gymnast does a roundoff onto the board, then jumps backward onto his hands on the vault, and then flips backward off the vault

12 Return to Play in Gymnastics

Table 12.8 Range of motion of the lumbar spine for male and female artistic gymnasts

Lumbar motion	ROM (open chain)
Lumbar flexion	Hands to floor
Lumbar extension	>35°
Lumbar side bending	Fingertips > crease of knee
Lumbar rotation	>18°

Table 12.9 The Total Functional Motion for open-chain and closed-chain movements in male and female gymnasts [29]

Total functional motion	ROM (open chain)	ROM (closed chain)
Thoracic extension	45°	NA
Thoracic rotation	45°	NA
Posterior pelvic tilt/sacral nutation	45°	NA
Anterior pelvic tilt/sacral counter-nutation	60°	NA
Shoulder flexion	>190°	>220°
Hip extension	>30°	>30°
Hip flexion	Thigh to torso	NA

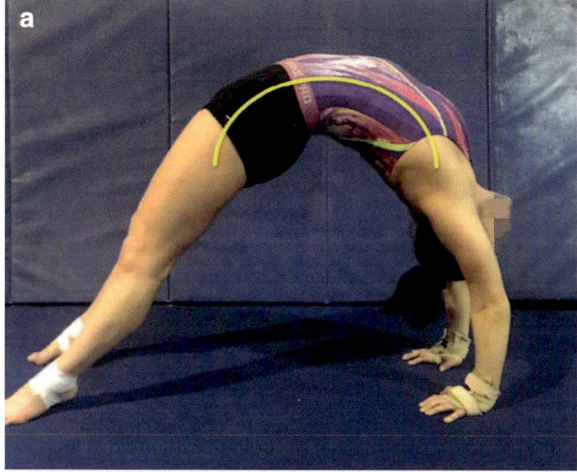

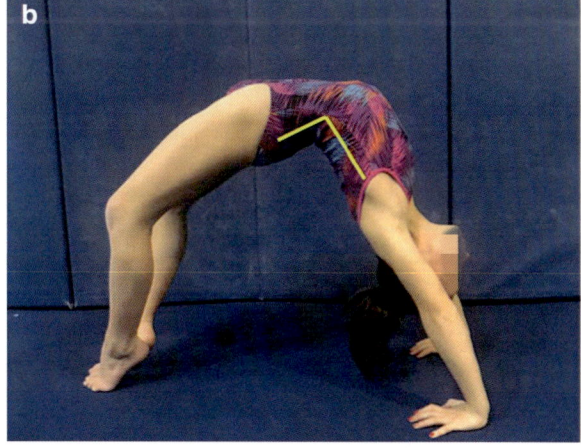

Fig. 12.6 Bridge position with proper (**a**) and improper (**b**) shoulder flexion, thoracic extension, hip extension, and pelvic tilt mobility

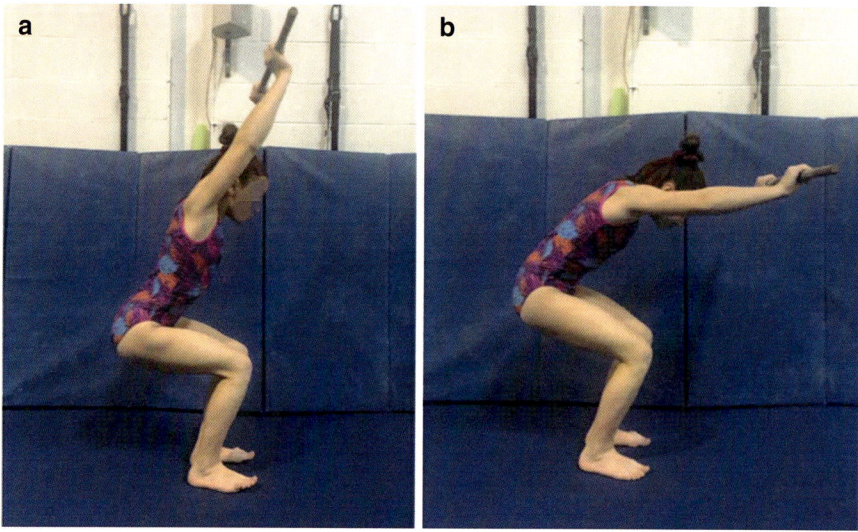

Fig. 12.7 Overhead squat position with proper (**a**) and improper (**b**) shoulder flexion, thoracic extension, hip flexion/lumbopelvic dissociation, and pelvic tilt mobility

squat position (especially for FBSI) (Fig. 12.7). If the athlete is unable to obtain proper shoulder flexion, thoracic extension, hip flexion that dissociates from the low back, and anterior pelvic tilt mobility, then an increase in lumbar flexion will occur with additional loads placed on the lumbar spine.

Once the athlete is able to show proper TFM throughout their joints combined with strength and stability within these ranges of motion, then the athlete is ready to perform low repetitions (3–8 repetitions) of neutral, nonimpact gymnastics skills in a progressive manner such as handstands, cartwheels, pirouettes, squatting, lunging conditioning exercises, and swinging on bars.

12.4.2 Posture: Upper and Lower Crossed Body Syndromes

Teaching proper posture positioning is the most important basic skill a gymnast can learn, and proper posture must be obtained prior to returning to gymnastics. A gymnast's posture becomes the building blocks of a handstand, a giant, a roundoff, and all other successive skills. Poor posture has been correlated with an increased risk for LBP in gymnasts [86]. There are two common postural deficits seen in gymnasts that should be evaluated in the RTP process. The first is the hyperlordotic posture that correlates with rounded upper back (increased kyphosis), rounded shoulders (internally rotated humerus), arched lower back (anterior tilted pelvis), hyperextended knees, and pronated feet. This posture is commonly associated with EBSI. The second type of posture is the swayback posture that correlates with a flat back (decreased lumbar and thoracic curvatures), rounded lower back (posterior tilted pelvis), and tight hamstrings. This posture is more commonly associated with FBSI. Both types of postural deficits also known as "Lower Crossed Syndrome" and "Upper Crossed Syndrome" [87] lead to muscle imbalances and can lead to pain and poor mechanics during gymnastics skills [87]. Postural deficits can lead to weak or inhibited muscles (such as gluteal, abdominal, and periscapular muscles) and tight or over activated muscles (such as pectoral, erector spinae, and iliopsoas muscles) [88]. These muscle imbalances lead to asymmetrical transmission of ground reaction forces through the pelvis and the lumbar spine [89, 90], leading to biomechanical changes in performance, and thereby contribute to injury and pain [4, 91]. Once an athlete is able to maintain proper posture, defined by the Watson and Mac Donncha Posture Analysis [92], in standing and sitting for 50% of the day, they can increase their number of repetitions (e.g., 10–15) of neutral, nonimpact gymnastics skills.

12.4.3 Core Stability and Functional Progression

Functional progression of core stability is one of the most important aspects of RTP after a low back injury because core strength and stability are responsible for maintaining a neutral position of the pelvis to receive trunk forces [90] and to stabilize the spine to decrease repetitive torsional stresses and microtraumas incurred during gymnastics skills [89]. Retraining the core muscles is vital in the rehabilitation process and in the prevention of low back injuries [93–95].

During the healing/resting phase of a spine injury, core stability should be a primary focus. An athlete can be cued to engage the deeper abdominal muscles (transversus abdominis) by bracing or pulling their belly button into their spine (also known as an abdominal set) and once that can be maintained, exercises can be initiated on top of the abdominal set. However, it is challenging to learn how to engage the core muscles in functional positions and even harder to learn how to maintain appropriate core control in gymnastics skills. Therefore, it is important to use a functional progression of positions in retraining the appropriate activation of these muscles (Fig. 12.8). The functional progression includes performing core stabilization exercises in supine, prone, quadruped, kneeling, standing, functional movement patterns (such as squatting and lunging), handstand position, and then during specific gymnastics skills (such as leaps, jumps, and flips).

Functional tests appropriate for assessing core stability sufficient for RTP progression are the prone instability test [96], balance ball test [97], plank holds [63], hollow holds, and double-leg lower test [60]. Gymnasts should be able to pass these tests before returning to neutral-impact gymnastics skills such as sprinting, jumping, flipping, roundoffs, and dismounts. A "pass" requires proper alignment of the spine while holding a plank, side plank, hollow hold, and arch hold for a minute for a high-level gymnast.

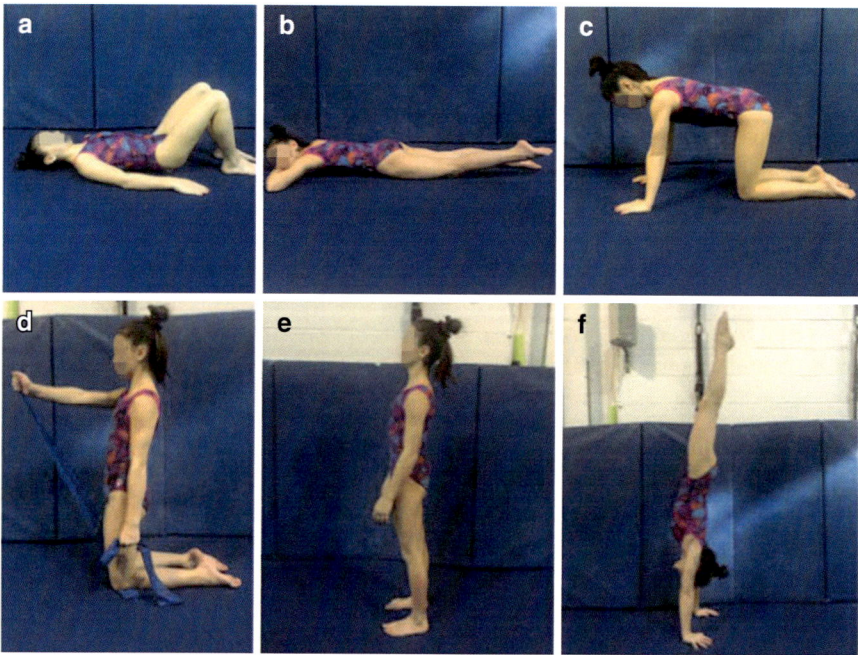

Fig. 12.8 Functional progression for core stabilization exercises while supine (**a**), prone (**b**), quadruped (**c**), kneeling (**d**), standing (**e**), and in handstand (**f**)

12.4.4 Glute Activation

The gluteal muscles are large contributors to proper rehabilitation and RTP of low back, hip, and knee injuries, as well as for forming proper posture. In general, this muscle group contributes to the propulsion and deceleration from explosive take-offs, landings, and directional changes. During the healing and resting phase of a spine injury, in addition to the RTP phase, it is important to continue to monitor glute activation in conjunction with core strength. A common pattern of imbalances that is seen regularly is tightness in the back extensor and the hip flexor musculature, coupled with deep abdominal and gluteal muscle group weaknesses as discussed in the "Lower Body Crossed Syndromes" [98].

Adequate muscle length and flexibility are necessary for proper joint function and efficiency of movement. If there is any imbalance occurring where agonist muscles become dominant and short, while antagonists become inhibited and weak, reinjury may occur. One example of a muscle imbalance pattern includes tightness and overactivity of the primary hip flexor (iliopsoas), which in turn causes reciprocal inhibition of the primary hip extensor (gluteus maximus).

It is important to pay attention to the muscles that are being used during exercises to identify if proper technique is being used. If an athlete feels the anterior thigh during gluteal exercises, they are often overcompensating and using the quadriceps

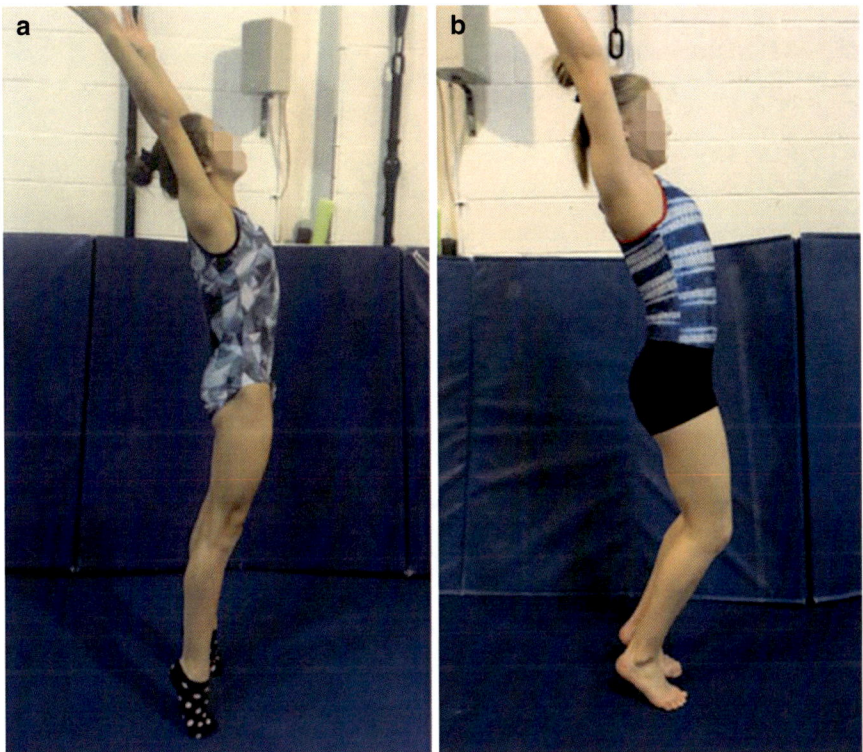

Fig. 12.9 Proper (**a**) and improper (**b**) gluteal activation seen during the "set" or takeoff position of tumbling

muscles in the front instead of the gluteal muscles in the back. If an athlete is unable to open through the hips and fire the gluteal muscles during a jump, they will hinge at the back causing increased pressure and leading to injury. This improper movement and firing pattern are commonly seen in the "set" or takeoff position of tumbling (Fig. 12.9).

Weak gluteal muscles can be caused by tight hamstrings, chronic tight hip flexors, low back pain, and knee injuries. If the pelvis is not in a "neutral" position, then access to gluteal muscles is inhibited. It is important to identify all underlying causes of gluteal inactivation in the rehabilitation process and make sure the gluteal muscles are firing appropriately during gluteal strengthening exercises in the RTP progression by asking the athletes where they feel the workload of the exercise occurring. Gymnasts should feel their gluteal muscles firing first rather than the anterior or lateral leg muscles.

Functional tests appropriate for assessing proper gluteal activation sufficient for RTP are prone hip extension test, single-leg bridge test, single-leg squat test, single-leg balance test, lateral step down test, and star excursion balance test [99–102]. Gymnasts should be able to pass these tests by exhibiting controlled movement without pain before returning to low repetitions of gymnastics skills that require jumping and landing, in addition to extension-based gymnastics skills such as back handsprings, front handsprings, and front layouts.

12.4.5 Lumbopelvic Dissociation

The lumbopelvic-hip complex includes the core, lumbar spine, pelvic girdle, and hip joint. Lumbopelvic dissociation is independent motion about the hips or lumbar spine without directly changing the movements at the other joints. During gymnastics, which requires squatting, jumping, and landing, the concept of lumbopelvic dissociation is very important, especially for FBSI. The hips influence motion at the low back and if hamstring flexibility and pelvic control are lacking, then it is common to see posterior pelvic tilting or lumbopelvic dysfunction with hip flexion activities such as squatting, jumping, and landing. Exercises to help retrain lumbopelvic dissociation should move from a static position to a dynamic multijoint motion. A functional lumbopelvic dissociation progression includes isolated hip movements without associated low back motion starting in supine position and progressing to quadruped, kneeling, squatting, and then jumping and landing positions (Fig. 12.10).

When a gymnast is able to dissociate the hips from the low back in functional movements such as squatting, jumping, and landing, then he/she is ready to return to low repetitions of dismounting and landing higher-level gymnastics skills.

12.4.6 Muscular Endurance

Gymnasts should score a 5/5 on the manual muscle test for all lumbar, thoracic, UE, and LE-related strength tests before beginning the RTP progression [64]. However, this test does not indicate that a gymnast is ready to perform full gymnastics skills as it lacks the endurance component of strength, which is imperative to gymnastics. Research has suggested that reduced endurance of trunk muscles plays an important role in the development of low back pain, lumbar-related injuries, and stress fractures [89, 103, 104]. Therefore, a total fitness program that includes endurance of specific spinal stabilization exercises and general conditioning exercises is important to include.

The Functional Measurement Tool developed by Sleeper et al., discussed in the UE section, can also be used to measure abdominal strength in female [65] and male [66] gymnasts. The rope climb test, the hanging pike test, the agility test, and the STAR excursion balance test can be used as benchmarks for the RTP progression for low back injuries as they give normative values for strength and endurance during functional gymnastics moves (Table 12.10). Other important trunk muscle

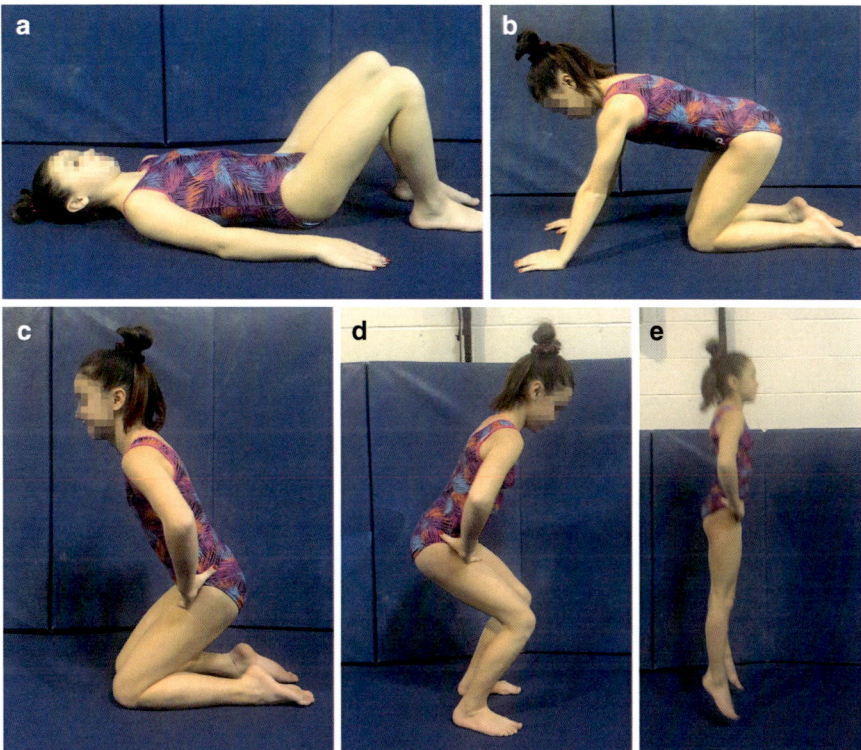

Fig. 12.10 A functional lumbopelvic dissociation progression includes isolated hip movements without associated low back motion in supine (**a**), quadruped (**b**), kneeling (**c**), squatting (**d**), and jumping (**e**)

endurance tests found reliable and effective are the side bridge endurance test, the trunk flexor endurance test, and the trunk extensor test [105, 106]. When a gymnast is able to pass these core endurance tests, he or she is ready to start increasing the number of repetitions of skills performed in practice, in addition to start putting skills together in combinations and routines.

12.4.7 Plyometric Power

Plyometric training exerts maximum force in a short amount of time with a goal of increasing power. These exercises help develop speed, strength, and endurance which is necessary for advancement in the sport. Gymnastics requires plyometric power in tumbling and vaulting; therefore, an enormous amount of speed and power is necessary for acceleration for height and distance. Tumbling runs and sprints to

Table 12.10 Mean scores for functional tests for gymnasts competing between levels 4 and 10 for females [65] and males [66]

	The rope climb test (secs)	The hanging pike test (reps)	Agility test (secs)	The STAR excursion balance test (total distance/leg length *100)
Mean scores (sd) in females [67]	12.40 (6.9)	17.62 (10.6)	19.12 (1.3)	–
Mean scores in males [68]	–	17.8 (10.3)	19.84 (2.1)	767 (89.5)

Adapted from Sleeper et al. [65, 66] and used with permission of the International Journal of Sports Physical Therapy

the vault can be greatly enhanced by improving muscle balance, core strength, and neuromuscular control. For example, a sport-specific physical therapy intervention improved handspring vault performance measures and functional power when added to the habitual training of youth female gymnasts [107]. The additional 2 hours of plyometric training seemingly improved the power generating capacity of movement-specific musculature, which consequently improved aspects of vaulting performance [107].

Maffiuletti et al. suggest that the application of a 12-week plyometric training program with high intensity and loads improves the performance of overhead athletes who perform highly intensive exercises regularly [108]. This type of training should be cautioned in gymnasts with spine injuries until the athlete is completely pain-free and in the strengthening phase. It is only at that point that a plyometric program can be added safely. Excessive increases in intensity, repetitions, or weight during a plyometric session can have detrimental effects on the body leading to further injury if not supervised. Nevertheless, when used correctly, plyometrics are a great tool for creating an increase in explosiveness during a RTP protocol.

One other functional test appropriate for assessing core plyometric power and speed in gymnasts is the medicine ball explosive power test [109, 110] which includes the overhead medicine ball throw test, the side medicine ball throw test, and the trunk flexion medicine ball throw. When gymnasts are able to complete these tests with quality, control, and no complaints of pain, then they are able to continue the progression toward low repetitions of plyometric gymnastics activities such as tumbling, vaulting, and dismounts.

12.4.8 Mechanics of Skill

While advancing through the RTP progression, it is crucial to make sure the form and mechanics of skills are executed correctly [73]. The athlete must be able to take what he or she learned (TFM, corrected posture, gluteal activation, core strength, and ability to dissociate the hips) and transfer it into skill acquisition in

12 Return to Play in Gymnastics

Table 12.11 Skill modifications for extension-based and flexion-based spine injuries

Extension injury	Suggestion	Flexion injury	Suggestion
Bridges	Avoid if possible or perform with legs up on panel mat	Piked stretch	Avoid or perform by bending at the hips and not by rounding the low back
Vault	Have gymnast perform Tsuk-type vault instead of Yurchenko-type vault	Vault	Decrease repetitions of hard landings by utilizing foam pit and soft mats
Floor	Avoid back handsprings and front handsprings in tumbling by doing roundoff directly into skill and doing front tumbling directly from a punch	Floor	Avoid piked skills such as double pikes and choose tucked or layout skills instead. Decrease repetitions of hard landings by utilizing foam pit and soft mats
Beam	Perform a series without back handsprings such as back tuck, back tuck, or aerial layout. Avoid extension-based jumps such as sheep jumps and ring jumps and choose flexion-based jumps such as wolf jump or tuck jumps	Beam	Decrease repetitions of hard landings on dismounts by utilizing foam pit and soft mats. Avoid flexion-based jumps such as wolf or piked jumps, and choose straight jump fulls, tour jete, or split jumps
Bars	Avoid jaeger or hecht release moves, teach Gienger or Ray instead	Bars	Avoid toe-on and stalder skills. Decrease repetitions of dismount landings by utilizing foam pits and soft mats

order to reduce the risk of reinjury. Therefore, a key step in the RTP process after a lumbar injury is to ensure proper form in basic skills, such as a handstand, a bridge, and an overhead squat. Basic form must also be maintained throughout the progression into harder skills such as giants on bars, back walkovers/back handsprings, the set into a tumbling pass, and landing position after a dismount or tumbling pass. Video recordings can be used to assess the mechanics of a skill at a slower rate. When assessing the mechanics, the load of the skill must be shared throughout the entire body (TFM), and there should not be hinging at one segment of the low back for an EBSI. For an FBSI, the athlete should be able to bend at their hips properly while squatting, jumping, landing, and dismounting. If a gymnast has difficulty with proper skill mechanics, then it is advised to structure the routines in a way to avoid high repetitions of extension or flexion skills. Suggestions are stated in Table 12.11. When gymnasts are able to display appropriate mechanics of skill, they are ready to increase the repetitions of the skills they are performing, progress toward combining skills in a routine, and performing the skills in competitions.

In conclusion, there are many factors to consider during the RTP progression of a lumbar spine injury. Gymnasts should be working on their TFM, posture, core strength, gluteal strength, and lumbopelvic dissociation throughout the rehabilitation phase and should continue to work on these areas during the RTP phase. When creating the RTP program, make sure to consider appropriate muscular endurance, plyometric power, and mechanics of skill. As these areas start to improve, the gymnast's skill level and number of repetitions of skills can start to progress as well.

12.5 RTP After Lower Extremity (LE) Injuries

Developing a RTP progression for LE injuries in gymnastics is important since LE injuries make up 60% of all gymnastics injuries [111]. Clinicians and coaches responsible for the RTP protocol should be cognizant of the forces that occur during recovery [112]. Once the injury has healed and the athlete has been cleared by the medical team to start the RTP progression in the gym, the following areas must be understood and integrated into the RTP program: LE weight-bearing progression, LE range of motion and mobility, LE strength and stability, muscular endurance, plyometric power, and mechanics of skill.

12.5.1 Lower Extremity Weight-Bearing Progression

A common RTP error is immediate return to high-impact training. Gymnasts should not be permitted to begin their RTP with an immediate return to takeoffs, landings, and dismounts. Tissues must gradually adapt to the high-impact demands of skills, and the proper foundation for skills must be reestablished to prevent reinjury. There must be a functional weight-bearing progression in place, with each successive progression being pain-free. A functional LE weight-bearing progression involves standing, squatting, forward step up, forward step down, running, jumping up, jumping down, and rebounding. Throughout these weight-bearing progressions, the athlete may be challenged in the following ways:

1. With eyes open and eyes closed
2. Using a stable surface and a nonstable surface (such as foam, trampoline, or Bosu ball)
3. From bilateral LE weight-bearing to tandem stance (beam stance) to unilateral LE weight-bearing (single-leg stance, single-leg squat, etc.)
4. Moving in the sagittal plane (forward and back) to the frontal plane (side to side) to multiplanar directions (diagonal positions, jump with turns, etc.)
5. Increasing endurance, time of weight-bearing, and repetitions
6. Increasing speed, power, and plyometric activity in each position

Sweeney et al. have developed a detailed return to gymnastics skill progression for LE injuries for female (Table 12.12) and male gymnasts (Table 12.13) that correlates well with the above functional weight-bearing progression [1].

Clinicians, coaches, parents, and athletes must remember that every LE injury is different, and the same injury may be unique in each athlete. As such, there is no

Table 12.12 Return to gymnastics skill progression for LE injuries for females [1]

Step	Vault	Uneven bars	Balance beam	Floor	Tumble track
Women: Lower extremity *impact-related pathology*					
1		Strap bar and pit bar without dismounts Basic skills on regular bars	Balance work Turns Straight jumps with good landing technique	Turns and low-impact choreography Straight jumps with good landing technique	Jumps Basic tumbling passes with landing in pit/resi-mat
2		Dismounts into pit All swinging skills	Low beam jumps and leaps Low beam cartwheels, handstands, and walkovers	Leaps and jumps Roundoff back handsprings Front handsprings (use rod floor if possible)[e]	Standing individual skills (handsprings, tucks, etc.) Twisting skills
3	Run-throughs	Release moves over pit	High beam: Balance work, jumps, and leaps; Cartwheels, handstands, and walkovers Floor beam: flight series with hands	Individual skills Roundoff back handsprings to single salto[a] onto soft mat Front handsprings and front saltos[a]	Double salto[a] skills on soft mat
4	Limited volume running and board drills Handspring and Tsuk[c] timers	Low-level dismount to mat in the pit Release moves (with spotter as needed)	Tumbling (acro) series on low beam	Basic tumbling/twisting skills onto regular floor Front tumbling passes	
5	Yurchenko[d] timers	Full dismount to mat in pit Single salto[c] dismount to regular landing mat	High beam tumbling (acro) series Dismounts into pit/resi-mat	Double saltos[a]	
6	Flipping onto soft mat without twists	Dismounts onto regular mats	Dismounts onto regular mats	Full progression	
7	Full vault onto regular mat	Front giant[b] Pirouetting skills			
Women: Lower extremity *stability-related pathology*					
1		Strap bar and pit bar; no dismounts Basic skills on regular bars	Balance work Turns Jumps with 2-foot landings without turns Handstands, cartwheels, and walkovers	Leaps and jumps without turns Standing back handsprings	Jumps Jump to firm surface with good landing technique

(continued)

Table 12.12 (continued)

Step	Vault	Uneven bars	Balance beam	Floor	Tumble track
2		Non-twisting dismounts to regular mat	Low beam single-leg landing leaps Back and front handsprings	Front handsprings Roundoff back handsprings	
3	Run-throughs	Increasing difficulty of skills, spotted if needed to avoid unstable landings	High beam balance Skills, jumps, and leaps Tumbling (acro) series on low beam	Single saltos[a] without twisting on regular floor	
4	Tsuk[c], handspring, and Yurchenko[d] timers to back	Progress to regular dismounts and release moves	Tumbling (acro) series on high beam Roundoff rebound off beam	Basic twisting and double saltos[a] skills	
5	Basic flipping vaults (no twisting)	Increasing difficulty of skills and dismounts with twisting	Dismounts without twisting to regular mat	Gradually increase to full skills	
6	Full vaults		Twisting dismounts		

[a]Salto: A front or back flip without hands in a tuck, pike, or straight position
[b]Giants: Circling backward or forward around the bar with the body extended straight in a handstand position
[c]Tsuk: (Tsukahara) A vault in which the gymnast hits the springboard, then does a half-turn (roundoff) onto the vault, and then flips backward off the vault
[d]Yurchenko: A vault in which the gymnast does a roundoff onto the board, then jumps backward onto her hands on the vault, and then flips backward off the vault
[e]Rod floor: A rod floor is slightly bouncier and has more compliance than a competitive floor, but has less compliance than a tumble track or a trampoline

guideline or time component related to how quickly or slowly to move through these functional progressions. Quality is more important than quantity, and therefore, control, stability, and lack of pain are the guide to progressing.

12.5.2 Lower Extremity Mobility

Whether the athlete endures an ankle, a knee, or a hip injury, mobility of the entire LE complex must be taken into consideration. Restoration of AROM and PROM in open chain and closed chain of the entire LE is necessary as body segments are interdependent.

12 Return to Play in Gymnastics

Table 12.13 Return to gymnastics skill progression for LE injuries for males [1]

Step	Floor	Pommel horse	Rings	Vault	Parallel bars	High bar	Tumble track
Men: Lower extremity *impact-related pathology*							
1	Flare/circle[b], and handstand skills Straight jumps with good landing technique	Basics without dismounts	Basics without dismounts Strength skills		Basics without dismounts	Strap bar and pit bar basics without dismounts	Jumps Roundoff back handsprings (add single salto[a]) Front handsprings
2	Jumps with good landing technique Roundoff back handsprings Front handsprings	Full skills with dismounts	Full-swing skills Dismounts into pit		Full-swing work Dismounts into pit	Full-swing skills Release moves over pit Dismounts into pit	Standing skills (back handsprings, tucks) Twisting saltos[a]
3	Standing back handspring and tucks Add single saltos[a] to tumbling passes onto a soft mat		Basic dismounts onto regular mat	Run through	Basic dismounts onto regular mat		Add double salto[a] skills onto soft mat
	Twisting saltos[c] All front tumbling			Handsprings and Tsuk[c] timers		Dismounts onto mat in pit	
5	Double saltos[a]		Full dismounts	Yurchenko[d] timers	Releases and dismounts without twisting	Basic dismounts onto regular mat	
6				Flip vault onto soft mat without twisting	Twisting releases and dismounts	Full dismounts	
7				Vault to regular mat			

(continued)

Table 12.13 (continued)

Step	Floor	Pommel horse	Rings	Vault	Parallel bars	High bar	Tumble track
Men: Lower extremity *stability-related pathology*							
1	Jumps with good landing technique Standing back handsprings	Basic skills without dismounts	Basic skills without dismounts		Basic skills without dismounts	Strap bar and pit bar basics without dismounts	Jump to firm surface with good landing technique
2	Front handsprings Roundoff back handsprings Standing back tucks	All skills with dismounts	Basic (no twisting) dismounts to regular mat More difficult skills (spot as needed)		More difficult skills (spot as needed)	Basic (no twisting) dismounts to pit Releases over pit	
3	Single, non-twisting saltos[a]			Run through	Basic (no twisting) dismounts to regular mat	More difficult skills (spot as needed) Full releases	Twisting and double salto[a] skills to firm surface
4	Basic twisting and double saltos[a] skills		Double salto dismounts	Tsuk[c], handspring and Yurchenko[d], timers	More difficult dismounts	Dismounts to mat without twisting	
5	More difficult tumbling passes		Twisting dismounts	Flip vaults without twisting		Dismounts with twisting	
6				Regular vault			

[a]Salto: A front or back flip without hands in a tuck, pike, or straight position
[b]Flare/circle: Gymnast circles legs around torso/shoulders while weight-bearing only on the hands
[c]Tsuk: (Tsukahara) A vault in which the gymnast hits the springboard, then does a half-turn (roundoff) onto the vault, and then flips backward off the vault
[d]Yurchenko: A vault in which the gymnast does a roundoff onto the board, then jumps backward onto his hands on the vault, and then flips backward off the vault

For example, lack of full ankle dorsiflexion will lead to excessive foot pronation [113], which will lead to increased knee valgus position, increased medial knee displacement, and increased quadriceps activation. This faulty movement pattern will put the athlete at risk for reinjury and/or future injuries, as research supports that lack of ankle dorsiflexion in impact sports can lead to ankle, Achilles, lower leg, knee, and hip injuries [113–122]. In addition, proper hip mobility is important for open kinetic chain splits, split leaps, walkovers, jumps, setting for a tumbling pass, as well as aesthetically pleasing airborne

Table 12.14 Normative values specific to male and female gymnasts for the UE joints [34, 129, 130]

Motion	ROM (open chain)	ROM (closed chain)
Great toe extension	90°	90°+
Ankle dorsiflexion	15°	45+
Ankle plantar flexion	75–90°	NA
Knee flexion	140–150°	Approximation of leg to thigh
Knee extension	0°	0°
Hip flexion	Thigh to torso	NA
Hip extension	20–40°	NA
Hip external rotation	75°	N/A
Hip internal rotation	45–65°	N/A
Hip flexor flexibility	(−) Thomas Test, 0° degrees of hip extension	Ability to maintain neutral pelvis (0° hip extension) in standing

positions. Researchers note that a lack of lumbopelvic-hip stability (especially hip extension and external rotation) or uneven hip mobility can place the athlete at risk for lumbar, sacral, hip, and knee injuries [123–127].

It is imperative to restore normative motion specific to male and female gymnasts for the LE joints. Gymnasts have different requirements for LE range of motion than standardized normative values for a generic population due to the demands of their sport [128]. Table 12.14 presents normative values specific to healthy male and female gymnasts for the LE joints. When these range of motion values are obtained, the gymnast will have the appropriate range of motion to move his/her LE through the air in non-weight-bearing positions. This means a gymnast can start performing swinging skills on bars, pommel horse, or rings, and other skills that do not require weight-bearing through the LE such as press handstands. For some LE injuries, athletes may be able to start these skills prior to having full motion (e.g., a gymnast may be able to perform giants if wearing a lace-up ankle brace after a mild sprain as long as this skill has previously been mastered). However, it is important to be mindful that each LE injury and athlete is unique and simply having full motion does not mean that the athlete is ready for full RTP status. In addition, the risk of fall or awkward landing must be accounted for when progressing athletes back to LE non-weight-bearing skills.

12.5.3 Lower Extremity Strength and Stability

When discussing the stability of the LE, the role of the core, hip, knee, and foot has a pivotal role in the RTP progression. For the athlete to have achieved optimal muscle strength, he/she must demonstrate strength and control of the LE in functional

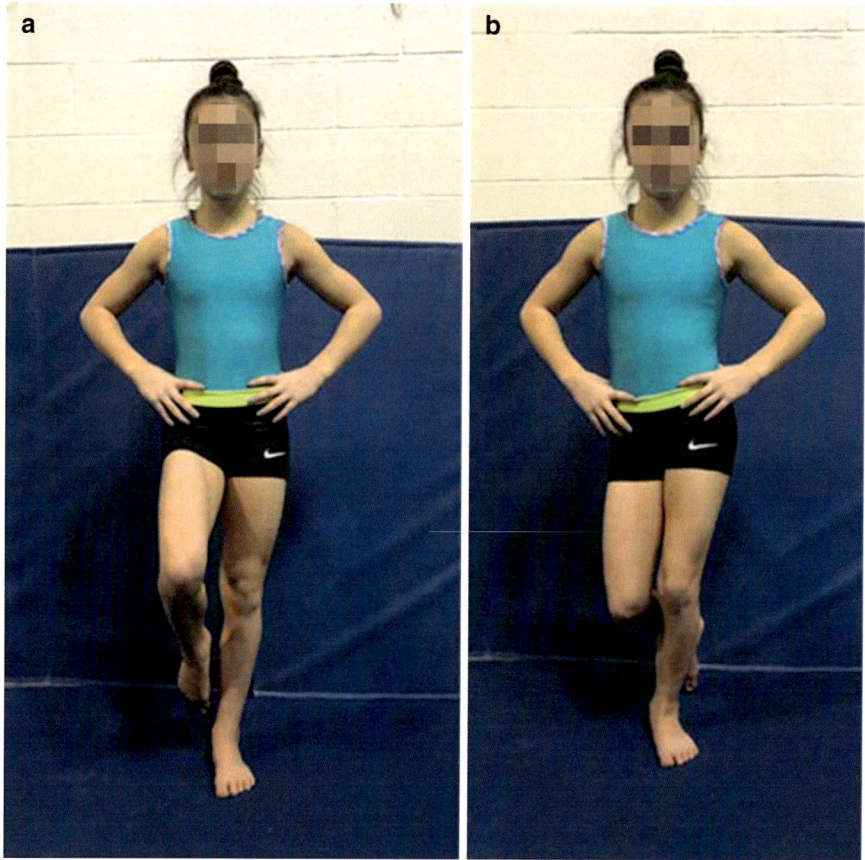

Fig. 12.11 Single-leg balance with proper alignment (**a**) and nonoptimal alignment (**b**) with pronated foot, valgus knee, internally rotated femur, and anteriorly pelvic tilt

activities. Proper alignment as seen in a single-leg stance (Fig. 12.11) must be achieved from the feet up to the hips no matter what LE injury occurred. During the RTP progression, it is common to see a gymnast with pronated feet, valgus knees, hyperextended knees, internally rotated femurs, and anterior pelvic tilt. These deficits occur due to a lack of stability and strength in multiple areas of the LE. Focus should be placed on building the strength and stability of all these combined joints, in addition to regaining proper strength ratios in opposing muscle groups such as the quadriceps to hamstring strength ratio [123].

Core stability and gluteal strength have been discussed multiple times in this chapter, and they are equally important in relation to LE injuries. Many studies have cited a relationship between core weakness and risk for LE injury and/or reinjury [124, 131–133] and gluteal weakness and its impact on knee control and LE injury [123, 133–135]. Core stability and gluteal strength both assist in maintaining a neutral pelvis during single-leg stance. Further, research has shown that when pelvic alignment is not maintained during functional activities, then there is a greater chance of injury and/or reinjury [133, 136]. Therefore, core stability and gluteal strength must be regained before the initiation of RTP.

Knee strength and stability can be observed during single-leg stance positions. When greater than zero degrees of knee extension (or hyperextension) is observed, measures should be taken to encourage the gymnast to stand, walk, run, and land with "soft" knees and avoid locking the knees out into end range motion. Unmediated hyperextended knees result in excessive forces on joint surfaces and ligamentous structures. Increased knee extension is also commonly associated with pelvic rotation anomalies that can impact distribution of injurious forces up the kinetic chain. Other abnormal knee alignments such as valgus knees can also be seen in the single-leg stance position. Most of the time, this position stems from weakness in the hips, quadriceps, or feet and needs to be corrected. Lastly, optimal quadriceps to hamstring strength ratios must be obtained in a gymnast as quadriceps dominance predisposes athletes to knee injuries. Thus, it is prudent to incorporate strength and conditioning programs targeting the hamstring in the RTP for LE [137–139].

Foot strength and stability is evident by the ability to maintain an arch under increasing weight-bearing forces without collapsing into pronation. Abnormal pronation causes increased knee valgus, increased hip internal rotation position, and increased anterior pelvic tilt. This change in position leads to greater mean peak forces through the joints of the LE during gymnastics skill landings. Increases in peak forces through nonoptimal LE alignment place the foot, ankle, knee, hip, and back at risk for reinjury or future injury [140–143]. Therefore, regaining foot stability and strength is important in RTP of the LE.

Functional tests appropriate for assessing LE strength and stability are the STAR excursion balance test, squat test, single-leg balance test, and step down test with a focus of maintaining equal pelvis height, soft knees, proper knee alignment, and foot control [144–147]. Gymnasts should pass these tests before returning to non-plyometric LE weight-bearing skills such as handstands, cartwheels, and back walkovers, and before returning to running and jumping.

12.5.4 Muscular Endurance

Gymnasts should score a 5/5 on the manual muscle test [64] for all LE strength tests before beginning the RTP progression. Manual muscle testing is a basic way to determine that the gymnast has recovered strength sufficient for daily activities. It is also a good test to indicate if a gymnast is ready to start performing progressive weight-bearing strengthening exercises. However, as described previously, this test does not indicate that a gymnast is ready to perform full gymnastics skills, as it lacks the functional weight-bearing and endurance component of strength, which is imperative in gymnastics. A floor routine may last up to 90 seconds, which requires not only strength but also endurance of the LE muscles. For this reason, the RTP protocol for LE must progressively build muscle endurance in non-weight-bearing and weight-bearing positions.

There are multiple ways to challenge the body to meet muscular endurance goals by increasing resistance, increasing repetitions, or decreasing rest between sets. LE strength and conditioning circuits should be developed with gymnastics-specific exercises included in the circuit. The circuit should last for the duration of a floor routine and include endurance type and plyometric type exercises with small rests between each exercise. Special tests for LE endurance include 30 single-leg heel raises, 30 single-leg supine bridges, 30 single-leg squat test, 30-second endurance jump test, 30-second quadrant jump test, multistage hurdle jump test, and 30 repetitions of the STAR excursion balance test [148]. These tests can be used as benchmarks for the RTP protocol of gymnasts as they help give normative values for strength and endurance during functional gymnastics moves. When a gymnast can pass these fitness tests, it shows he/she is ready to start increasing the number of repetitions of skills performed in practice, in addition to start putting skills together in combinations.

12.5.5 Plyometric Power

Return to full gymnastics participation requires repetitive jumping, landing, and rebounding requiring involvement of the entire LE chain. Ensuring that the gymnast has the power and control to execute symmetrical jumping and landings is critical to the success of a RTP for LE [149, 150]. Plyometric power exercise progressions and plyometric power tests should also be incorporated into the LE RTP progression.

In preparation for tumbling and apparatus landings, a jump progression should be included in the RTP process [151]. The jump progression may include:

1. Jumping up progressive heights (up to 36 inches) with proper landing mechanics
2. Jumping down forward, backward, and sideways from progressive heights (up to 48 inches) with proper landing mechanics
3. Single-leg jumping up progressive heights (up to 18 inches) with proper landing mechanics
4. Single-leg jumping down progressive heights (up to 12 inches) with proper landing mechanics

Once steps 1–4 are completed, the gymnast should repeat the steps and may also add a backward or forward flipping component with proper landing mechanics. Next, the gymnast should add a twisting component with proper landing mechanics, and finally, the gymnast should add a rebound component from progressive heights. When the athlete has completed these steps with safe and appropriate landing mechanics [150], he/she can return to tumbling, vaulting, and dismounting skills in a progressive manner.

Other functional tests appropriate for assessing plyometric power are single-leg hop test, triple hop test, agility test [65, 66], 20-yard sprint test [65, 66], and vertical jump test [152]. When a gymnast can complete the jump progression, in addition to the functional tests, with quality control and no complaints of pain, he/she can continue the progression toward LE plyometric gymnastics activities such as tumbling and vaulting.

12.5.6 Mechanics of Skill

RTP protocols are challenging as multiple factors contribute to a successful outcome. Even though a gymnast might have demonstrated perfect step down, squatting, and jumping mechanics with proper hip, knee, and foot control, he/she must also be able to demonstrate this control during skill performance such as landing a layout step-out on beam, landing a tumbling pass on floor, or a skill on vault. If the root problem is improper skill acquisition and this has not been addressed during the RTP protocol, then the repetitive motion of that skill will lead to future injury or reinjury. The athlete and coach should consider the time of rehabilitation to relearn LE movement patterns and skill acquisitions with special attention on jumping, leaps, tumbling, and dismounts. When mechanics of skill are consistent, then gymnasts are ready to combine skills in practice and work toward competition.

12.6 Conclusion

In conclusion, there are many factors to consider during the RTP progression after an UE, back, or LE injury or after a concussion. Gymnasts should be working on their core strength, flexibility, strength, and stability throughout their rehabilitation phase and should continue to work on these areas during the RTP phase. When creating the RTP program, proper weight-bearing progressions, as well as strength and stability, appropriate muscular endurance, proper plyometric power progression, and appropriately learned mechanics of skills are all incorporated. As these areas start to improve, the athlete's skill level and repetitions of skills can start to progress as well.

Understanding the many changing rules and demands of gymnastics is crucial when creating a RTP program for gymnasts. Clinicians should be guided by the basic principles of restoration of the injured tissue, developing the ability of restored tissue to withstand the rigors of gymnastics, and the readiness of the gymnast to return to competition. More effort must be placed in creating safe and effective RTP protocols that incorporate the different injuries and apparatuses seen in gymnastics. Research must be done frequently given the changes in the Code of Points every 4 years. For now, clinicians, coaches, and gymnasts must be able to dictate a plan with clear guidelines on navigating through the stepwise process of a RTP progression. Clear communication between medical providers, coaches, athletes, and parents is necessary in order to make any necessary changes or adaptations to the RTP protocol based on day-to-day performance and ability of the athlete.

References

1. Sweeney EA, Howell DR, James DA, Potter MN, Provance AJ. Returning to sport after gymnastics injuries. Curr Sports Med Rep. 2018;17:376–90. https://doi.org/10.1249/JSR.0000000000000533.
2. Sands WA. Injury prevention in women's gymnastics. Sports Med. 2000;30:359–73. https://doi.org/10.2165/00007256-200030050-00004.
3. Wade M, Campbell A, Smith A, Norcott J, O'Sullivan P. Investigation of spinal posture signatures and ground reaction forces during landing in elite female gymnasts. J Appl Biomech. 2012;28:677–86.
4. Kruse D, Lemmen B. Spine injuries in the sport of gymnastics. Curr Sports Med Rep. 2009;8:20–8. https://doi.org/10.1249/JSR.0b013e3181967ca6.
5. Ardern CL, Glasgow P, Schneiders A, Witvrouw E, Clarsen B, Cools A, et al. 2016 Consensus statement on return to sport from the First World Congress in Sports Physical Therapy, Bern. Br J Sports Med. 2016;50:853–64. https://doi.org/10.1136/bjsports-2016-096278.
6. Fournier M. Principles of rehabilitation and return to sports following injury. Clin Podiatr Med Surg. 2015;32:261–8. https://doi.org/10.1016/j.cpm.2014.11.009.
7. Sclafani MP, Davis CC. Return to play progression for rugby following injury to the lower extremity: a clinical commentary and review of the literature. Int J Sports Phys Ther. 2016;11:302–20.
8. McCrory P, Meeuwisse W, Dvorak J, Aubry M, Bailes J, Broglio S, et al. Consensus statement on concussion in sport—the 5th international conference on concussion in sport held in Berlin, October 2016. Br J Sports Med. 2017;51:838–47. https://doi.org/10.1136/bjsports-2017-097699.
9. Hsu C-J, Meierbachtol A, George SZ, Chmielewski TL. Fear of reinjury in athletes. Sports Health. 2016;9:162–7. https://doi.org/10.1177/1941738116666813.
10. Podlog L, Dimmock J, Miller J. A review of return to sport concerns following injury rehabilitation: practitioner strategies for enhancing recovery outcomes. Phys Ther Sport. 2011;12:36–42. https://doi.org/10.1016/j.ptsp.2010.07.005.
11. Collins MW, Kontos AP, Okonkwo DO, Almquist J, Bailes J, Barisa M, et al. Concussion is Treatable: Statements of Agreement from the Targeted Evaluation and Active Management (TEAM) Approaches to Treating Concussion Meeting held in Pittsburgh, October 15–16, 2015. Neurosurgery. 2016;79:912–29. https://doi.org/10.1227/NEU.0000000000001447.
12. Grool AM, Aglipay M, Momoli F, Meehan WP, Freedman SB, Yeates KO, et al. Association between early participation in physical activity following acute concussion and persistent postconcussive symptoms in children and adolescents. JAMA. 2016;316:2504–14. https://doi.org/10.1001/jama.2016.17396.
13. Meske S, Hazzard JB, Ni M, Hanson T, Van Horn L, Smith J. The prevalence of traumatic brain injury and on-campus service utilization among undergraduate students. J Head Trauma Rehabil. 2019;34:E18. https://doi.org/10.1097/HTR.0000000000000407.
14. Leddy JJ, Baker JG, Willer B. Active rehabilitation of concussion and post-concussion syndrome. Phys Med Rehabil Clin N Am. 2016;27:437–54. https://doi.org/10.1016/j.pmr.2015.12.003.
15. May KH, Marshall DL, Burns TG, Popoli DM, Polikandriotis JA. Pediatric sports specific return to play guidelines following concussion. Int J Sports Phys Ther. 2014;9:242–55.

16. Corwin DJ, Wiebe DJ, Zonfrillo MR, Grady MF, Robinson RL, Goodman AM, et al. Vestibular deficits following youth concussion. J Pediatr. 2015;166:1221–5. https://doi.org/10.1016/j.jpeds.2015.01.039.
17. Zuckerman SL, Brett BL, Jeckell AS, Yengo-Kahn AM, Solomon GS. Prognostic factors in pediatric sport-related concussion. Curr Neurol Neurosci Rep. 2018;18:104. https://doi.org/10.1007/s11910-018-0909-4.
18. Park K, Ksiazek T, Olson B. Effectiveness of vestibular rehabilitation therapy for treatment of concussed adolescents with persistent symptoms of dizziness and imbalance. J Sport Rehabil. 2018;27:485–90. https://doi.org/10.1123/jsr.2016-0222.
19. Beidler E, Bretzin AC, Hanock C, Covassin T. Sport-related concussion: knowledge and reporting behaviors among collegiate club-sport athletes. J Athl Train. 2018;53:866–72. https://doi.org/10.4085/1062-6050-266-17.
20. Vaughan CG, Gerst EH, Sady MD, Newman JB, Gioia GA. The relation between testing environment and baseline performance in child and adolescent concussion assessment. Am J Sports Med. 2014;42:1716–23. https://doi.org/10.1177/0363546514531732.
21. Bonci CM, Bonci LJ, Granger LR, Johnson CL, Malina RM, Milne LW, et al. National athletic trainers' association position statement: preventing, detecting, and managing disordered eating in athletes. J Athl Train. 2008;43:80–108.
22. Meier TB, Brummel BJ, Singh R, Nerio CJ, Polanski DW, Bellgowan PSF. The under-reporting of self-reported symptoms following sports-related concussion. J Sci Med Sport. 2015;18:507–11. https://doi.org/10.1016/j.jsams.2014.07.008.
23. Caine DJ. Injury epidemiology. Sci Asp Womens Gymnast. 2003;45:72–109. https://doi.org/10.1159/000067494.
24. Meeusen R, Borms J. Gymnastic Injuries. Sports Med. 1992;13:337–56. https://doi.org/10.2165/00007256-199213050-00004.
25. Kegerreis S. The construction and implementation of functional progressions as a component of athletic rehabilitation. J Orthop Sports Phys Ther. 1983;5:14–9. https://doi.org/10.2519/jospt.1983.5.1.14.
26. Andrew TL. Closed kinetic chain exercise. A comprehensive guide to multiple-joint exercises. J Chiropr Med. 2002;1:200. https://doi.org/10.1016/S0899-3467(07)60039-1.
27. McLaren K, Byrd E, Herzog M, Polikandriotis JA, Willimon SC. Impact shoulder angles correlate with impact wrist angles in standing back handsprings in preadolescent and adolescent female gymnasts. Int J Sports Phys Ther. 2015;10:341–6.
28. Bahr R, Engebretsen L, IOC Medical Commission, editors. Sports injury prevention. Chichester, UK/Hoboken, NJ: Wiley-Blackwell; 2009.
29. Sands WA, Shultz BB, Newman AP. Women's gymnastics injuries. A 5-year study. Am J Sports Med. 1993;21:271–6. https://doi.org/10.1177/036354659302100218.
30. Nelson NG, Metzing M. Joint mobility and force application during the thrust phase of the front handspring on floor exercise. ISBS - Conf Proc Arch 1994;1.
31. Wadley GH, Albright JP. Women's intercollegiate gymnastics. Injury patterns and "permanent" medical disability. Am J Sports Med. 1993;21:314–20. https://doi.org/10.1177/036354659302100224.
32. Berryman, Reese N, Bandy WD. Joint range of motion and muscle length testing. 3rd ed. St. Louis, MO: Elsevier; 2017.
33. Guerra MRV, Estelles JRD, Abdouni YA, Falcochio DF, Rosa JRP, Catani LH. Frequency of wrist growth plate injury in young gymnasts at a training center. Acta Ortop Bras. 2016;24:204–7. https://doi.org/10.1590/1413-785220162404157422.
34. Pongetti Angeletti G. Gymnastics medicine for you. Gina Pongetti Angeletti and MedGym LLC; 2012
35. Sands WA. Lowering to a back bend. Technique. 1994;14:8.
36. Horsley I, Herrington L, Hoyle R, Prescott E, Bellamy N. Do changes in hand grip strength correlate with shoulder rotator cuff function? Shoulder Elbow. 2016;8:124–9. https://doi.org/10.1177/1758573215626103.

37. Mandalidis D, O'Brien M. Relationship between hand-grip isometric strength and isokinetic moment data of the shoulder stabilisers. J Bodyw Mov Ther. 2010;14:19–26. https://doi.org/10.1016/j.jbmt.2008.05.001.
38. Balogun JA, Akomolafe CT, Amusa LO. Grip strength: effects of testing posture and elbow position. Arch Phys Med Rehabil. 1991;72:280–3.
39. Alizadehkhaiyat O, Fisher AC, Kemp GJ, Vishwanathan K, Frostick SP. Shoulder muscle activation and fatigue during a controlled forceful hand grip task. J Electromyogr Kinesiol. 2011;21:478–82. https://doi.org/10.1016/j.jelekin.2011.03.002.
40. Mathiowetz V, Weber K, Volland G, Kashman N. Reliability and validity of grip and pinch strength evaluations. J Hand Surg. 1984;9:222–6.
41. Petersen P, Petrick M, Connor H, Conklin D. Grip strength and hand dominance: challenging the 10% rule. Am J Occup Ther. 1989;43:444–7.
42. Weiss JM. Hypermobility and specific joint pathology in young competitive gymnasts; n.d., p. 49.
43. Myers TW. Anatomy trains: myofascial meridians for manual and movement therapists. 3rd ed. Edinburgh, Churchill Livingstone; 2014.
44. Cook G, Burton L, Kiesel K, Rose G, Byrant MF. Movement functional movement systems: screening, assessment, corrective strategies. 1st ed. Santa Cruz, CA: On Target Publications; 2011.
45. Sahrmann S. Diagnosis and treatment of movement impairment syndromes. 1st ed. St. Louis, MO: Mosby; 2001.
46. Tucci HT, Martins J, Sposito G de C, Camarini PMF, de Oliveira AS. Closed Kinetic Chain Upper Extremity Stability test (CKCUES test): a reliability study in persons with and without shoulder impingement syndrome. BMC Musculoskelet Disord. 2014;15(1) https://doi.org/10.1186/1471-2474-15-1.
47. Westrick RB, Miller JM, Carow SD, Gerber JP. Exploration of the y-balance test for assessment of upper quarter closed kinetic chain performance. Int J Sports Phys Ther. 2012;7:139–47.
48. Huxel Bliven KC, Anderson BE. Core stability training for injury prevention. Sports Health. 2013;5:514–22. https://doi.org/10.1177/1941738113481200.
49. Silfies SP, Ebaugh D, Pontillo M, Butowicz CM. Critical review of the impact of core stability on upper extremity athletic injury and performance. Braz J Phys Ther. 2015;19:360–8. https://doi.org/10.1590/bjpt-rbf.2014.0108.
50. Radwan A, Francis J, Green A, Kahl E, Maciurzynski D, Quartulli A, et al. Is there a relation between shoulder dysfunction and core instability? Int J Sports Phys Ther. 2014;9:8–13.
51. Kibler WB, Press J, Sciascia A. The role of core stability in athletic function. Sports Med. 2006;36:189–98.
52. Burkhart SS, Morgan CD, Kibler WB. The disabled throwing shoulder: spectrum of pathology part I: pathoanatomy and biomechanics. Arthrosc J Arthrosc Relat Surg. 2003;19:404–20. https://doi.org/10.1053/jars.2003.50128.
53. Davies GJ, Dickoff-Hoffman S. Neuromuscular testing and rehabilitation of the shoulder complex. J Orthop Sports Phys Ther. 1993;18:449–58. https://doi.org/10.2519/jospt.1993.18.2.449.
54. Kibler BW, Sciascia A. Kinetic chain contributions to elbow function and dysfunction in sports. Clin Sports Med. 2004;23:545–52, viii. https://doi.org/10.1016/j.csm.2004.04.010.
55. Meister K. Injuries to the shoulder in the throwing athlete. Part one: biomechanics/pathophysiology/classification of injury. Am J Sports Med. 2000;28:265–75. https://doi.org/10.1177/03635465000280022301.
56. Kibler WB, Sciascia A. Current concepts: scapular dyskinesis. Br J Sports Med. 2010;44:300–5. https://doi.org/10.1136/bjsm.2009.058834.
57. Paine R, Voight ML. The role of the scapula. Int J Sports Phys Ther. 2013;8:617–29.
58. Paine RM, Voight M. The role of the scapula. J Orthop Sports Phys Ther. 1993;18:386–91. https://doi.org/10.2519/jospt.1993.18.1.386.

59. Cools AM, Geerooms E, Van den Berghe DFM, Cambier DC, Witvrouw EE. Isokinetic scapular muscle performance in young elite gymnasts. J Athl Train. 2007;42: 458–63.
60. Krause DA, Youdas JW, Hollman JH, Smith J. Abdominal muscle performance as measured by the double leg-lowering test. Arch Phys Med Rehabil. 2005;86:1345–8. https://doi.org/10.1016/j.apmr.2004.12.020.
61. Latimer J, Maher CG, Refshauge K, Colaco I. The reliability and validity of the Biering–Sorensen test in asymptomatic subjects and subjects reporting current or previous nonspecific low Back pain. Spine. 1999;24:2085.
62. McGill SM, Childs A, Liebenson C. Endurance times for low back stabilization exercises: clinical targets for testing and training from a normal database. Arch Phys Med Rehabil. 1999;80:941–4. https://doi.org/10.1016/S0003-9993(99)90087-4.
63. Tong TK, Wu S, Nie J. Sport-specific endurance plank test for evaluation of global core muscle function. Phys Ther Sport. 2014;15:58–63. https://doi.org/10.1016/j.ptsp.2013.03.003.
64. Cuthbert SC, Goodheart GJ. On the reliability and validity of manual muscle testing: a literature review. Chiropr Osteopat. 2007;15:4. https://doi.org/10.1186/1746-1340-15-4.
65. Sleeper MD, Kenyon LK, Casey E. Measuring fitness in female gymnasts: the gymnastics functional measurement tool. Int J Sports Phys Ther. 2012;7(2):124–38.
66. Sleeper MD, Kenyon LK, Elliott JM, Cheng MS. Measuring sport-specific physical abilities in male gymnasts: the men's gymnastics functional measurement tool. Int J Sports Phys Ther. 2016;11(7):1082–100.
67. Penitente G, Merni F, Sands W. Kinematic analysis of the centre of mass in the back handspring: a case study. Gym Coach. 2011;4:1–11.
68. Penitente G, Sands WA. Exploratory investigation of impact loads during the forward handspring vault. J Hum Kinet. 2015;46:59–68. https://doi.org/10.1515/hukin-2015-0034.
69. Hogarth LW, Deakin G, Sinclair W. Are plyometric push-ups a reliable power assessment tool? JASC. 2013;21:4.
70. Falsone SA, Gross MT, Guskiewicz KM, Schneider RA. One-arm hop test: reliability and effects of arm dominance. J Orthop Sports Phys Ther. 2002;32:98–103. https://doi.org/10.2519/jospt.2002.32.3.98.
71. Harris C, Wattles AP, DeBeliso M, Sevene-Adams PG, Berning JM, Adams KJ. The seated medicine ball throw as a test of upper body power in older adults. J Strength Cond Res. 2011;25:2344. https://doi.org/10.1519/JSC.0b013e3181ecd27b.
72. Negrete RJ, Hanney WJ, Kolber MJ, Davies GJ, Ansley MK, McBride AB, et al. Reliability, minimal detectable change, and normative values for tests of upper extremity function and power. J Strength Cond Res. 2010;24:3318–25. https://doi.org/10.1519/JSC.0b013e3181e7259c.
73. Zetaruk MN. The young gymnast. Clin Sports Med. 2000;19:757–80. https://doi.org/10.1016/S0278-5919(05)70236-2.
74. Caine D, Cochrane B, Caine C, Zemper E. An epidemiologic investigation of injuries affecting young competitive female gymnasts. Am J Sports Med. 1989;17:811–20. https://doi.org/10.1177/036354658901700616.
75. Hall SJ. Mechanical contribution to lumbar stress injuries in female gymnasts. Med Sci Sports Exerc. 1986;18:599–602.
76. Kujala UM, Taimela S, Oksanen A, Salminen JJ. Lumbar mobility and low back pain during adolescence. A longitudinal three-year follow-up study in athletes and controls. Am J Sports Med. 1997;25:363–8. https://doi.org/10.1177/036354659702500316.
77. Caine DJ, Maffulli N. Epidemiology of children's individual sports injuries. An important area of medicine and sport science research. Med Sport Sci. 2005;48:1–7. https://doi.org/10.1159/000084274.

78. Panzer V, Wood GA, Bates BT, Mason BR. Lower extremity loads in landings of elite gymnasts. In: de Groot G, et al., editors. Biomechanics XI-B. Amsterdam: Free University Press; 1988. p. 727–35.
79. Kerr ZY, Hayden R, Barr M, Klossner DA, Dompier TP. Epidemiology of National Collegiate Athletic Association Women's Gymnastics Injuries, 2009–2010 Through 2013–2014. J Athl Train. 2015;50:870–8. https://doi.org/10.4085/1062-6050-50.7.02.
80. Gittoes M, Irwin G. Biomechanical approaches to understanding the potentially injurious demands of gymnastic-style impact landings. Sports Med Arthrosc Rehabil Ther Technol. 2012;4:4. https://doi.org/10.1186/1758-2555-4-4.
81. Micheli LJ. Back injuries in gymnastics. Clin Sports Med. 1985;4:85–93.
82. Standaert C, Herring S. Spondylolysis: a critical review. Br J Sports Med. 2000;34:415–22. https://doi.org/10.1136/bjsm.34.6.415.
83. Jackson DW, Wiltse LL, Cirincoine RJ. Spondylolysis in the female gymnast. Clin Orthop. 1976:68–73.
84. Cooke PM, Lutz GE. Internal disc disruption and axial back pain in the athlete. Phys Med Rehabil Clin N Am. 2000;11:837–65.
85. Sands WA, McNeal JR, Penitente G, Murray SR, Nassar L, Jemni M, et al. Stretching the spines of gymnasts: a review. Sports Med. 2016;46:315–27. https://doi.org/10.1007/s40279-015-0424-6.
86. Sarkar DA, Sarkar DMD. Early low back pain caused by bad posture and weak back and abdominal muscles. Int J Sci Res. 2018;7
87. Liebenson C. Rehabilitation of the spine: a practitioner's manual. Philadelphia: Lippincott Williams & Wilkins; 2007.
88. Page MP, Frank CC, Lardner R. Assessment and treatment of muscle imbalance: the Janda Approach. 1st ed. Champaign, IL: Human Kinetics; 2010.
89. Weber MD, Woodall WR. Spondylogenic disorders in gymnasts. J Orthop Sports Phys Ther. 1991;14:6–13. https://doi.org/10.2519/jospt.1991.14.1.6.
90. Gould J, Davies G. Orthopaedic and sports physical therapy. 2nd ed. St. Louis: C.V. Mosby Co; 1985.
91. Kenworthy KL. Global Posture of Female Collegiate Gymnasts and Their Peers [Internet]. [California, PA]: California University of Pennsylvania; 2008. Available from: http://libweb.calu.edu/thesis/umi-cup-1063.pdf.
92. Watson AW, Mac Donncha C. A reliable technique for the assessment of posture: assessment criteria for aspects of posture. J Sports Med Phys Fitness. 2000;40:260–70.
93. Chang W-D, Lin H-Y, Lai P-T. Core strength training for patients with chronic low back pain. J Phys Ther Sci. 2015;27:619–22. https://doi.org/10.1589/jpts.27.619.
94. Akuthota V, Ferreiro A, Moore T, Fredericson M. Core stability exercise principles. Curr Sports Med Rep. 2008;7:39–44. https://doi.org/10.1097/01.CSMR.0000308663.13278.69.
95. Coulombe BJ, Games KE, Neil ER, Eberman LE. Core stability exercise versus general exercise for chronic low back pain. J Athl Train. 2017;52:71–2. https://doi.org/10.4085/1062-6050-51.11.16.
96. Alqarni AM, Schneiders AG, Hendrick PA. Clinical tests to diagnose lumbar segmental instability: a systematic review. J Orthop Sports Phys Ther. 2011;41:130–40. https://doi.org/10.2519/jospt.2011.3457.
97. Tidstrand J, Horneij E. Inter-rater reliability of three standardized functional tests in patients with low back pain. BMC Musculoskelet Disord. 2009;10:58. https://doi.org/10.1186/1471-2474-10-58.
98. Youdas JW, Hartman JP, Murphy BA, Rundle AM, Ugorowski JM, Hollman JH. Magnitudes of muscle activation of spine stabilizers, gluteals, and hamstrings during supine bridge to neutral position. Physiother Theory Pract. 2015;31:418–27. https://doi.org/10.3109/09593985.2015.1010672.
99. Kivlan BR, Martin RL. Functional performance testing of the hip in athletes: a systematic review for reliability and validity. Int J Sports Phys Ther. 2012;7:402–12.

100. Norris B, Trudelle-Jackson E. Hip- and thigh-muscle activation during the star excursion balance test. J Sport Rehabil. 2011;20:428–41.
101. Crossley KM, Zhang W-J, Schache AG, Bryant A, Cowan SM. Performance on the single-leg squat task indicates hip abductor muscle function. Am J Sports Med. 2011;39:866–73. https://doi.org/10.1177/0363546510395456.
102. Suehiro T, Mizutani M, Ishida H, Kobara K, Osaka H, Watanabe S. Individuals with chronic low back pain demonstrate delayed onset of the back muscle activity during prone hip extension. J Electromyogr Kinesiol. 2015;25:675–80. https://doi.org/10.1016/j.jelekin.2015.04.013.
103. Clement DB. Tibial stress syndrome in athletes. J Sports Med. 1974;2:81–5.
104. Swain C, Redding E. Trunk muscle endurance and low back pain in female dance students. J Dance Med Sci. 2014;18:62–6. https://doi.org/10.12678/1089-313X.18.2.62.
105. Evans K, Refshauge KM, Adams R. Trunk muscle endurance tests: reliability, and gender differences in athletes. J Sci Med Sport. 2007;10:447–55. https://doi.org/10.1016/j.jsams.2006.09.003.
106. Waldhelm A, Li L. Endurance tests are the most reliable core stability related measurements. J Sport Health Sci. 2012;1:121–8. https://doi.org/10.1016/j.jshs.2012.07.007.
107. Hall E, Bishop DC, Gee TI. Effect of plyometric training on handspring vault performance and functional power in youth female gymnasts. PLoS One. 2016;11:e0148790. https://doi.org/10.1371/journal.pone.0148790.
108. Maffiuletti NA, Aagaard P, Blazevich AJ, Folland J, Tillin N, Duchateau J. Rate of force development: physiological and methodological considerations. Eur J Appl Physiol. 2016;116:1091–116. https://doi.org/10.1007/s00421-016-3346-6.
109. Stockbrugger BA, Haennel RG. Validity and reliability of a medicine ball explosive power test. J Strength Cond Res. 2001;15:431–8.
110. Ikeda Y, Miyatsuji K, Kawabata K, Fuchimoto T, Ito A. Analysis of trunk muscle activity in the side medicine-ball throw. J Strength Cond Res. 2009;23:2231. https://doi.org/10.1519/JSC.0b013e3181b8676f.
111. Saluan P, Styron J, Ackley JF, Prinzbach A, Billow D. Injury types and incidence rates in precollegiate female gymnasts. Orthop J Sports Med. 2015;3:232596711557759. https://doi.org/10.1177/2325967115577596.
112. Kirialanis P, Malliou P, Beneka A, Giannakopoulos K. Occurrence of acute lower limb injuries in artistic gymnasts in relation to event and exercise phase. Br J Sports Med. 2003;37:137–9. https://doi.org/10.1136/bjsm.37.2.137.
113. Hughes LY. Biomechanical analysis of the foot and ankle for predisposition to developing stress fractures. J Orthop Sports Phys Ther. 1985;7:96–101.
114. Dill KE, Begalle RL, Frank BS, Zinder SM, Padua DA. Altered knee and ankle kinematics during squatting in those with limited weight-bearing-lunge ankle-dorsiflexion range of motion. J Athl Train. 2014;49:723–32. https://doi.org/10.4085/1062-6050-49.3.29.
115. Bell-Jenje T, Olivier B, Wood W, Rogers S, Green A, McKinon W. The association between loss of ankle dorsiflexion range of movement, and hip adduction and internal rotation during a step down test. Man Ther. 2016;21:256–61. https://doi.org/10.1016/j.math.2015.09.010.
116. Mason-Mackay AR, Whatman C, Reid D. The effect of reduced ankle dorsiflexion on lower extremity mechanics during landing: a systematic review. J Sci Med Sport. 2017;20:451–8. https://doi.org/10.1016/j.jsams.2015.06.006.
117. Lima YL, Ferreira VMLM, de Paula Lima PO, Bezerra MA, de Oliveira RR, Almeida GPL. The association of ankle dorsiflexion and dynamic knee valgus: a systematic review and meta-analysis. Phys Ther Sport. 2018;29:61–9. https://doi.org/10.1016/j.ptsp.2017.07.003.
118. Neely FG. Biomechanical risk factors for exercise-related lower limb injuries. Sports Med. 1998;26:395–413. https://doi.org/10.2165/00007256-199826060-00003.
119. Fong C-M, Blackburn JT, Norcross MF, McGrath M, Padua DA. Ankle-dorsiflexion range of motion and landing biomechanics. J Athl Train. 2011;46:5–10. https://doi.org/10.4085/1062-6050-46.1.5.

120. Pope R, Herbert R, Kirwan J. Effects of ankle dorsiflexion range and pre-exercise calf muscle stretching on injury risk in Army recruits. Aust J Physiother. 1998;44:165–72. https://doi.org/10.1016/S0004-9514(14)60376-7.
121. Youdas JW, McLean TJ, Krause DA, Hollman JH. Changes in active ankle dorsiflexion range of motion after acute inversion ankle sprain. J Sport Rehabil. 2009;18:358–74.
122. Rabin A, Kozol Z, Finestone AS. Limited ankle dorsiflexion increases the risk for midportion Achilles tendinopathy in infantry recruits: a prospective cohort study. J Foot Ankle Res. 2014;7:48. https://doi.org/10.1186/s13047-014-0048-3.
123. Hewett TE, Lindenfeld TN, Riccobene JV, Noyes FR. The effect of neuromuscular training on the incidence of knee injury in female athletes. A prospective study. Am J Sports Med. 1999;27:699–706. https://doi.org/10.1177/03635465990270060301.
124. Willson JD, Dougherty CP, Ireland ML, Davis IM. Core stability and its relationship to lower extremity function and injury. J Am Acad Orthop Surg. 2005;13:316–25.
125. Pool-Goudzwaard AL, Vleeming A, Stoeckart R, Snijders CJ, Mens JMA. Insufficient lumbopelvic stability: a clinical, anatomical and biomechanical approach to 'a-specific' low back pain. Man Ther. 1998;3:12–20. https://doi.org/10.1054/math.1998.0311.
126. Prather H. Pelvis and sacral dysfunction in sports and exercise. Phys Med Rehabil Clin N Am. 2000;11:805–36, viii.
127. Reid DC, Burnham RS, Saboe LA, Kushner SF. Lower extremity flexibility patterns in classical ballet dancers and their correlation to lateral hip and knee injuries. Am J Sports Med. 1987;15:347–52. https://doi.org/10.1177/036354658701500409.
128. Kim M-K, Kong B-S, Yoo K-T. Effects of open and closed kinetic-chain exercises on the muscle strength and muscle activity of the ankle joint in young healthy women. J Phys Ther Sci. 2017;29:1903–6. https://doi.org/10.1589/jpts.29.1903.
129. Prisk VR, O'Loughlin PF, Kennedy JG. Forefoot injuries in dancers. Clin Sports Med. 2008;27:305–20. https://doi.org/10.1016/j.csm.2007.12.005.
130. Steinberg N, Siev-Ner I, Peleg S, Dar G, Masharawi Y, Zeev A, et al. Joint range of motion and patellofemoral pain in dancers. Int J Sports Med. 2012;33:561–6. https://doi.org/10.1055/s-0031-1301330.
131. Bliss LS, Teeple P. Core stability: the centerpiece of any training program. Curr Sports Med Rep. 2005;4:179. https://doi.org/10.1097/01.CSMR.0000306203.26444.4e.
132. Rickman AM, Ambegaonkar JP, Cortes N. Core stability: implications for dance injuries. Med Probl Perform Art. 2012;27:159–64.
133. Leetun DT, Ireland ML, Willson JD, Ballantyne BT, Davis IM. Core stability measures as risk factors for lower extremity injury in athletes. Med Sci Sports Exerc. 2004;36:926–34.
134. Khayambashi K, Ghoddosi N, Straub RK, Powers CM. Hip muscle strength predicts noncontact anterior cruciate ligament injury in male and female athletes: a prospective study. Am J Sports Med. 2016;44:355–61. https://doi.org/10.1177/0363546515616237.
135. Hansberger BL, Acocello S, Slater LV, Hart JM, Ambegaonkar JP. Peak lower extremity landing kinematics in dancers and nondancers. J Athl Train. 2018;53:379–85. https://doi.org/10.4085/1062-6050-465-16.
136. Cichanowski HR, Schmitt JS, Johnson RJ, Niemuth PE. Hip strength in collegiate female athletes with patellofemoral pain. Med Sci Sports Exerc. 2007;39:1227–32. https://doi.org/10.1249/mss.0b013e3180601109.
137. Rosene JM, Fogarty TD, Mahaffey BL. Isokinetic hamstrings:quadriceps ratios in intercollegiate athletes. J Athl Train. 2001;36:378–83.
138. Vogelpohl R, Wolz L, Neltner T, Burkhardt Z, Bonner T, Ericksen H. Comparison of isokinetic knee flexion and extension strength between trained dancers and traditional sport female collegiate athletes. Int J Exerc Sci. 2017;10:1196–207.
139. Jaiyesimi AO, Jegede JA. Hamstring and quadriceps strength ratio: effect of age and gender. J Niger Soc Physiother. 2005;15:54–8.
140. Murphy DF, Connolly DA, Beynnon BD. Risk factors for lower extremity injury: a review of the literature. Br J Sports Med. 2003;37:13–29. https://doi.org/10.1136/bjsm.37.1.13.

141. Dahle LK, Mueller M, Delitto A, Diamond JE. Visual assessment of foot type and relationship of foot type to lower extremity injury. J Orthop Sports Phys Ther. 1991;14:70–4. https://doi.org/10.2519/jospt.1991.14.2.70.
142. Beckett ME, Massie DL, Bowers KD, Stoll DA. Incidence of hyperpronation in the ACL injured knee: a clinical perspective. J Athl Train. 1992;27:58–62.
143. Allen MK, Glasoe WM. Metrecom measurement of navicular drop in subjects with anterior cruciate ligament injury. J Athl Train. 2000;35:403–6.
144. Gribble PA, Hertel J, Plisky P. Using the star excursion balance test to assess dynamic postural-control deficits and outcomes in lower extremity injury: a literature and systematic review. J Athl Train. 2012;47:339–57.
145. Birmingham TB. Test-retest reliability of lower extremity functional instability measures. Clin J Sport Med. 2000;10:264–8.
146. Kim S-H, Kwon O-Y, Park K-N, Jeon I-C, Weon J-H. Lower extremity strength and the range of motion in relation to squat depth. J Hum Kinet. 2015;45:59–69. https://doi.org/10.1515/hukin-2015-0007.
147. Herman G, Nakdimon O, Levinger P, Springer S. The forward step-down test evaluation by a broad cohort clinician agreement. J Sport Rehabil. 2015;25:227. https://doi.org/10.1123/jsr.2014-0319.
148. Ioan-Sabin S, Marcel P. Testing agility skill at a basketball team (10-12 years old); 2015
149. Čuk I, Marinšek M. Landing quality in artistic gymnastics is related to landing symmetry. Biol Sport. 2013;30:29–33. https://doi.org/10.5604/20831862.1029818.
150. Christoforidou A, Patikas DA, Bassa E, Paraschos I, Lazaridis S, Christoforidis C, et al. Landing from different heights: biomechanical and neuromuscular strategies in trained gymnasts and untrained prepubescent girls. J Electromyogr Kinesiol. 2017;32:1–8. https://doi.org/10.1016/j.jelekin.2016.11.003.
151. Colclough A, Munro AG, Herrington LC, McMahon JJ, Comfort P. The effects of a four week jump-training program on frontal plane projection angle in female gymnasts. Phys Ther Sport. 2018;30:29–33. https://doi.org/10.1016/j.ptsp.2017.11.003.
152. Manske R, Reiman M. Functional performance testing for power and return to sports. Sports Health. 2013;5:244–50. https://doi.org/10.1177/1941738113479925.

Index

A
Acetaminophen, 122
Achilles musculotendinous complex, 225
Achilles tendinopathy, 225
Achilles tendon injuries, 210, 225
ACL rupture, 219
Acrobatic gymnastics, 7, 8
Acromioclavicular (AC) joint sprain, 180
Active range of motion (AROM), 299, 328
Active rest, 293
Activities of daily living (ADL), 66
Adam's forward bend test, 151, 152
Aerobic gymnastics, 10, 11
The agility test, 322
Allostatic load, 239
Allostatic overload, 243
Amenorrhea, 109, 110
American Parkour (APK), 12
Andersen, M.B., 76–80
Andrews, J. R., 244
Ankle sprains, 210, 223, 224
Anorexia nervosa, 108, 109
Anterior cruciate ligament (ACL)
    injury, 269
    rupture, 218
Anterior inferior iliac spine (AIIS), 214, 215
Anterior knee pain, 220
Anterior labral pathology, 262
Anterior ring apophysis fracture, 150
Anterior superior iliac spine (ASIS), 215
Apophysitis, 192, 215, 225, 256
Apophysitis and avulsion fractures, 215, 216
Appaneal, R.N., 78, 79
Arm bar test for posterior elbow pathology, 193
Atlanto-axial instability, 129
Avulsion fractures, 188

B
Balance ball test, 319
Bartlett, M., 88
Basal metabolic rate (BMR), 66
Batatinha, 68
Beck, C., 2
Beighton criteria, 186
Belle, R., 12
Biomarkers, 121
Biomechanically sound landing technique, 235
Biomechanics
    acute and chronic force mitigation, 27
    anatomical variability, 30
    axes of rotation, 32
    Bankart lesion, 30
    baseline knowledge, 30
    cardinal planes, 32
    close-packed positions, 36
    compression, 34
    contact stress, 35
    contemporary research, 48, 49
    coordinate reference system, 33
    evidence-based medicine paradigm, 30
    footwear, 48
    gymnastics equipment and matting, 42, 43, 45, 46
    high peak (and chronic) joint loading, 46
    impulse, 37
    joint congruency, 35
    joint laxity, extreme ROM and propensity for, 47, 48
    joint moments, 33

Biomechanics (*cont.*)
  kinematics, 32
  kinetics and kinematics, 27
  leaps and bounds, 28
  material fatigue, 37
  material properties, 34
  mechanical stress and strain, 34
  men's high bar, 30
  mitigation, 37
  moment arm component, 35
  momentum, 37
  musculoskeletal anatomy, 27
  musculoskeletal system, 30, 35
    airborne saltos and twisting skills, 41
    arm-supported skill performance, 41–42
    jumping, 39
    landing, 40
    running, 39
    women's floor exercise, 38
  N∗m^{-1} (torque), 33
  Newton's laws, 36
  Newtons (linear force), 33
  olympic weightlifting, 30
  open chain activities, 36
  open-packed positions, 36
  orthopedic biomechanics, 29
  "overhead" mechanisms, 30
  parallel bars, 30
  proximal tibial geometric anomalies, 31
  PSI (pressure), 33
  qualitative assessment and record-keeping, 35
  research knowledge acquisition, 30
  rings, 30
  shared surface contact area, 36
  shear force, 34
  shoulder complex injuries, 30
  sport protocol phases of healing, 29
  "swinging"/"pirouetting" skill, 30
  system of levers, 35
  tension, 34
  third-class lever system, 35
  unique sport-specific biomechanics, 29
  vector forces, 33
  weight-bearing status, 36
  women's uneven bars, 30
  yields shoulder injuries, 30
  Young's modulus, 34
Bone mineral density (BMD), 106
Borelli, G., 28
Brewer, B.W., 80, 90
Bulimia nervosa, 108, 109

C
Calcium, 71
Cam-type FAI, 213
Cardiopulmonary resuscitation (CPR), 126
Cartesian coordinate system, 33
"Cat twist" technique, 41
Centers for Disease Control (CDC), 55
Certified mental performance consultant (CMPC), 86
Cervical cord neuropraxia, *see* Transient quadriparesis
Cervical musculature, 123
Cervical spine injuries
  anatomy, 123–125
  epidemiology, 123–125
  history and diagnosis, 125–127
  management, 128–129
  pathophysiology, 123–125
  treatment and return to play, 127, 130
Cervical stenosis, 128
Chronic inflammation, 215
Chronically untreated ligament tears, 201
Cirque gymnastics, 13
Closed kinetic chain upper extremity stability test (CKCUEST), 254, 309, 310
Coakley, J., 81
Cobb angle, 153
Cognitive behavioral therapy, 122
Cognitive rest, 121
Compression-type stress fracture, 215
Concussion
  definition of, 119
  epidemiology, 119, 120
  gymnastics return-to-play, 122
  history and diagnosis, 120, 121
  pathophysiology, 119, 120
  prognosis, 123
  return to play (RTP) protocols, 293, 294
    clearance & final follow up, 296, 297
    return-to-gymnastics (RTG) assessment, 294–296
    return-to-learn, 294
  treatment, 121–123
Core stability, 309, 310, 319, 332
C-reactive protein (CRP), 140
Crossed pelvic syndrome, 167
Cupal, D.D., 90

D
da Vinci, L., 28
de Coubertin, P., 28
Delayed puberty, 58

Diabetes mellitus (DM), 105, 106
Diaphragmatic breathing, 90
Dietary reference intake (DRI), 71
Distal radial physis injury, 194, 195
Distal radioulnar joint (DRUJ), 196
Dorsal wrist impingement, 202
Double Leg Lowering test (DLL), 310, 319
Double mini-trampoline, 9
Drop sign, 193
Dual x-ray absorptiometry (DXA), 65
Dynamic shear test for labral pathology, 185
Dynamic stability, 248

E
Elbow hypermobility, 308
Elbow injuries, 249, 250
    elbow dislocation, 192, 193
    lateral elbow
        olecranon apophysits/stress
            fracture, 192
        osteochondritis dissecans, 190–192
        Panner disease, 189, 190
    medial elbow
        Little League elbow, 187
        medial epicondyle avulsion
            fractures, 188
        ulnar collateral ligament
            injury, 188, 189
    OCD, 250
    return to weight-bearing and traction force
        progressions, 251, 252
Elbow stability, 308, 309
Electromyography (EMG), 28
Elite, 63
Epstein-Barr virus (EBV), 102
Erythrocyte sedimentation rate (ESR), 140
Exercise induced bronchoconstriction
    (EIB), 105
Exercise-induced amenorrhea, 110
Exertional rhabdomyolysis (ER), 106
Extension-based spine injuries (EBSI), 313
External workload, 239, 240
Extra-articular hip injuries, 214
Extra-articular impingement, 214

F
Facet joint anatomy, 158
Facet pain, 157–159
Farana, R., 178
Federation of International Gymnastics
    (FIG), 4, 63

Female Athlete Triad, 215, 222, 223
Femoral acetabular impingement (FAI), 31, 262
Femoral neck stress fractures, 215
Femoral stress fractures, 215
Femoroacetabular impingement (FAI), 213
Fibula fractures, 224
Flexion-based spine injuries (FBSI), 313, 322
Follen, C., 2
Follicle-stimulating hormone (FSH), 108
Food item, 70
Foot strength and stability, 333
Force transfer, 43
Fredericson grading system, 222
Functional hypothalamic amenorrhea, 110
Functional measurement tool, 311, 322
Functional progression, 319
Functional weight-bearing progression, 297

G
Gabbett, T., 237
Ganglion cysts, 201
General ballistic training, 255
General physical preparation (GPP), 236
Generalized ligamentous laxity, 186
Glasgow coma scale (GCS) score, 119, 120
Glenohumeral laxity, 185
Glute activation, 320–322
Gonadotropin-releasing hormone
    (GnRH), 108
Grade IV spondylolisthesis, 147
Grip lock injuries, 202
Grip strength, 307
Ground reaction force (GRF), 37
Growth plate fractures, 224
Gymnast's wrist, *see* Distal radial physis
    injury
Gymnastics
    body composition and anthropometrics,
        65, 66
    current regulations, 4
    definition, 1
    disciplines
        acrobatic gymnastics, 5, 7
        aerobic gymnastics, 5, 10, 11
        cirque gymnastics, 13
        Gymnastics for All, 5, 11
        men's artistic gymnastics, 5–7
        parkour, 5, 11, 12
        rhythmic gymnastics, 5, 10
        T&T, 9
        tumbling and trampoline, 5
        women's artistic gymnastics, 5, 6

Gymnastics (cont.)
    history, 1, 2, 4
    injuries
        acute vs. overuse injuries, 21
        altered/poor biomechanics, 23
        catastrophic injuries, 21–22
        club level gymnasts, 18, 19
        elite gymnasts, 20
        evaluation of injuries, ED, 22
        high school and club competition seasons, 24
        high school gymnastics, 19
        immature musculoskeletal systems, 22
        injury differences in disciplines, 20, 21
        injury rates, 19
        lower extremity injuries, female gymnasts, 18
        multiple risk factors, 23
        NCAA gymnastics, 19, 20
        overall injury rate, 17
        practice vs. competition, 23–24
        shoulder injuries, 23
        strains/sprains, 18
        tumbling and dismount/landing, 23
        upper extremity injuries, male gymnasts, 18
    injury epidemiology, 17
    normal puberty, 55, 58, 59
    nutrition
        energy needs of gymnasts, 66, 67
        macronutrients, 67–69
        micronutrients, 69, 71
    participation, 15, 16
    training, growth, and development
        catch up growth, 65
        chronological age, 63, 64
        delayed skeletal age/bone age, 63
        genetic predisposition, 65
        lagging bone age, 64
        lower and upper extremity injuries, 64
        optimal somatotype, 63
        pubertal maturation, 64
        training time and intensity, 63
Gymnastics for All, 11

H
Hamstring injuries, 216
Hand placement in back handsprings, 178
The handstand push up test, 311
The handstand test, 311
The hanging pike test, 322
Harringe, M. L., 211
Hawkins-Kennedy sign, 183

Head and neck injuries in gymnasts
    cervical spine injuries
        anatomy, 123–125
        epidemiology, 123–125
        history and diagnosis, 125–127
        management, 128–129
        pathophysiology, 123–125
        treatment and return to play, 127, 130
    concussion
        epidemiology, 119, 120
        gymnastics return-to-play, 122
        history and diagnosis, 120, 121
        pathophysiology, 119, 120
        prognosis, 123
        treatment, 121–123
Healing imagery, 92
Hébert, G., 12
Heerey, J., 262
Hepatitis B virus (HBV), 103
Hepatitis C virus (HCV), 103
Herman, M.J., 87
High hamstring tendinopathy, 216
Hill-Sachs/bony Bankart lesions, 181
Hip and thigh injuries
    apophysitis and avulsion fractures, 215, 216
    femoroacetabular impingement, 213
    hip dysplasia, 213, 214
    impingement and labral pathology, 261–263
    impingement of the hip, 214
    labral tears, 213, 214
    soft tissue and overuse injuries, 263–265, 268
    stress fractures, 214, 215
    tendon injuries, 216, 217
Hip dysplasia, 213, 214
Hip thrusters, 270
Hollenberg MRI classification, 143
Hollow holds, 319
Hudash, G. W., 210
Hughes, R., 81
Human immunodeficiency virus (HIV), 103
Hunt, K. J., 210
Hunter, L. Y., 212
Hypertrophy, 247

I
Ibuprofen, 122
Iliopsoas tendinopathy, 216
Immediate post-concussion assessment and cognitive testing (ImPACT) scores, 121

Impingement injuries, 182, 183
Incomplete ligament injuries, 201
Individual trampoline, 9
Individualized education plan (IEP), 294
Inferior shoulder instability, 186
Internal workload, 239, 240
International Olympic Committee (IOC), 4, 113
International Parkour Federation (IPF), 12
Intra- and extra-articular hip injuries, 214
Intracranial injury (ICI), 120
Iron, 69

J
Jahn, J.F., 1
Jobe (empty can) test, 182
Junior olympic levels (Levels 1-10), 63

K
Kerr, G., 225
Kibler dynamic labral shear, 183
Kim's biceps load test I and II, 183
Kinematics, 32
Kinetic chain theory, 308
Knee injuries, 267
　　anterior knee pain, 220
　　ligamentous and instability injuries, 269, 270
　　ligamentous and meniscus tears, 217, 218
　　osteochondritis dissecans (OCD), 221
　　patellar instability, 219, 220
　　repetitive tissue stress injuries, 270
Knee joint, 210
Knee strength and stability, 333
Kolt, G.S., 80
Korbut, O., 4
Kubler-Ross model, 82

L
Labral pathology, 261–263
Labral tears, 183, 184, 213, 214
Landing error scoring system (LESS), 269
Lax shoulder, 180
Leather dowel grips, 180
Legg-Calve-Perthes disease, 189
Leiber, F., 2
Ligamentous and instability injuries, 269, 270
Ligamentous and meniscus tears, 217, 218
Ligamentous injury considerations, 271, 272
Ling, P.H., 2
Little League elbow, 187

Lorenz, D., 238
Low bone mass, 111–113
Lower body crossed syndromes, 320
Lower crossed syndrome, 319
Lower extremity injury, 177
　　ballistic training, 255
　　clinical approach, 212, 213
　　definition, 210
　　epidemiology, 210–212
　　　　acute injuries, 211, 212
　　　　ankle injuries, 210
　　　　chronic injuries, 211
　　　　floor exercise, 212
　　　　knee joint, 210
　　hip and thigh injuries (*see* Hip and thigh injuries)
　　knee injuries, 267
　　　　anterior knee pain, 220
　　　　ligamentous and instability injuries, 269, 270
　　　　ligamentous and meniscus tears, 217, 218
　　　　osteochondritis dissecans (OCD), 221
　　　　patellar instability, 219, 220
　　　　repetitive tissue stress injuries, 270
　　lower legs, ankles, and feet injuries
　　　　Achilles tendon, 225
　　　　ankle sprains, 223, 224
　　　　apophysitis, 225
　　　　fractures, 224
　　　　ligamentous injury considerations, 271, 272
　　　　repetitive tissue stress injuries, 272
　　　　shin and calf injuries, 222, 223
　　plyometric training, 256
　　return to play (RTP) protocols, 326
　　　　mechanics of skill, 335
　　　　mobility, 328, 330, 331
　　　　muscular endurance, 333, 334
　　　　plyometric power, 334, 335
　　　　strength and stability, 331–333
　　　　weight bearing progression, 326–330
　　soft landing, 255
Lower legs, ankles, and feet injuries
　　Achilles tendon, 225
　　ankle sprains, 223, 224
　　apophysitis, 225
　　fractures, 224
　　ligamentous injury considerations, 271, 272
　　repetitive tissue stress injuries, 272
　　shin and calf injuries, 222, 223

Lumbar spine injuries
   compression and traction pathologies, 281–283
   compression loading during tumbling take off, 273
   extension and/or rotation pathologies, 279–281
   flexion and/or rotation pathologies, 281, 282
   general spine rehabilitation based on five-stage progression, 276–279
   return to play (RTP) protocols, 313
      core stability and functional progression, 319
      EBSI, 313
      glute activation, 320–322
      lumbopelvic dissociation, 322
      mechanics of skill, 324–326
      muscular endurance, 322–324
      plyometric power, 323, 324
      return to gymnastics skill progression, 314–316
      total functional range of motion, 315, 317, 318
      upper and lower crossed body syndromes, 318, 319
   skill profiles for accurate diagnosis and treatment programs, 274–276
Lumbopelvic dissociation, 322
Luteinizing hormone (LH), 108

M
Macrina, L. C., 244
Macronutrients, 67–69
Maffiuletti, N. A., 324
McGill, S., 262
McKenzie method, 157
McMurray's, Thessaly's and Apley's tests, 217
McNitt-Gray, J., 211
Mechanical diagnosis and therapy (MDT), 157
Mechanical strain, 34
Mechanical stress, 34
Mechanotransduction, 241
Medial epicondylar physis, 187
Medial epicondyle avulsion fractures, 188
Medial patellofemoral ligament (MPFL), 219
Medial tibial stress syndrome (MTSS), 222
Medical illness
   diabetes mellitus, 105, 106
   exertional rhabdomyolysis, 106
   female athlete triad
      abnormal eating behaviors, 107
      anorexia nervosa, 107–109
      bulimia nervosa, 108, 109
      eating disorders, 107
      energy availability, 107
      initial laboratory studies, 109
      low bone mass, 111–113
      low energy availability, 109
      menstrual dysfunction, 109–111
      RED-S, 113, 114
   infectious diseases, 101–103
   non-infectious skin conditions, 103, 104
   respiratory conditions, 105
   Vitamin D deficiency, 115, 116
Men's artistic gymnastics, 6, 7
Menstrual abnormalities, 110
Menstrual dysfunction, 110
Mental toughness, 250
Mental vs. physical readiness, 293
Methicillin-resistant *staphylococcus aureus* (MRSA), 102
Microinstability, 262
Mild head injury, *see* Concussion
Mild traumatic brain injury (mTBI), *see* Concussion
Mindfulness based stress reduction (MBSR), 92
Mohammed, W.A., 93
Morrison, S., 238
Multidirectional instability (MDI), 184–187
Muscular endurance, 310, 311, 322–324, 333, 334
Muybridge, E., 28

N
The National Collegiate Athletic Association (NCAA), 5
NCAA injury surveillance systems, 177
Neer sign, 183
Newton, I., 33
Nonsteroidal anti-inflammatories (NSAIDS), 127

O
O'Brien test, 183, 184
O'Kane, J. W., 210
Objective return to sports programs for shoulder-specific skills, 249
Olecranon apophysits/stress fracture, 192
Olympic weightlifting, 30

Index

One arm hop test, 311
Open and closed chain dynamic stability
   training, 248
Osgood-Schlatter disease, 220
Osteochondritis dissecans (OCD), 189–192,
   221, 249, 250
Ottawa ankle rules, 223
The over grip pull up test, 311

P

Pain management imagery, 92
Palpation, 126, 180, 188
Panner disease, 189, 190
Paoli, A., 68
Parallel bars, 3
Parathyroid hormone (PTH), 115
Parkour, 11, 12
Passive range of motion (PROM), 299, 328
Passive relaxation, 90
Patellar instability, 219, 220
Patellofemoral pain (PFP), 220
Patellofemoral pain syndrome (PFRS), 270
Pelée, M., 12
Performance imagery, 92
Perna, F.M., 80
Physical therapy, 194, 201, 214, 216, 217,
   223–225
Pincer-type FAI, 213
Plank holds, 319
Plank test, 310
Plexopathy, 127
Plyometric power, 311, 323, 324, 334, 335
Plyometric push up test, 311
Plyometric training, 255, 256, 271, 323
Plyometric weight bearing
   progressions, 298
Pommel horse, 2
Positive ulnar variance, 196
Post-concussive syndrome (PCS), 294
Potential (stored) energy, 43
Potential energy, 43
Precocious puberty, 58
Progressive muscle relaxation (PMR), 90
Progressive single arm loading programs,
   248, 249
Prone instability test, 319
Proximal femur/acetabulum, 31
Proximal hamstring tendinopathy, 216
Pseudodefect, 191
Psychological interventions box, 80
The push up test, 311

R

Radiculopathy, 127
Range of motion exercises, 181, 193
Ray, R., 76
"Red flag" symptoms, 137
Redmond, C.J., 80
Rehabilitation imagery, 92
Rehabilitation process, 233
   challenge of skill and force variability,
      234–236
   lower extremity (*see* Lower extremity
      injury)
   lumbar spine injuries
      compression and traction pathologies,
         281–283
      compression loading during tumbling
         take off, 273
      extension and/or rotation pathologies,
         279–281
      flexion and/or rotation pathologies,
         281, 282
      general spine rehabilitation based on
         five-stage progression, 276–279
      skill profiles for accurate diagnosis and
         treatment programs, 274–276
   upper extremity
      elbow injuries, 249–252
      shoulder injuries, 243–249
      wrist injuries, 252–254
   workload ratios, 237
      acute to chronic workload ratios and
         rolling averages, 237, 238
      five-stage rehabilitation process,
         240, 241
      inverted U curve and fitness being
         protective, 238, 239
      rationale for the five-stage progression,
         241–243
      sports psychology, 243
      tracking external and internal
         workloads, 239, 240
Rehabilitation program, 181, 182
Reinold, M. M., 244, 248
Relative energy deficiency in sports (RED-S)
   model, 113, 114
Repetitive tissue stress injuries,
   270, 272
Response to intervention
   protocol, 294
Return to gymnastics, 300–306, 314–315,
   327–330
Return to learn protocol, 294

Return to play (RTP) protocols, 122
    after concussion, 293, 294
        clearance & final follow up, 296, 297
        return-to-Gymnastics (RTG) assessment, 294–296
        return-to-learn, 294
    lower extremity injuries, 326
        mechanics of skill, 335
        mobility, 328, 330, 331
        muscular endurance, 333–334
        plyometric power, 334, 335
        strength and stability, 331–333
        weight bearing progression, 326–330
    lumbar spine injuries, 313
        core stability and functional progression, 319
        EBSI, 313
        glute activation, 320–322
        lumbopelvic dissociation, 322
        mechanics of skill, 324–326
        muscular endurance, 322–324
        plyometric power, 323, 324
        return to gymnastics skill progression, 314–316
        total functional range of motion, 315, 317, 318
        upper and lower crossed body syndromes, 318, 319
    principles, 292, 293
    unique demands of gymnastics, 292
    upper extremity (UE) injuries
        core stability, 309, 310
        elbow stability, 308, 309
        grip strength, 307
        mechanics of skill, 311–313
        mobility, 299, 307
        muscular endurance, 310, 311
        plyometric power, 311
        scapula stability, 309, 310
        weight bearing progression, 297, 298, 300–306
Return to sport, 296
Return-to-gymnastics (RTG) assessment, 294–296
Return-to-sport protocol, 122
Rhythmic gymnastics, 10
Rings hold test, 311
Rips injuries, 203
Roman Empire, 1
The rope climb test, 311, 322
Rotator cuff, 180, 181
Rotator cuff and parascapular muscle training programs, 247
Rotator cuff injuries, 182, 183
Round-offs and back handsprings, 178

S
Salter-Harris fractures of the proximal humeral physis, 180
Salters Harris fractures, 224
Sands, W. A., 28, 235
Scaphoid fracture, 199
Scaphoid impaction syndrome, 200
Scaphoid injuries, 199, 200
Scapholunate ligament injury/dissociation, 200, 201
Scapula stability, 309, 310
Scapular dyskinesis, 180
Scapular instability, 310
Scapular stabilization exercises, 181
Scheuermann's disease, 147–149
Scheuermann's kyphosis, 148
Schroth method, 154
Sclerosis, 190
Scoliosis, 151–154
Seated medicine ball throw, 311
Seated slump test, 139
Segond fracture, 217, 219
Shapiro, J.L., 93
Shin and calf injuries, 222, 223
Shoulder injuries, 243, 244
    clinical approach
        exam, 180, 181
        history, 180
        imaging, 181
        treatment, 181, 182
    impingement and rotator cuff, 182, 183
    labral tears, 183, 184
    leather dowel grips, 180
    MDI, 184–187
    objective return to sports programs for shoulder-specific skills, 249
    open and closed chain dynamic stability training, 248
    pathomechanics, 244
    progressive single arm loading programs, 248, 249
    rotator cuff and parascapular muscle training programs, 247
    soft tissue flexibility, management of, 245–247
Side bridge endurance test, 323
Side bridge test, 310
Sinding-Larsen-Johansson syndrome, 220
Single arm seated shot put test, 311
Single leg balance test, 333
Single-photon emission CT (SPECT), 142, 143
Skill profile, 274–276
SLAP lesions, 183
SLAP tears, 183, 184

Sleep disturbance, 122
Sleeper, M. D., 311, 322
Soft landing, 255
Soft landing' technique, 268
Soft tissue and overuse injuries, 263–265, 268
Soft tissue flexibility, management of, 245–247
Sorensen test, 310
Specific physical preparation (SPP), 236
Speed and Yergason tests, 183
Spinal cord concussion, *see* Transient quadriparesis
Spine injuries
  diagnostics and imaging, 138, 140
  gymnast's spine, 165–168
  history and examination, 137, 138
  psychosocial factors, 168
  sacrum and sacroiliac joints
    fibrous capsule, 161
    history and diagnosis, 162, 163
    sexual dimorphism, 162
    structural ligaments and myofascial structures, 162
    treatment, 164, 165
  Scheuermann's disease, 148
  spondylolysis and spondylolisthesis
    bone scans, 142
    clinical presentation, 141
    CT scans, 142
    Hollenberg MRI classification, 143
    kyphotic posture, 142
    MRI, 143
    prognosis of, 144, 145
    SPECT, 143
    standing anteroposterior and lateral radiographs, 142
    stress fracture, 141
    stress reactions, 141
    traumatic microfracture, 140
    treatment of, 145, 146
    types, 140
    VIBE sequences, 143
  thoracic and lumbar spine
    biomechanics, 136, 137
    CT scans, 143
    discogenic pain and radiculopathy, 154–157
    epidemiology, 135, 136
    facet pain, 157–159
    imaging for, 142–144
    MRI, 143
    multiple algorithms, 142
    myofascial pain, 160
    prognosis of, 144–145
    Scheuermann's disease, 147–149
    scoliosis, 151–154
    SPECT, 143
    spondylolysis and spondylolisthesis treatment of, 145–147
    vertebral ring apophysis fracture, 149–151
Sport Concussion Assessment Tool Version 5 (SCAT5), 120
Sport injury
  environmental factors, 76
  musculoskeletal imbalances, 76
  psychological antecedents
    psychological stress, 76
    stress and injury model (*see* Stress and injury model)
  psychological aspects of returning from injury
    achieving return-to-sport goals, 95
    autonomy, 94
    competence, 93, 94
    holistic recovery approach, 95–96
    psychological readiness, 95
    relatedness, 94, 95
    social support, 95
  psychological interventions, goal setting, 90
  psychological response
    biological factors, 84
    biopsychosocial approach, 84
    cognitive appraisal, 83
    emotional and behavioral responses, 81
    grief-response models, 82
    integrated model, 82
    intermediate biopsychological outcomes, 85
    multidisciplinary team, 85–88
    negative emotions, 81
    physical therapy, 81
    positive/adaptive emotions and outcomes, 82
    social/contextual factors, 85
    sociodemographic factors, 84
    sport injury rehabilitation outcomes, 85
    stage models, 82
    stress-related growth, 82
  rehabilitation, psychological interventions
    goal setting, 89, 90
    imagery, 91
    mindfulness, 92, 93
    relaxation training, 90
    self-talk, 91
    social support, 88, 89
  sociocultural antecedents, 81
  training load and subsequent load, 76

Sport Parkour League, 12
Sports medicine, 234, 236
Spring coefficients, 43
Spurling's test, 126
Squat test, 333
Standardized assessment of concussion (SAC), 120
STAR excursion balance test, 322, 333, 334
Star excursion balance test (SEBT), 269
Step down test, 333
Steroid, 181
Stiff leg, 255
Stinger, 124, 128
Stress and injury model
　anxiety, 78
　athlete's attentional field, 77
　cognitive appraisal, 77
　cognitive interventions, 77
　coping resources, 77, 80
　daily hassles, 79
　history of stressors, 77
　locus of control, 78, 79
　major life events, 79
　moderator, 78
　mood, 79
　personality, 77, 78
　previous injury, 80
　psychological stress, 76
　social support, 80
Stress fractures, 192, 214, 215, 222
Stress fractures in the clavicles, 180
Stress Response box, 80
Stress-injury relationship, 78
Stress-related growth, 82
Stress-shielding, 34
Strug, K., 81
Stuck landing, 40
Subspine and iliopsoas impingement, 214
Sweeney, E. A., 38, 298, 313, 326
Synchronized trampoline, 9

T
Tanner, J.M., 59
Tanner staging, 59
Tendinopathy, 216
Tendon injuries, 216, 217
Thermic effect of food (TEF), 66
Thompson test, 225
3D volumetric interpolated breath hold examination (VIBE), 143
Thyroid stimulating hormone (TSH), 111
Tibial stress fractures, 222, 223
Torgan, C., 212

Total functional motion (TFM), 315, 317, 318, 325
Toxic stress, 238, 243
Trampoline gymnastics, 9
Transient quadriparesis, 124, 129
Traumatic brain injury (TBI), 120
Triangular fibrocartilage complex (TFCC)
　injuries, 197–199
　tears, 195, 197, 198
Trochanteric-pelvic impingement (TPI), 214
The trunk extensor test, 323
Trunk flexor endurance test, 323
T-shape technique, 178
Tumbl Trak, 179
Tumbling, 9
Tumbling and trampoline (T&T), 9
Turner syndrome, 59

U
Ulnar collateral ligament (UCL) injury, 187–189
Ulnar impaction syndrome, 195, 196
Upper and lower crossed body syndromes, 318, 319
Upper extremity injuries
　elbow (*see* Elbow injuries)
　evaluation, 179
　gymnastics technique, 178, 179
　incidence of upper, 177
　return to play (RTP) protocols
　　core stability, 309, 310
　　elbow stability, 308, 309
　　grip strength, 307
　　mechanics of skill, 311–313
　　mobility, 299, 307
　　muscular endurance, 310, 311
　　plyometric power, 311
　　scapula stability, 309, 310
　　weight bearing progression, 297, 298, 300–306
　treatment, 179
　wrist injuries, 252
　　objective return to impact programs, 254
　　screening and management of radiocarpal extension range of motion, 253, 254
Upper Quarter Y Balance Test (UQYBT), 309, 310
Upper respiratory infections (URIs), 102
USA Gymnastics (USAG), 4
USA Gymnastics Junior Olympic (USAG JO) program, 15

Index

V
Valgus stress test, 188
Varus and valgus stress testing, 217
Vertebral ring apophysis fracture, 149–151
Vitamin D, 69
Vitamin D deficiency, 115, 116
Vocal cord dysfunction (VCD), 105

W
Wahoff, M. S., 262
Watson Mac Donncha Posture analysis, 319
Westermann, R. W., 211
Wiese-Bjornstal, 76
Wilk, K. E., 244, 248
Williams, J.M., 76–80
Wolff's law, 38, 241
Women's artistic gymnastics, 5, 6
Workload ratios, 237
    acute to chronic workload ratios and rolling averages, 237, 238
    five-stage rehabilitation process, 240, 241
    inverted U curve and fitness being protective, 238, 239
    rationale for the five-stage progression, 241–243
    sports psychology, 243
    tracking external and internal workloads, 239, 240
World Freerunning Parkour Federation, 12
Wrist and hand injuries
    distal radial physis injury, 194, 195
    dorsal wrist impingement, 202
    ganglion cysts, 201
    grip lock injuries, 202
    objective return to impact programs, 254
    rips, 203
    scaphoid injuries, 199, 200
    scapholunate ligament injury/dissociation, 200, 201
    screening and management of radiocarpal extension range of motion, 253, 254
    TFCC injuries, 197–199
    ulnar impaction syndrome, 195, 196

Y
Young's modulus, 34